DEAF EPISTEMOLOGIES

DEAF EPISTEMOLOGIES

Multiple Perspectives on the Acquisition of Knowledge

Peter V. Paul
Donald F. Moores

EDITORS

Gallaudet University Press
Washington, DC

Gallaudet University Press

Washington, DC 20002

http://gupress.gallaudet.edu

Printed in the United States of America

Library of Congress Cataloging-in-Publication Data

Deaf epistemologies : multiple perspectives on the acquisition of knowledge / Peter V. Paul, Donald F. Moores, editors.

p. cm.

Includes index.

ISBN 978-1-56368-525-5 (hbk. : alk. paper) – ISBN 1-56368-525-6 (hbk. : alk. paper) – ISBN 978-1-56368-526-2 (e-book) – ISBN 1-56368-526-4 (e-book)

1. Deaf. 2. Knowledge, Theory of. 3. Deafness–Psychological aspects. I. Paul, Peter V. II. Moores, Donald F.

HV2395.D43 2012

001'.01–dc23

2011051062

∞ The paper used in this publication meets the minimum requirements of American National Standard for Information Sciences–Permanence of Paper for Printed Library Materials, ANSI Z39.48-1984.

Contents

Contributors

Rachel Cooper
Politics, Philosophy, and Religion
Lancaster University
Lancaster, United Kingdom

Goedele A. M. De Clerck
International Institute for Sign Languages and Deaf Studies
University of Central Lancashire
Preston, United Kingdom

Peter C. Hauser
Department of Research and Teacher Education
National Technical Institute for the Deaf
Rochester Institute of Technology
Rochester, New York

Thomas K. Holcomb
Division of Deaf Studies
Ohlone College
Fremont, California

Donna M. McDonald
Disability Studies
School of Human Services and Social Work
Griffith University
Queensland, Australia

Michael M. McKee
Family Medicine Research Programs
Department of Family Medicine
University of Rochester School of Medicine and Dentistry
Rochester, New York

Margery Miller
New Leadership Alliance for Student Learning and Accountability
Washington, DC

Donald F. Moores
Department of Exceptional Student and Deaf Education
University of North Florida
Jacksonville, Florida

Ila Parasnis
Department of Research and Teacher Education
National Technical Institute for the Deaf, Rochester Institute of Technology
Rochester, New York

Peter V. Paul
College of Education and Human Ecology
Ohio State University
Columbus, Ohio

Antti Raike
Student Services at University Level
Aalto University
Helsinki, Finland

Ye Wang
Communication Sciences and Disorders
Missouri State University
Springfield, Missouri

PART I

INTRODUCTION

1

Toward an Understanding of Epistemology and Deafness

Peter V. Paul and Donald F. Moores

The title of this chapter contains two provocative constructs, *epistemology* and *deafness*, which have been the implicit or explicit topics in numerous publications on the social and educational welfare of individuals who are d/Deaf or hard of hearing (d/Dhh) (e.g., Paul & Moores, 2010; Moores & Paul, 2010). What is epistemology? What is deafness? How does the construct of epistemology relate to that of deafness? Are answers to these questions relevant for developing explanatory theories, conducting rigorous research, or engaging in effective practices?

Perspectives on these questions are examined throughout *Deaf Epistemologies*. We remove some suspense by immediately proffering one of our convictions (that is, one conviction on which we both agree!): *There is no God's eye view of either epistemology or deafness.* It might be counterproductive or perhaps nearly impossible to attempt to reach a consensus on the meaning of these terms or others, as argued by several scholars (e.g., Bernecker & Dretske, 2000; Noddings, 2007; Pring, 2004; Ritzer, 2001). Nevertheless, it is critical to strive for conceptual clarity of what it means, for example, to improve the educational or social welfare of or to empower individuals who are d/Dhh. Even *improvement* and *empowerment* are arbitrary constructs, perhaps even social constructs, that are open to interpretation and debate.

In addressing these questions, we consider the range of views proffered by the contributors to this book. These views can be categorized with respect to three major themes or groups of perspectives: sociological and anthropological, historical/psychological and literary, and educational and philosophical. Neither the views nor the categories are exhaustive, nor are they mutually exclusive; however, readers should understand a few possible approaches to exploring the construct of deaf epistemologies.

This includes exposure to ideas such as the adoption of a naturalized, critical epistemological stance (De Clerck, Chapter 2), the juxtaposition (or hybrid) of deaf epistemologies and the standard epistemology of science (Holcomb, Chapter 7), and the possibility of understanding deafness or Deafhood via literature (McDonald, Chapter 9). Perhaps the construct of deaf epistemologies requires an examination of acquisition and learning (e.g., of literacy) from a metaparadigmatic stance (Wang, Chapter 11) or the use of insights from the development of a personal epistemology by d/Dhh individuals (Raike, Chapter 12), especially a personal epistemology informed by the integration of gender, sexuality, race, ethnicity, and class (Parasnis, Chapter 4).

From another standpoint, it might be feasible to view this construct within the context of dueling or competing epistemologies, considering the historical perspectives of the education of d/Dhh children and adolescents (Moores, Chapter 6). For some scholars, deaf epistemologies exemplify the development of a Deaf identity (a positive entity) and not a focus on deafness (a negative entity) (McKee & Hauser, Chapter 3; Parasnis, Chapter 4). Within this purview, such individuals are predominantly visually oriented or predominantly shaped or enculturated by the use of vision more than that of individuals who have typical hearing.

The nature of this Deaf identity or related terms such as *Deafhood* or *Deaf-World*, including the composition of the members, becomes more complex upon further perusal (Miller, Chapter 8) and should be more diverse than portrayed in practice by educators and others, who often fixate on studying the effects of deafness or the *experience-with-deafness* notion (Parasnis, Chapter 4). Others believe that exploring the effects of deafness on learning is not necessarily restrictive, degrading, or negative. In fact, it might contribute to our understanding of the acquisition of knowledge in the content areas, especially in comparison with other learners, such as English language learners, those with disabilities, or those who are typical or without disabilities (Paul, Chapter 10).

Focusing on both the notion of Deafhood and on the experience-with-deafness construct might provide deep insights into the question: Can it be a good thing to be deaf? (Cooper, Chapter 13). Not surprisingly, the answer to this question is not absolute and cannot be separated from a context that relates deafness or Deafhood to some other phenomenon, such as learning a language, crossing a noisy street, or concentrating on a visual task.

In addition to exploring the constructs of epistemology and deafness, we examine the validity of the following statements, which are not only influenced by these aforementioned constructs but also have engendered numerous debates in the scholarly literature on deafness (Paul & Moore, 2010, p. 418):

- Individuals who are d/Deaf are visual learners.
- Individuals who are d/Deaf learn differently from hearing individuals.
- Anything based on sound/speech is not appropriate for d/Deaf learners.
- American Sign Language (or any sign language) is the natural language of d/Deaf individuals.
- The Deaf brain or the Deaf mind is different from the hearing brain or the hearing mind.
- Mainstream theories and research are inappropriate or not sufficient for understanding d/Deaf individuals.

As we have argued elsewhere (Paul & Moores, 2010), research on these statements is influenced by one's implicit or explicit epistemology, which drives not only the selection or development of a theoretical framework but also every aspect of the process, from the formulation of questions to the interpretations of results. There might be intense disagreements on the means and the ends of research investigations, making it a challenge to increase understanding the issues (e.g., Noddings, 2007; Pring, 2004; see also an interesting accessible account in Blackburn, 2005).

EPISTEMOLOGY

As a branch of philosophy, epistemology entails the study of a construct labeled *knowledge* (Bernecker & Dretske, 2000; Noddings, 2007; Moser, Mulder, & Trout, 1998). Traditionally, the foci have been on the conditions, sources, and limits of knowledge. Debate has centered on perspectives involving the relationship between the knower and what is known—between subject/agent and object or between the observer and the object of observation (see also the discussions in De Clerck, Chapter 2; Miller, Chapter 8; Wang, Chapter 11). Pertinent questions include the following: Is there a separation of the two entities such that what is known can be shared with and agreed upon by others regardless of conditions (or qualifications) such as location or time? Are these two entities so intertwined that insights can only be personally or socially constructed, influenced by time or context? Is the framing of this issue erroneous, limited, or simply meaningless with no true or specific response or resolution (e.g., Nagel, 1986, 1987)?

In essence, the debate on the relationship between the knower and what is known has engendered dissension with respect to the notions of objectivity and subjectivity as well as approaches to combine the two or to address the dichotomy that exists (e.g., Blackburn, 2005; Nagel, 1986, 1987; Ritzer, 2001; see also, De Clerck, Chapter 2; Miller, Chapter 8; Wang, Chapter 11). There is no consensus on the most constructive manner in which to frame this debate; however, the following passage provides a representative (albeit dramatic) description:

> The sides in this conflict have various names: absolutists versus relativists, traditionalists versus postmodernists, realists versus idealists, objectivists versus subjectivists, rationalists versus social constructivists, universalists versus contextualists, Platonists versus pragmatists. These do not all mean the same, and some people who stand on one side or the other would be choosy about allowing them to apply to themselves. So for the moment they simply act as pointers. (Blackburn, 2005, p. xiii)

This relationship between the knower and what is known has been debated since the beginnings of philosophy and has also been operationalized as epistemological debates on the mind–body problem (e.g., Bernecker & Dretske, 2000; Blackburn, 1999, 2005) and other phenomena, most notably the constructs of teaching and learning (e.g., Phillips & Soltis, 2004; see also, Raike, Chapter 12). This debate has led to varying perspectives on the meanings and effects of the constructs of metatheories, paradigms, and worldviews and ways to address differences (e.g., see Holcomb, Chapter 7; Wang, Chapter 11).

METATHEORIES AND PARADIGMS

For an in-depth discussion of metatheories and paradigms, see the work of Ritzer (2001). In short, metatheories—resulting from metatheorizing—are based on analyses of extant theories and are well grounded in the interpretations of empirical research, such as introspectionism, behaviorism, cognitivism, socioculturalism, and combinations. As argued by Ritzer (2001), it is not possible to do research—logically or empirically—to compare or evaluate metatheories because they are grounded in different worldviews. Thus, it can be argued that the adoption of a metatheory, albeit influenced by one's education and experiences, is actually a metaphysical choice—that is, based on one's conception of or approach to understanding the nature of reality or knowledge (e.g., see basic descriptions of metaphysical terms in Beebee, Effingham, & Goff, 2011).

These assertions also apply to the construct of paradigm, although paradigms are quite different from metatheories (e.g., Ritzer, 2001). A *paradigm* is a belief system that guides the manner in which one should do science or conduct scholarly inquiries (Ritzer, 2001; see also Wang, Chapter 11). Arguments are essentially metaphysical dissensions (e.g., Taylor, 1983) ranging from the nature of science or the scientific method to whether a discipline can be studied within a scientific framework or must be examined within a multiparadigmatic framework.

The overarching perspective (i.e., the paradigm) exists on a macro level, whereas on the micro level are examinations of specific items, views, and methods within a discipline (e.g., the best inquiry or behavioral approach within either constructivism or behaviorism, respectively). A paradigmatic analysis is also a form of a meta-analysis (see Wang, Chapter 11). Similar to metatheories, there is no scientific (i.e., objective) way to argue that one paradigm is better than another because paradigms reflect the tenets of different epistemologies (i.e., different worldviews).

In the field of deafness (and even in disability studies), it is possible to argue that there are two major paradigms—clinical (medical or pathological) and cultural or sociocultural (e.g., see Paul, 2001, 2009; Paul & Moores, 2010). These broad dichotomies are also known as the medical and social views of disability (e.g., see Oliver, 1992; Thomas & Vaughn, 2004).

Concluding Remarks on Epistemology

Before we proceed to the issues of research on individuals who are d/Dhh, we should emphasize again the complexity of the meaning of knowledge, especially with respect to *conducting research.* In fact, as we mentioned previously, it is not simply to assert what it means to engage in scholarly endeavors such as conducting research, advancing knowledge, or improving the welfare of individuals who are d/Dhh. All aspects of scholarly inquiry require incessant examinations ranging from the formulation of questions to the adoption of methods to the contents of analyses and, most important, the nature of the epistemology (e.g., Paul & Moores, 2010; see also Blackburn, 2005; Noddings, 2007). This ongoing process is so controversial that it is difficult to reach a consensus—although some philosophers have argued that reaching a consensus is not the goal (e.g., Pring, 2004). Rather, the goal is to obtain an understanding of the variety of perspectives that emerge at every stage, from the development of questions to the proffering of conclusions or interpretations.

In essence, the adoption of an epistemology or a *way of knowing* is a metaphysical choice (e.g., Eacker, 1983; Taylor, 1983; see also Beebee at al., 2011). "To think metaphysically is to think, without arbitrariness and dogmatism, on the most basic problems of existence" (Taylor, 1983, p. 1). To adopt a position—even an epistemological one—is not based on empiricism per se. The formulation of the epistemological question may not only be a metaphysical decision but also an indication of the methodology to be employed and the boundary of the interpretation of the findings (see Wang, Chapter 11).

Without oversimplifying further, we feel that an epistemological inclination is related to the relationship between the knower and what is known. To obtain a nuanced version of our epistemologic positions, it is best to read our individual chapters in this book (Moores, Chapter 6; Paul, Chapter 10). In some cases, the epistemology of the other contributors has been made explicit—that is, the particular contributor has labeled his or her epistemological approach.

STANDARD EPISTEMOLOGY AND RESEARCH

If scholars believe that there is a distinct or strict separation between the knower and the known, then it should be possible to examine what is purported to be known (i.e., the object of study) in an objective manner such that the same findings would be reached, regardless of physical or mental constitution, time, or context (e.g., Lehrer, 2000; Noddings, 2007; Ritzer, 2001). In essence, what is known is out there to be discovered and is called *mind independent*.

The strict view of this separation has been related to the construct of the standard epistemology, fueled by the traditional view of knowledge as justified true belief and buttressed by the assumption that there is an absolute toward which one is striving (e.g., Bernecker & Dretske, 2000; Lehrer, 2000; Moser et al., 1998; Noddings, 2007). Standard epistemology implies there is a foundation to empiricism (i.e., similar frame of reference), which should lead to a mutual understanding of events often connected with and driven by constructs such as truth, reason, and objectivity. Striving toward mutual understanding (or consensus) involves the reduction of theories to an ultimate one often characterized as elegant and simple, at least in some disciplines (e.g., Ritzer, 2001; see also a popular account in Hawking & Mlodinow, 2010).

In short, the traditional view of standard epistemology asserts that there is a foundation for knowledge that transcends situations, cultures, and time. This should not be construed to mean that there are no social, cultural, or historical influences on what is known. In any case, there is an incessant need to refine previous claims of knowledge with closer and closer approximations of *truth* or *reality* (e.g., see Lehrer, 2000; Noddings, 1995, 2007; Ritzer, 2001). Despite biases due to culture, the use of language, or even to theory-laden approaches, it is possible to proffer generalizations, laws, or theories as accurate or complete for a particular point in time—but *not for all time.*

This is a brief—admittedly simplified—description of the standard epistemology, which exemplifies what it means to *do science* or *scientific-based research*. Although this form has been debated, the basic principles of doing science such as observation, prediction, control, and generalization are still widely accepted and utilized (e.g., see Bernecker & Dretske, 2000; Moser et al., 1998; Noddings, 2007; Ritzer, 2001; for popular accounts, see Blackburn, 2005; Medawar, 1984). Even challenges to the basic assumptions of mind-independent realism in the standard epistemology (e.g., see the popular account in Hawking & Mlodinow, 2010), resulting in notions such as mode-dependent realism and variations, do not advocate the abandonment of the basic principles of doing science. These challenges underscore the notion that there might be more than one theory (or a group of theories) to explain *reality*; nevertheless, all of these theories are scientifically based.

What it means to do science has been debated by numerous philosophers, several of whom have responded to the assertions of Popper (Miller, 1985; see also, Raike, Chapter 12) and Kuhn (Kuhn, 1996; Nickles, 2003; see also De Clerck, Chapter 2; Wang, Chapter 11). However, it should be possible to obtain some agreement on the basic principles. That is, the task of doing science is to generate and test hypotheses that discover the causes and nature of phenomena. If a deep understanding is obtained, then it should be possible to predict future events or behaviors.

In some cases, the examination of phenomena is undertaken by proposing interventions (e.g., treatments, approaches) and assessing their effects, as might be the case in the health and educational sciences or research endeavors (e.g., Gay & Airasian, 2000). Other disciplines, most notably physics and economics, use complex mathematics to test hypotheses on phenomena quite distant or estranged from our everyday physical reality that are mostly outside of our realm of experience. For example, think about arguments associated with the beginning of the universe, whether the universe had a beginning (as we know that word), and even whether there is one universe (e.g., see Hawking & Mlodinow, 2010).

The adoption of a hypothesis (or theory) in science is dependent on an objective assessment of the evidence. However, what constitutes data and the methods for ascertaining the connection between theory and data are debatable and complex (e.g., Pring, 2004; Ritzer, 2001; see also De Clerck, Chapter 2; Raike, Chapter 12). It is unlikely that scientific researchers (of the standard epistemology) would promote hypotheses that are ad hoc—that is, tailor-made principles that are not generalizable and are confined to a specific situation or context.

Our contention is that most scientific theories produce generalizations. For example, can we generalize from the findings on children who are typical to those who are not (e.g., see Paul & Wang, 2012)? Can we generalize from children who are hearing to those who are d/Dhh (e.g., see Paul, 2009; Paul & Wang, 2012; see also Paul, Chapter 10; Wang, Chapter 11)? Can we discover generalizations within a specific population, for example, children with specific disabilities or in special education? Should scientific research predominantly guide theorizing and practice for children with disabilities or conditions? Individuals who espouse a strict description of multiple epistemologies (MEs) would most likely respond in the negative to nearly all of those questions (e.g., Guess, 1981; Horkheimer, 1995; Noddings, 2007; Ritzer, 2001; Tanesini, 1999).

MULTIPLE EPISTEMOLOGIES AND RESEARCH

If the standard epistemology (and its variations) anchor one end of a continuum, then Multiple Epistemologies (MEs) and variations are situated at the other end (e.g., Ritzer, 2001). The fun begins as one travels along the continuum and encounters phrases such as *critical positivism* or *multiparadigmatic science* (e.g., Ritzer, 2001). However, the real challenge is to describe what is meant by multiple epistemologies—which should take the plural form of epistemology.

Blackburn (2005) offers an eloquent description of this conceptual scheme (or schemes):

> We confront the idea of the Other: the person or persons whose minds are shaped so differently—by language, experience, culture or beliefs—that interpretation and understanding are baffled by them. Their entire way of thinking is different. The same stimuli provoke entirely different reactions. The world as they apprehend it is different from the world as we [*i.e., those who espouse the standard epistemology*; words and italics added] apprehend it. Here the "diversity of subjectivities" . . . engulfs so much that mutual understanding is impossible. Their whole "conceptual scheme" is different. . . . Attempts to understand others, they say, are exercises of power: We [*i.e., those who use the standard epistemology*; words and italics added] impose them, trample on their difference, and force them into our own mould. (p. 199)

In short, the concept of MEs can be operationalized by many forms such as feminist epistemologies, black epistemologies, queer epistemologies, and deaf epistemologies (e.g., see also Bauman, 2008; Ladd, 2003). As indicated by the passage, this construct implies that there are multiple ways of knowing influenced by a number of factors in the experience of an individual. These factors include education, familial/home experiences, ethnicity, history, sociocultural factors such as the prestige and power associated with various authorities and institutions, and the beliefs and mores connected to a particular geography (e.g., the location of one's residence) (see also Parasnis, Chapter 4; Miller, Chapter 8).

Proponents of MEs do not embrace the indiscriminate use of the scientific approach as described previously (e.g., Lehrer, 2000; Noddings, 1995, 2007; Tanesini, 1999). They react against the positivistic and objective underpinnings of the standard epistemology (or variants) and move toward situated or critical stances (e.g., see De Clerck, Chapter 2; Wang, Chapter 11). Proponents of the strict view of MEs may respond in a mode similar to strict proponents of critical metatheories, which provide the underpinnings of such approaches. For example, they may argue that the scientific approach is a limited or distorted view of reality, suggesting that nonscientific, even literary, approaches have much to offer in the way of understanding, for example, the development of individuals who are d/Dhh (e.g., see McDonald, Chapter 9; Parasnis, Chapter 4).

Perhaps, the strongest assertions are the following. There is no value-free knowledge because there is no real separation of the knower and the known. It is simply not possible to express this knowledge (i.e., on the object of study) with the use of any language that is neutral and objective (see also the discussion in De Clerck, Chapter 2, and

Raike, Chapter 12). As argued by Horkheimer (1995) and others (e.g., Noddings, 2007; Ritzer, 2001), objectivity is a construct that is agreed upon, typically by individuals or groups in power. Objectivity is not really objective in the absolute or even neutral sense. Thus, subjectivity and relativity are acceptable, unavoidable, and necessary because they are intertwined—and dependent on power (e.g., Nagel, 1986, 1987).

This does not mean that it is not possible to do science—assuming that there is an agreement on what it means to do science within the MEs framework (e.g., see McKee & Hauser, Chapter 3) or in conjunction with MEs' approaches/perspectives (e.g., see Holcomb, Chapter 7; Wang, Chapter 11). Nevertheless, the application of the so-called scientific approach within the purview of MEs might be conditioned by a priori principles or assumptions associated with the population under study. For example, researchers might have decided that d/Deaf individuals are visual learners whose epistemology is inherently or implicitly shaped by the use of vision. If this is the case, then it is not likely that researchers will examine the use, effect, or development of audition or speech. Furthermore, scholars may invoke the label of *audism* because the previously mentioned factors produce negative consequences such as low self-esteem or an external locus of control (e.g., Lane, 1992; Paul, 2009; Paul & Whitelaw, 2011; see also McKee & Hauser, Chapter 3).

In essence, the metaphysics of MEs involve the use of nonscientific or limited scientific approaches typically associated with those of critical theories and even cultural theories (e.g., Guess, 1981; Horkheimer, 1995; Noddings, 2007; Ritzer, 2001; Tanesini, 1999). In conducting scholarly inquires, there are basic assumptions and values that are personally or socially constructed in a nonscientific manner by elite members or representatives of this group (e.g., Noddings, 1995, 2007; Ritzer, 2001; Tanesini, 1999). These basic *axioms* preserve the integrity and identity of the group and postulate that the appropriate developmental procedures are contingent on the group's centerness, constitution, or framework.

In the field of deafness, a preponderant amount of controversy exists regarding attempts to provide descriptions of the *groupness* associated with deafness, Deaf identity, or Deaf-World (see also McDonald, Chapter 9; Miller, Chapter 8; Parasnis, Chapter 4), especially with respect to education and interactions involving the larger population of individuals who are typical (e.g., Moores, Chapter 6). This can lead to restricted use of a wide range of research paradigms or, more negatively, the adoption of a paradigm that does not reflect the heterogeneity of the population of d/Dhh children and adolescents (see Moores, Chapter 6; Wang, Chapter 11).

One of the most beneficial aspects of MEs has been the inclusion of voices and perspectives (not to mention an array of role models) in our understanding of the wide variations in physical and mental constitutions associated with the human condition (e.g., Noddings, 1995; Pring, 2004; Ritzer, 2001; Tanesini, 1999). The benefits of culturally relevant pedagogy and other related concepts are also evident from a critical, reflective stance. However, it is an open question whether the best or most effective teachers (clinicians, parents, or whoever!) are those that match the agreed-upon characteristics of the *group*. That is, it is not clear that the best teachers of women are other women or that the best teachers of lesbians are other lesbians.

Another major assumption of MEs of interest is that it is unrealistic or not possible to compare the educational and social development of one group (e.g., d/Dhh individuals) with that of another (e.g., individuals who are typical or hearing)—this is comparing apples with oranges. In other words, the characteristics of one group are shaped by the group's centerness or constitution, resulting in learning that is qualitatively differentiated from that of other groups. The influence of social and cultural factors notwithstanding, there is research that documents similarities in developmental trajectories, albeit much more work needs to be done (e.g., Paul & Lee, 2010; Paul & Wang, 2012; Paul, Chapter 10; Wang, Chapter 11). Part of the reason for these dissensions might be the implicit assumptions associated with the description of deafness (or Deaf identity or Deafhood).

d/DEAF OR HARD OF HEARING

Now let us examine our second major construct, which can be construed as a question that can take any number of forms:

- What is deafness?
- What is Deafhood?
- What is a Deaf identity?
- What is this thing or condition call deafness?

Deafness and the Medical/Clinical View

Several contributors to this book would argue that the use of the word *deafness* is negative because the main focus (i.e., theorizing, research, practice) is on what are considered the deleterious or negative effects of this condition on development and learning (e.g., McKee & Hauser, Chapter 3; Parasnis, Chapter 4). In short, the use of the word *deafness* is often associated with the medical or clinical view, which is deemed to be negative because of its emphasis on finding a cure or engaging in prevention (e.g., Lane, 1992; Paul, 2009). The medical/clinical view seems to be grounded in the beliefs, values, and mores of individuals who are hearing or do not have disabilities (see also Paul & Moores, 2010).

Within this framework, it would not be a gross overgeneralization to state that mainstream theories, research, and practices are applied, at least initially, to theorizing, research, and practice with individuals who are d/Dhh as well as to individuals with other conditions (Paul & Jackson, 1993; Paul & Moores, 2010). Research seems to require the documentation of characteristics that impact development—for example, degree of hearing impairment, age at onset, etiology (cause), location of the impairment, parental hearing status, and the presence of additional disabilities.

As a caveat, the application of mainstream models does or should not preclude specific research on d/Dhh individuals, and the research findings need to be considered in the development or refinement of the models (e.g., Paul, Chapter 10; Wang, Chapter 11). Nevertheless, mainstream models do serve as a barometer for interpretation, and these models might argue against radical MEs' views, which propose strict frameworks that vary according to social conditions such as race, gender, ethnicity, sexual orientation, and disability.

Deaf Mind/Brain

The positive phrases to use to formulate questions about d/Dhh individuals are those that contain words such as *Deafhood* or *Deaf identity* and refer to members of Deaf culture or the Deaf-World. The employment of these phrases acknowledges the contributions of vision and the use of a sign language in conjunction with other social and cultural factors (e.g., status of parents, gender, ethnicity, race, etc.) to cognitive and socioemotional development. The intertwinement of these factors might produce an entity such as a Deaf Mind or Deaf Brain and render moot (e.g., as examples of audism) the consideration of inappropriate theories, research, practices, or attributes (e.g., audition, speech, nonvisual learning strategies) that do not conform to the centerness or groupness of individuals in a visual-oriented world.

In short, scholars should not discuss such individuals with reference to the norms, values, or beliefs of individuals with typical hearing. With reference to centerness or groupness—in this case, the Deaf center—the grounding for this framework is based on the mores and beliefs of members of a sociological or cultural group, that is, members of the Deaf-World. This cultural or sociological model has been endorsed vehemently:

> To apply a cultural model to a group is to invoke quite a different conceptual framework. Implicit in this posture are issues such as: What are the interdependent values, mores, art forms, traditions, organizations, and language that characterize this culture? How is it influenced by the physical and social environment in which it is embedded? Such questions are, in principle, value neutral, although of course some people are ill-disposed to cultural diversity, while others prize it. The institutions invoked by a cultural model of a group include the social sciences; professions in a mediating role between cultures, such as simultaneous interpretation; and the schools, an important locus of cultural transmission.
>
> I maintain that the vocabulary and conceptual framework our society has customarily used with regard to deaf people, based as it is on infirmity, serves us and the members of the deaf community less well than a vocabulary and framework of cultural relativity. I want to replace the normativeness of medicine with the curiosity of ethnography. (Lane, 1992, pp. 18–19)

The focus on centerness or groupness is critical for understanding the development and growth of a personal and social epistemology (McKee & Hauser, Chapter 3; Raike, Chapter 12)—albeit an array of historical, educational, social, and cultural attributes and influences and their interwinement—need to be considered. (De Clerck, Chapter 2; Holcomb, Chapter 7; Miller, Chapter 8; Moores, Chapter 6; Parasnis, Chapter 4). Attention to these areas might improve academic achievement and literacy (Holcomb, Chapter 7; Moores, Chapter 6; Wang, Chapter 11). However, it still might be the case that d/Dhh individuals' acquisition of knowledge is not qualitatively different, cognitively, when compared to that of hearing or typical individuals, with respect to content areas such as English language, literacy, and others (Paul, Chapter 10; Wang, Chapter 11).

Epistemology and d/Deaf or Hard of Hearing Individuals

Regardless of the phrases used in describing Deafhood or deafness, an in-depth analysis still must ascertain whether there are positive or negative consequences, especially with respect to specific agreed-upon outcomes such as academic achievement and socioemotional development. The debate centers on the nature and comparison reference point (or group) of the outcomes, which can be influenced by attempts to define Deafhood or deafness as well as by the nature of an individual's epistemology.

If, as we have stated elsewhere (e.g., Paul & Moores, 2010; Moores & Paul, 2010), there is no God's eye view of deafness, then there should be no attempt to restrict or confine the nature of the questions and consequently the nature of research endeavors (e.g., Pring, 2004). It should be acceptable to examine individuals who are d/Dhh from a clinical/deafness or a cultural/sociological/Deafhood framework (see also Holcomb, Chapter 7; Wang, Chapter 11). Exploring the behavior of individuals who are d/Dhh from multiple perspectives, including the standard epistemology and MEs, should be encouraged. There should be no restrictions on the *means* with respect to understanding the *ends*, although reaching a consensus on everything from research questions to data interpretations and the nature of the outcomes will be considerably difficult (Pring, 2004).

We are sensitive to the negative consequences of audism, but we think that scholars and researchers should consider the changing demographics of d/Dhh individuals as a result of the continuing development of assistive devices such as digital hearing aids and cochlear implants (e.g., Mayer & Leigh, 2010; Paul & Whitelaw, 2011). Dissensions on the positive effects of these devices notwithstanding (e.g., Paul, 2009; Paul & Whitelaw, 2011), there does seem to be a cohort of individuals that may challenge and refine our assumptions of the construct of deaf epistemologies as discussed in this book. We are confident that such changes will produce new perspectives and a range of answers to the question: Can it be a good thing to be deaf? (Cooper, Chapter 13).

CONCLUSION: WHAT NOW, WHAT NEXT, WHERE TO?

Let us assume that we are correct that it is a metaphysical decision to adopt an epistemology and a description of deafness or Deafhood to guide theorizing, conducting research, and implementing practice. Should we permit this decision to be made on a national, state, local, or personal/parental level? Examples include No Child Left Behind, states' graduation examinations, local school board control, parental choice, and children's rights. Is this a decision to employ the standard epistemology, MEs, some combination, or something different?

It is one thing to state that there is no God's eye view of a particular entity, for example, epistemology, deafness, or Deafhood. It is quite another to come to an agreement to move forward. Perhaps agreement is not necessary, only understanding. We are certain that additional perspectives can be gleaned from our contributors. All of us are concerned with the educational and social welfare of individuals who are d/Dhh, although we might quibble over the means as well as the ends.

Understanding reality is a lifelong quest filled with challenges:

> The harmony between our thoughts and the world, the bridge we build between past and future, the sense of what the physical world contains and how our minds fit into it, are all topics on which the finest thinkers have hurled themselves, only to be frustrated. There always seem to be better worlds, if only we could find them, just over the horizon. (Blackburn, 1999, p. 298)

REFERENCES

Bauman, H.-D. (Ed.). (2008). *Open your eyes: Deaf studies talking.* Minneapolis, MN: University of Minnesota Press.

Beebee, H., Effingham, N., & Goff, P. (2011). *Metaphysics: The key concepts.* New York, NY: Routledge.

Bernecker, S., & Dretske, F. (Eds.). (2000). *Knowledge: Readings in contemporary epistemology.* New York, NY: Oxford University Press.

Blackburn, S. (1999). *Think: A compelling introduction to philosophy.* New York, NY: Oxford University Press.

Blackburn, S. (2005). *Truth: A guide.* New York, NY: Oxford University Press.

Eacker, J. (1983). *Problems of metaphysics and psychology.* Chicago, IL: Nelson-Hall.

Gay, L., & Airasian, P. (2000). *Educational research: Competencies for analysis and application* (6th ed.). Upper Saddle River, NJ: Merrill/Prentice-Hall.

Guess, R. (1981). *The idea of a critical theory: Habermas and the Frankfurt school.* New York, NY: Cambridge University Press.

Hawking, S., & Mlodinow, L. (2010). *The grand design.* New York, NY: Bantam Books.

Horkheimer, M. (1995). *Critical theory: Selected essays* (M. J. O'Connell et al., Trans.). New York, NY: Continuum.

Kuhn, T. (1996). *The structure of scientific revolutions* (3rd ed.). Chicago, IL: University of Chicago Press.

Ladd, P. (2003). *Understanding Deaf culture: In search of Deafhood.* Buffalo, NY: Multilingual Matters.

Lane, H. (1992). *The mask of benevolence: Disabling the Deaf community.* New York, NY: Vintage.

Lehrer, K. (2000). *Theory of knowledge* (2nd ed.). Boulder, CO: Westview.

Mayer, C., & Leigh, G. (2010). The changing context for sign bilingual education programs: Issues in language and the development of literacy. *International Journal of Bilingual Education and Bilingualism, 13*(2), 175–186.

Medawar, P. B. (1984). *The limits of science.* New York, NY: Harper & Row.

Miller, D. (Ed.). (1985). *Popper selections.* Princeton, NJ: Princeton University Press.

Moores, D., & Paul, P. (2010). Summary and prologue. *American Annals of the Deaf, 154*(5), 493–496.

Moser, P., Mulder, D., & Trout, J. (1998). *The theory of knowledge: A thematic introduction.* New York, NY: Oxford University Press.

Nagel, T. (1986). *The view from nowhere.* New York, NY: Oxford University Press.

Nagel, T. (1987). *What does it all mean? A very short introduction to philosophy.* New York, NY: Oxford University Press.

Nickles, T. (Ed.). (2003). *Thomas Kuhn.* New York, NY: Cambridge University Press.

Noddings, N. (1995). *Philosophy of education.* Boulder, CO: Westview.

Noddings, N. (2007). *Philosophy of education* (2nd ed.). Boulder, CO: Westview.

Oliver, M. (1992). Changing the social relations of research production. *Disability, Handicap, and Society, 7*(2), 101–114.

Paul, P. (2001). *Language and deafness* (3rd ed.). San Diego, CA: Singular/Thomson Learning.

Paul, P. (2009). *Language and deafness* (4th ed.). Sunbury, MA: Jones & Bartlett.

Paul, P., & Jackson, D. (1993). *Toward a psychology of deafness: Theoretical and empirical perspectives.* Needham Heights, MA: Allyn & Bacon.
Paul, P., & Lee, C. (2010). The qualitative similarity hypothesis. *American Annals of the Deaf, 154*(5), 456–462.
Paul, P., & Moores, D. (2010). Toward an understanding of epistemology and deafness. *American Annals of the Deaf, 154*(5), 417–420.
Paul, P., & Wang, Y. (2012). *Literate thought: Understanding comprehension and literacy.* Sudbury, MA. Jones & Bartlett Learning.
Paul, P., & Whitelaw, G. (2011). *Hearing and deafness: An introduction for health and education professionals.* Sudbury, MA: Jones & Bartlett Learning.
Phillips, D., & Soltis, J. (2004). *Perspectives on learning.* New York, NY: Teachers College Press.
Pring, R. (2004). *Philosophy of educational research* (2nd ed.). New York, NY: Continuum.
Ritzer, G. (2001). *Explorations in social theory: From metatheorizing to rationalization.* Thousand Oaks, CA: Sage.
Tanesini, A. (1999). *An introduction to feminist epistemologies.* Malden, MA: Blackwell.
Taylor, R. (1983). *Metaphysics* (3rd ed.). Englewood Cliffs, NJ: Prentice-Hall.
Thomas, G., & Vaughn, M. (2004). *Inclusive education: Readings and reflections.* Maidenhead, NJ: Open University Press.

SUGGESTIONS FOR FURTHER READING

Blackmore, S. (2004). *Consciousness: An introduction.* New York, NY: Oxford University Press.
Eacker, J. (1975). *Problems of philosophy and psychology.* Chicago, IL: Nelson-Hall.
Harris, J. (1992). *Against relativism: A philosophical defense of method.* LaSalle, IL: Open Court.
Hofstadter, D., & Dennett, D. (2000). *The mind's I: Fantasies and reflections on self and soul.* New York, NY: Basic Books.
Isaacson, W. (2007). *Einstein: His life and universe.* New York, NY: Simon & Schuster.

PART II

SOCIOLOGICAL AND ANTHROPOLOGICAL PERSPECTIVES

2

Contributing to an Era of Epistemological Equity: A Critique and an Alternative to the Practice of Science

Goedele A. M. De Clerck

In July 2010, the Organizing Committee of the International Congress on the Education of the Deaf (ICED) rejected the resolutions of the 1880 ICED conference that excluded sign language in deaf education, apologized for the negative consequences of these resolutions for deaf[1] people worldwide, and agreed to work toward "a new era of deaf participation and collaboration" (see Jamieson & Moores, 2011). The promising "rebirth of Deaf communities worldwide" is also reflected by the "global Deaf renaissance" theme of the World Congress of the World Federation of the Deaf held in Durban, South Africa, in July 2011. The congress's aim was to "demonstrate that we are an essential part of human diversity in the world and its development" (World Federation of the Deaf, 2010).[2]

This "new era" should also be an era of intellectual emancipation of deaf people around the world. How, after a long period of epistemic violence (Spivak, 1995), can the new era be an era of "epistemological equity" (Dei, 2010, p. 98)? Conceptualizing and continuing this reflection from an epistemic stance involves raising questions:

> What is the status of (indigenous) deaf knowledge(s) versus science?
> How can deaf knowers be conceptualized in science?
> In what context are science and knowledge produced, and what is the value of science?
> How do deaf people construct their knowledge?

This project has been supported by a postdoctoral research grant from the Research Foundation-Flanders. I give special thanks to Donald F. Moores and Peter V. Paul for their encouragement and constructive feedback during the writing of this essay. I also thank Rik Pinxten for his inspiring scholarship and his generous support of my work through frequent discussions and Yerker Andersson for comments on an earlier version of this essay.

Is it legitimate for deaf people to claim knowledge, and why?
How can the wisdom and knowledge(s) of deaf people, which have been marginalized, contribute to the well-being of deaf people and all people around the world?
Can deaf knowledge(s) be a source of inspiration for educational and social transformation?
How can research practice provide room for deaf knowledge and partnership?

Drawing on the field of anthropology, which has inspired and legitimated the cultural turn in deaf studies, and situating deaf epistemologies in the evolution of the philosophy of science, I argue that deaf epistemologies is a feasible alternative line of cognition and theorizing in an approach to science that is inclusive of gender, sexuality, class, race, culture, language, religion, and disability. In this chapter, I explore an interdisciplinary view of deaf studies and the social sciences and humanities from a naturalist and critical perspective, employing a practice that is both descriptive and normative.[3]

Deaf epistemologies challenge scholars and others to reflect on audism in the production of theory and knowledge. This is compatible with the radical stance toward science found in Marxist criticism, postcolonial and subaltern criticism, feminist criticism, and black/Afrocentric criticism that provides the basis for critical discussion of the social and cultural structure of knowledge production and the influence of epistemic theorizing on daily life (e.g., Aldridge & James, 2007; Ashcroft, Griffiths, & Tiffin, 1995; Collins, 1990; Dei, 2010; Higgs, 2008, 2010; Tanesini, 1999; Tyson, 1999; see also Paul & Moores, Chapter 1). As a young and interdisciplinary field, deaf studies has heavily relied on these disciplines. Deaf epistemologies are oriented toward emancipation and motivated by the wish of deaf people to live equal lives and to fulfill their potential.

Although the concept of deaf culture led to a deaf cultural critique of science, it was not until recently that epistemological issues were explicitly addressed in deaf studies. Further metatheorizing can contribute significantly to the development of this critical project. I contribute to this project by providing a culture-sensitive alternative in deaf studies. This is exemplified in a discussion of global-local dynamics in deaf identity, deaf culture, and deaf education. In this chapter, I argue for a naturalized epistemology that describes human practices and functions in the interest of humankind (Pinxten & Note, 2005; Tanesini, 1999).

Uniting in solidarity and enabling all deaf people to flourish necessarily implies taking into account the heterogeneity among deaf people and deaf communities, the complex and multiple identities of deaf people, differences in deaf people's sociocultural positions, and the "structural violence" (Farmer, 2010, p. 358) deaf people face. Deaf people in some parts of the world have little or no access to deaf education (see also Haualand & Allen, 2009). A new era of partnership and collaboration also means that rather than focus on individual problems, we should reframe these problems as a matter of social justice and collective responsibility (see also Dei, 2010; Nussbaum, 2006).

ANTHROPOLOGY AND THE DEVELOPMENT OF A NONCOLONIAL SCIENCE

For a broad anthropological and epistemological stance, I draw primarily on Pinxten (2006) and Pinxten and Note (2005). After decolonization, anthropology could no longer maintain its confidence in the objectivity of science. It has become a self-critical discipline (Ashcroft et al., 1995; Geertz, 1995; Nader, 2006; Said, 1995).

Pinxten (2006) argues that both the positivist and the phenomenological approaches in the social sciences are guilty of a colonial attitude: Research subjects are reduced to objects, and indigenous knowledge of the informants is granted secondary status in the production of scientific knowledge about indigenous knowledge. A bidirectional epistemological stance is needed to overcome the colonialist attitude: Research is a contextualized interactive and communicative process between the researchers and collaborators, who participate in a joint venture (see also Pinxten, 1997b).

Bourdieu's praxeology (Bourdieu, 1990, 1998; Bourdieu & Wacquant, 1992) analyzes both objective structures and the observational and attitudinal categories of agents. This epistemological stance grants equal roles to the researchers and collaborators in the study. Performance ethnography (Fabian, 1990) gains insight through experiencing, doing, and learning. Cultural knowledge is created and transmitted in and through events in a coproduction of anthropologists and informants, who guide the anthropologist.

Some argue that the debate on the status of indigenous knowledge[4] versus science has been settled (Pinxten, 2006; see also Nader, 2006; Pottier, Bicker, & Sillitoe, 2003; Sillitoe, 1998). On the one hand, research on ethnoscience (e.g., Pinxten, 1997a, 1997b) indicaties that indigenous thought systems use cognitive tools that had been supposed to be Western. On the other hand, some styles of everyday thought are close to scientific thinking (Crombie, 1994).

I take a naturalized epistemological stance. This stance focuses on the situatedness of knowledge, takes into account social factors in the study of knowledge, and is critical of "a God's eye view" of knowledge production (Pinxten & Note, 2005; Tanesini, 1999). The description of human practices aims to foster further understanding rather than provide an explanation only in causal terms. This chapter can be situated in an empirical and evolutionary epistemology (Campbell, 1989).

This epistemological contribution is also normative: It aims to contribute to an inclusive science and be supportive of the interests of humankind (Pinxten & Note, 2005): "Science should not be turned into a master narrative which provides the standards for its own agenda" (Tanesini, 1999, p. 117). Sensitivity to class, gender, race, ethnicity, culture, sex, disability, age, language, and audiological status appeals to social values. In this view, epistemology can be viewed as a "motor of change."

As an international and human practice, science needs to deal with researchers and subjects from a variety of local contexts (Pinxten & Note, 2005). Anthropological research has revealed a gradual transformation and hybridization of cultures (Appadurai, 2003; Hannerz, 2003; Young, 1995). Parallel to the growth of information technology and the marginalization of groups without technological access, local, regional, cultural, and religious identities have been mobilized (Massey & Jess, 1995; Pinxten & De Munter, 2006).

If the countermovement of postcolonial studies is taken into account, an open and non-exclusive view of science is highly relevant (Pinxten, 2006; Pinxten & Note, 2005).

The practice of "studying knowledge in terms of epistemic practices" (Tanesini, 1999, p. 116) and describing these epistemic practices as activities in a historical, cultural, and social context is illustrated by the Cameroonian case study in Chapter 5.

DEAF EPISTEMOLOGIES AND ALTERNATIVES TO THE PRACTICE OF SCIENCE

According to the *received view* of science, science is a cumulative enterprise to find a true theory that is the key to nature. The received view claims epistemic foundationalism in its efforts toward a logic of justification: Each scientific theory can be (re)formulated by rules of correspondence between the language of theory and the language of observation. The observer is distinguished from the object of observation: Any interference by the subject is eliminated, and theories are confirmed by empirical verification. This leads to a deductive certainty as far as is possible at a particular moment in time.

Critics in the 1950s and 1960s pointed out that science is conducted from within a weltanschauung and hence epistemological theorizing must pay attention to the dynamic historical and sociological context and the linguistic-conceptual frameworks that influence the production of science and knowledge. Kuhn (1962) points out the value of the notion of a consensus or shared research tradition (paradigm) that is the basis for scientific theorizing among the researchers in the same field. Observation is theory laden: Knowledge is reasonable for a particular subject in a particular context, while the meaning of *reasonable* depends on the conceptual and theoretical framework that influences the organization of the data. Feyerabend (1965) criticized science's language of neutral observation and acknowledged the need for theoretical pluralism.

This is relevant for deaf epistemologies because diverse philosophies of the various weltanschauungen reflect on the social construction of scientific practice.

OBJECTIVISM AND RELATIVISM

Situating knowledge production in a cultural, social, political, and historical context is often discussed as a form of cognitive relativism; this differs from objectivism that seeks universals (see Paul & Moores, Chapter 1). Pinxten (1991) distinguishes between a more traditional objectivism and a recent (post-Kantian) objectivism: Whereas traditional objectivism refers to an ontological foundation for the evaluation of statements about the world, post-Kantian objectivism situates the foundation for statements of truth in the theoretical consensus that scientists have reached. Pinxten distinguishes four versions of relativism:

1. *Kuhn's conception of the incommensurability of paradigms.* Because we do not have a universal language of observation, facts are theory-laden (see also Hesse, 1970; Wang, Chapter 11).

2. *Science is conducted from within a weltanshauung* (see Suppe, 1977).
3. *Worldviews and theories are relativistic.* Underneath these superficial differences, an a apriori criterion of universality (including truth and logic) is able to provide for cross-cultural understanding. Barnes (1994, in Pinxten, 1991, p. 184) states that this universal foundation cannot be found in truth or rationality; rather it can be found in "an unproblematice baseline of normality." This is problematic, because the concept of what is normal is relativistic.
4. *Science may have cultural components* (Pinxten, 1991, p. 184; see also Elzinga & Jamison, 1981; Needham, 1965). Values of the sociocultural context in which science is produced constitute knowledge production and need to be taken into account in the study of epistemic practices.

Perelman and Olbrechts-Tyteca (1957) found that speakers in philosophy of science focus on a universal audience, presenting rational and universal statements of truth. In sociological terms, a particular philosophical and scientific audience is identified as universal (standing for humankind), and a priori knowledge and "hard facts" are claimed to be true or highly probable. Calling these claims of objectivity and universality into question, Kuhn's relativistic stance shocked scientific traditions.

For ontological objectivists, there is correspondence between reality and the statement of truth; that is, critics need to be convinced that abstract values are well founded. Epistemological ontologists refer to a set of a priori statements (a theory). The relativists whom I have discussed all deal with epistemological issues and as such do not argue against realism. The second and third versions of relativism advanced by Pinxten focus on the type of correspondence theory. The first version (Kuhn's incommensurability) focuses on the question of whether we should share consistency as value in order to be a universal audience. The fourth version explores the question of an overarching set of values: "In what sense is science a cultural phenomenon (local knowledge), and if it is, how can universal truths be conceived?" (Pinxten, 1991, p. 189).

Pinxten concludes that none of the relativists actually argue against realism (i.e., ontological objectivism). Ontological objectivism and epistemological relativism discuss different things, and as such are not mutually exclusive. Rather there are "gradual diversifications" (Pinxten, 1991, p. 189); for example, Lukes's infrastructural basis of rationalism includes some objectivism; Kuhn's incommensurability and critique do not give up objectivity; and the weltanshauungen views diverse knowledge traditions as different but sharing the same rationality.

The epistemological argument of the present chapter are situated in this fourth version of cognitive relativism. From the description and comparison of diverse knowledge systems, "an empirical foundation for a possible relativitistic epistemology (of the fourth type)" may emerge that will be accepted as "an posteriori basis for the universals for an objectivist epistemology" (Pinxten, 1991, p. 191):

> We are able to communicate and interact with each other in order to arrive at some common understanding regarding the way we see and think about the world: about the limits and constraints on well-founded or dependable knowledge; perhaps even about "good" (i.e., commonly cherished) ways to use it. (Pinxten, 1991, p. 191)

This perspective on relativism is a heuristic epistemological process. Science is now localized "as a way of thinking and acting in the very broad context of one or more civilizations" (Pinxten & Note, 2005, p. 95).

The situatedness of science affects both the status and the contents of the knowledge that is produced. Social factors grant more authority to certain scholars, which may influence whether a certain theory is more acceptable than another (Bourdieu 1990, 1998; see also Addelson, as cited in Tanesini, 1991). For example, deaf scholars experience bias toward their work and have limited opportunities to conduct research. Standard views of knowledge may perceive the concept of deaf epistemologies as revolutionary and not open for critique and discussion. Deaf scholars, Third World criticism, and Third World deaf scholars are still scarce in the field.

Moores and Paul (2010) argue that the different positions of standard epistemology and d/Deaf epistemologies can be placed on "a continuum with a potentially infinite number of possibilities" (p. 494; see also Moores & Paul, Chapter 14). Consideration of this discussion as well as from analyses of feminist epistemologies (e.g., Code, 2006; Davis, Evans, & Lorber, 2006; Tanesini, 1999), a field in which metatheorizing has been further developed, raises the question of whether there is an endless range of possible positions in d/Deaf epistemologies. Further metatheorizing in the field will bring more clarity on these positions.

DEAF EPISTEMOLOGIES AS A CRITIQUE AND ALTERNATIVE TO THE PRACTICE OF SCIENCE

Stokoe, Casterline, and Croneberg's *Dictionary of American Sign Language on Linguistic Principles,* published in 1965, legitimized American Sign Language (ASL) as a bona fide language. Drawing on the fields of structural comparative linguistics and anthropology, the dictionary used a new vocabulary to describe the language of deaf people (Padden, 1980; Padden & Humphries, 2005).

"The Linguistic Community," an appendix to the dictionary, provides academic recognition and a description of "the social and cultural characteristics of the linguistic community" (Stokoe et al., 1965, p. 297). The text employs notions such as *minority group, community,* and *culture.*

This new perspective on deaf people as a cultural and linguistic minority group led to a paradigm shift in the field of deaf studies in the decades that followed: Sociological and anthropological studies (e.g., C. Erting, 1978; Higgins, 1980; Padden & Humphries, 1988; Woodward, 1982) employing qualitative and ethnographic research methods documented the lives of deaf people from an emic perspective. A deaf knowing subject emerged, and deaf ways of seeing and being were claimed.

Woodward (1982) conceptualized this focus, distinguishing between *deaf,* referring to the hearing status of deaf people (and how deaf people are viewed by hearing people) and *Deaf,* referring to the perspective of deaf people who view themselves as a group with a language and a culture.

Padden and Humphries noticed that deaf people's daily lives, values, myths, and art had escaped the focus of science. In their 1988 book *Deaf in America: Voices From a Culture,* they aimed not only to throw light on deaf culture from the inside but also to employ a deaf way of writing,[5] "in contrast to the long history of writing that treats [deaf people] as medical cases, or as people with 'disabilities,' who 'compensate' for their deafness by using sign language" (p. 1).

Padden and Humphries (2005, p. 2) subsequently drew on the work of George Veditz, who had described deaf people as "first, last, and for all time, people of the eye" in 1912, to emphasize that although the notion of culture may be new, deaf people have always viewed themselves as visually oriented and as such have developed knowledge about themselves and the world:

> Deaf people's practices of "seeing" are not necessarily natural or logical, in the sense that they have a heightened visual sense, but their ways of "seeing" follow from a long history of interacting with the world in certain ways—in cultural ways. (p. 2)

Woodward (1982) critiques of the practice of science. Not only had the experiences of deaf people been excluded from science (see also Higgins, 1980), but the epistemic foundationalism of science had been put into question: Science was perceived as a practice that was not value neutral, but instead influenced by "hearing ideology" (Woodward, 1982, p. 75). Markowicz and Woodward (1982) noticed that the literature on deafness was dominated by psychological studies that investigated the causal relationship between deaf people's behavior and intelligence while failing to take into account the possible influence of the deaf cultural experience in the testing situation and questioned the results of research on deaf community membership done by hearing researchers.

This line of criticism has been expanded in a postmodern stance in deaf studies. On a pragmatic level, Lane (1999) wrote that power and money are in play. He referred to Humphries's notion of *audism*: "In short, audism is the hearing way of dominating, restructuring, and exercising authority over the Deaf community" (p. 43).

Lane (2005) deconstructed social science research as an institution that objectifies and paternalizes deaf people. He also criticized the relationship between research and technology: The economic benefits of what Foucault called "bio-power," Lane wrote, are exemplified by the promotion of the cochlear implant. Genetic research is another example of Foucault's normalization technologies that are threatening the deaf world.

THE EMANCIPATORY VALUE OF THE DEAF CULTURE NOTION

Connected with deaf studies' criticism of science is deaf epistemology's concern with the emancipatory value of science. Initial anthropological and sociological studies have employed terms such as *Deaf culture* and *Deaf identity* as political tools that could contribute to the emancipation process of deaf people (Padden & Humphries, 2005). In 2005, Padden and Humphries reflected on their first book (1988), in which they were "writing not as anthropologists but as agents of a changing discourse and consciousness" (p. 2). Deaf people were still reluctant to have their language examined and publicized; debates with anthropologists concerned the question of whether deaf culture was a bona fide culture. Taxonomic descriptions and a search for definitions of *deaf culture, deaf community, membership,* and *ethnicity* mark this stage of research (e.g., Erting, 1978; Johnson & Erting, 1989; Kyle, 1990; Padden, 1980; Woodward, 1982).

A 1994 discussion in *Sign Language Studies* touched on epistemological perspectives in deaf studies. Turner (1994) questioned the circularity of definition seeking in the field of deaf studies, the homogeneous and static construction of the deaf culture concept, and the political motivation underlying the research studies aiming to document a distinct deaf culture. In critiques of his paper, researchers argued that *deaf culture* was originally an academic term that had been adopted by deaf people (Bahan, 1994; Stokoe, 1994) and that the use of categories developed by deaf people (e.g., *Deaf-World*) should be encouraged, with differences between terms critically examined (Andersson, 1994; Bahan, 1994). Recognizing the value of anthropological frameworks to the emancipation of deaf people (Monaghan, 1994), scholars called for critical reflection on the limits of general frameworks for understanding deaf culture. Johnston (1994) drew on the social sciences to legitimate deaf scholars' explicit support of the deaf cause: Criteria such as transparency on the position and motivation of the researcher were regarded as more appropriate than a standard notion of objectivity. Bahan (1994) suggested that "it may be productive to investigate how Deaf people see what unites and divides us" (p. 248).

This inward turn was developed by Ladd (2003). Dissatisfied with the medical term *deafness,* he conceptualized a deaf way of being and knowing in the epistemic notion of *Deafhood.* Deafhood

> represents a process—the struggle by each Deaf child, Deaf family, and Deaf adult to explain to themselves and each other their own existence in the world. In sharing their lives with each other as a community . . . Deaf people are engaged in a daily praxis, a continuing internal and external dialogue. (p. 3)

Providing a strong center, "which can then create new spaces for more sophisticated liberatory discourses to flourish" (Ladd, 2003, p. 81), the concept of Deafhood is necessarily strategically essentialist, a stance based on Spivak's subaltern theory (e.g., Spivak, 1995). Deafhood is expressed in the global connections of deaf people and shared deaf experience and sign language use. Deafhood allows for diverse readings.

GLOBAL PERSPECTIVE AND CULTURAL CRITIQUE IN DEAF STUDIES

Linguistic research has fostered the legitimization of sign languages and consciousness raising in deaf communities worldwide (Baker & Battison, 1980; Erting, Johnson, Smith, & Snider, 1994; Goodstein, 2006; Monaghan, Schmaling, Nakamura, & Turner, 2003). Monaghan (2003) distinguished some common patterns in deaf communities. The founding of deaf schools in Europe and the United States in the 19th century enabled deaf children to acquire sign language in interaction with deaf peers. Deaf schools have been considered root places of deaf culture; deaf adults have socialized in deaf clubs, often founded close to these schools (Fisher & Lane, 2003; Van Cleve & Crouch, 1989).

Deaf schools in developing countries were often established through the efforts of missionaries under colonial influences or under the auspices of programs to develop cooperation between countries. Consequently, schools adopted the philosophy and sign language of the founding or supporting country (Barcham, 1998; Erting et al., 1994; Goodstein, 2006). A general internationalism has fostered a growing recognition of deaf people's rights and has been beneficial to deaf people's empowerment (Monaghan et al., 2003).

These social developments have influenced deaf people's lives and identity construction. Deaf studies research and the emancipation movement of ethnic minorities and their discourses transformed deaf identities in the United States. Deaf people liberated themselves from medical discourses and identified themselves as members of a linguistic and cultural minority group (Jankowski, 1997). A review of literature on the dynamics of deaf identity in northwestern Europe (De Clerck, 2009b) indicates a three-stage model of emancipation: In the first stage, deaf people come under the influence of oralism, are subordinated, and withdraw from society. In the second stage, the legitimization of sign language through linguistic research politicizes deaf identities, with deaf people claiming a separate linguistic and cultural identity after the 1970s. In the third stage, young deaf people who have grown up in inclusive realms of life view sign language as a regular mode of communication; being deaf is an aspect of diversity in a pluralistic society. Although a political basis is maintained, the boundary between the hearing and deaf communities has weakened. Simultaneously, studies reveal that deaf people easily communicate transnationally, adapting their own sign language, using international sign, or picking up the local sign language. Benefiting from globalization and from technological and economic resources, some young deaf people develop transnational deaf identities (Breivik, 2005; De Clerck, 2007; Haualand, Gronningsaeter, & Hansen, 2003; Turner, 2004).

Apart from these trends, it is important to note that the construction of deaf identity is also related to local sociocultural, political, educational, and social policy constructions, and hence differs among countries. The politicization of deaf identity and the emancipation processes in deaf communities should also be interpreted against the background of historical and anthropological research that finds that deaf people are included in social life in some contexts (e.g., Groce, 1995; Johnson, 1994). This observation raises the question of whether unitary concepts such as *deaf culture* and *deaf identity* can be used to gain accurate insight into culturally constructed deaf identities.

Insight into the cultural construction of deaf identities is particularly relevant to understanding conflicts between identities and shifts in identities in a transnational and global context. Deaf people's transnational interaction has fostered the transfer of (culturally constructed) discourses on deaf identity, sign language, and deaf culture and raised deaf consciousness (Breivik, 2005; De Clerck, 2007; Le Master, 2003; Nakamura, 2005).

Nakamura's (2005) anthropological research in Japan reveals how conflicts have emerged between a younger generation of deaf people, who are inspired by presentations of American deaf activists and identify as culturally deaf, and a senior generation of deaf people, who also define themselves as culturally deaf without a capital "D" and in a different way. The older group of deaf people attended deaf schools and have continued to socialize in deaf organizations since graduation. Voicing while signing, they view sign language as a mode of communication that does not fundamentally differ from Japanese. The younger generation experienced linguistic and social exclusion in mainstreaming. Influenced by American discourses on deaf identity and deaf culture, they developed political deaf identities and advocate for a *pure* (unvoiced) sign language. Nakamura warns that in a homogeneous Japan, ethnolinguistic discourses will not easily receive government recognition, whereas deaf people have been able to receive recognition as a disability group.

Between 1984 and 1988 and again in 2000, Le Master (2003) did ethnographic research in the deaf community in Dublin, Ireland. Her study in linguistic anthropology found shifts in identity between a senior generation of deaf people who grew up in a signing educational environment and a younger generation of deaf people who did not experience educational inclusion. The older generation conceptualizes sign language as a regular mode of communication and is open to including hearing people in conversations. Enforced oralism has led to "oppositional Deaf identities" in young deaf people (Le Master, 2003, p. 168) and the adoption of cultural and political Deaf discourses that became available through transnational contacts. The differences between the two generations of deaf people have not led to a political separation. Few of the older people participate in ethnic-minority discourses. However, they have supported the political organization and promotion of Irish Sign Language led by the younger group.

I studied emancipation processes through the life stories of 25 international deaf people at Gallaudet University (De Clerck, 2009a). By applying a multidimensional analytical framework that conceptualizes identity dynamics as a complex of processes (Pinxten, Verstraete, & Longman, 2004), I gained insight into differences and conflicts in culturally situated constructions of deaf identity. Deaf people are exploring different ways to negotiate equal status for sign language and deaf people in local contexts. In my research, I deconstructed one-dimensional concepts of deaf identity and deaf culture, which are often employed in the field of deaf studies, as culturally situated (and Western) perspectives. If this theoretical operation is to be more fully developed and insight is to be gained into identity dynamics and processes of empowerment in deaf people and deaf communities in different localities, cross-cultural comparative research is necessary. In-depth understanding of culturally constructed identity dynamics can contribute significantly to successful contextualized intercultural negotiation (De Clerck, 2009b; see also Pinxten, 1999) of core constructs that are vital to deaf people.

To achieve this goal, the anthropological methods described earlier may be employed in the field of deaf studies as well. For a comparative perspective, Geertz's (1983) empirical study and cultural description of *fact and law* in different local contexts is inspiring. Geertz's methods are valuable for deaf researchers as well, who share cultural intuitions with the people who collaborate in their research.[7]

CULTURE-SENSITIVE AND INCLUSIVE VIEW ON LEARNING AND EDUCATION

The paradigm shift in deaf studies goes hand in hand with deaf-centered and bilingual-bicultural education, which provides deaf students with opportunities to learn sign language and deaf culture, to come into contact with deaf role models and teachers, and to become equipped with the knowledge and skills to negotiate core constructs in their identity and live equal lives. The question "Whose education?" (Simms, 2006) illustrates deaf people's claims to involvement in all aspects of deaf education.

Consistent with the anthropological framework of the present chapter, research methods and expertise from the field of ethnoscience (e.g., Pinxten, 1997a, 1997b) may be valuable to deaf education. Education, cognition, and learning processes are socioculturally specific phenomena (Cole, 1996; Daniels, Cole, & Wertsch, 2007; Vygotsky, 1978); therefore, it is important to develop concepts and terms within the vernacular language, categorization system, and learning strategies. Studies exploring visual learning strategies are in line with this research orientation. In a long-term interdisciplinary ethnographic study, Erting et al. (2006) investigated the development of American Sign Language (ASL) and English literacy learning strategies of deaf children in both the home and classroom environments. The interaction of the children with their deaf teachers, compared with the interaction with their deaf and hearing (sign language–learning) parents, reveals a rich variety of deaf knowledge. Another example is the research documenting how deaf parents and teachers mediate English in bilingual settings, moving back and forth among ASL, fingerspelling, and written English (Erting, Thumann-Prezioso, & Benedict, 2000; Padden, 1996a, 1996b).

In a study on deaf empowerment in Flemish deaf role models (De Clerck, 2007), I found that empowered deaf peers and barrier-free environments in the United Kingdom, the United States, and Nordic countries provided examples of possible and inspiring ways of living in comparison with the Flemish context. Global deaf identities, a common use of sign language, and a common experience of being deaf (Ladd, 2003) facilitate the transfer of empowering knowledge. The concept *deaf ways of education* was employed to refer to this informal networking and emancipatory information exchange among deaf people. Erting (1996), writing on "the Deaf way," said, "For as long as Deaf people have formed communities, a Deaf way of life has been recognized by Deaf people themselves. These patterns of behavior, attitudes, beliefs, and values have been referred to in American Sign Language as 'DEAF TEND (THEIRS)'" (p. xxiii). Reilly (1995) used the phrase "deaf way of education" in the title of his doctoral dissertation and explained visual modes of learning and communication among deaf students.

Western educational programs for deaf students in non-Western countries and education programs for deaf immigrant children that fail to take into account indigenous (deaf) knowledge(s)[8] may cause cultural and linguistic transformations, disruptions, and oppression. Anthropological studies call for a critical perspective.

Branson and Miller's (2004) study of the linguistic environment in northern Bali illustrates how education programs inspired by Western experts and concepts can be examples of neocolonialism. Deaf children from an inclusive signing environment are instructed in a national language (Indonesian) and sign language (i.e., a signed system) that is not used in their local environment. This is not only ineffective but also results in semilingualism and poor communication when deaf students return home. They may have lost their ability to speechread the Balinese language and communicate with non-Indonesian-speaking relatives; only strong signing environments provided by family members who have not lost their signing competence during their children's education guarantee appropriate communication. This situation challenges the deaf community concept, which originated in the development of Western deaf communities around deaf schools. The question is which community's sign language should be implemented in education: "The only communities of relevance to the deaf students in the schools are communities where local languages are spoken and where the signing used is thoroughly localized" (Branson and Miller, 2004, p. 32).

In Kano State, Nigeria, Schmaling (2003), an ethnographic researcher, found that the local inclusion of deaf people and the wide use of sign language as a mode of communication by both hearing and deaf people is threatened by urbanization and the implementation of ASL in education, which implies that the local sign language is inferior. This divides the deaf community into *educated* deaf people using ASL, on the one hand, and *uneducated* deaf people and hearing people using indigenous sign language, on the other hand.

A study by Branson and Miller (1998) on the education of deaf immigrant children in Australia indicated that the concept of bilingual-bicultural education can be exclusive if it does not include indigenous languages and indigenous sign languages. The researchers proposed an educational plan for deaf students of non-English-speaking and non-Australian Sign Language–using backgrounds to graduate as bilingual in two sign languages and two written sign languages at the end of secondary education.

Storbeck and Magongwa (2006) have developed a fruitful approach to a diverse deaf studies curriculum that can meet the needs of a heterogeneous deaf community. As exemplified in the learning situation of deaf Zulu children in South Africa, the scholars have employed the multiethnic educational framework of Banks (1994) to integrate deaf culture into the whole school and curriculum while paying attention to the mixed backgrounds of deaf children, "thus creating a Deaf-centric curriculum—including content, visual learning and teaching styles, and Deaf indigenous teaching and learning practices" (Storbeck & Magongwa, p. 121).

While similarities in deaf epistemologies suggest global learning strategies of visually oriented and signing people, sensitivity to different ways of indigenous deaf learning and the broader context in which this learning takes place is crucial. For deaf students, successful education necessarily involves multilingualism and an understanding of culturally situated meanings of education and emancipation.

CONCEPTUALIZING THE DEBATE ON ESSENTIALISM AS AN EPISTEMOLOGICAL DEBATE

Earlier in the present chapter, I described the adoption of academic terms such as *deaf culture, deaf community,* and *sign language* for use by increasing self-aware deaf communities. Humphries (2007) draws on the work of anthropologist James Clifford to describe this movement as the transition from *talking deaf culture* to *deaf culture talking*. Padden and Humphries (2005, p. 162) reflect on the adoption of the term *culture* by deaf people as an illustration of human diversity: "Perhaps this is the true lesson of human cultures and languages, that our common human nature is found not in how we are alike, but in how we are different, and how we have adapted to our differences in very human ways." De Clerck and Pinxten (2011a) noticed that human beings are intrinsically diverse clusters of identity: "deaf culture" has emerged as an instance of this human predicament. However, as the overview of research studies in this chapter and Chapter 5 on the Cameroonian deaf community illustrate, the notion of *deaf culture* is a complex one. The practice of studying deaf culture has evolved beyond a static, homogeneous conception of deaf culture that needs to be defined along a list of characteristcs. New theoretical and epistemological approaches are needed to gain insight into deaf indigenous practices and concept formation (see also De Clerck & Pinxten, 2011a).

The naturalized stance I take in this chapter in regard to studying deaf cultural practices differs from that described by Mindess (1999) and Ladd (2003). Mindess draws on the field of intercultural communication, founded on the work of anthropologist E. T. Hall, to study deaf culture. Intercultural communication was developed in the early 1950s as a means of training diplomats for interactions abroad. It was also used to prepare Americans to host foreign students and to help people admitted to the Peace Corps gain awareness about multiple cultural identities. Employing a categorical framework (e.g., collectivism–individualism, high culture–low culture, time orientation, and reasoning–rhetoric) from the point of view of interpreters moving between the American hearing and deaf cultures, Mindess described American deaf culture as collectivist, low culture, polychronic, and past oriented, and rhetorically moving from the specific to the general (in contrast to hearing culture). However, in intercultural negotiation (see also the criticism on Hofstede, 1991, whose model was based on empirical research in 50 countries), the challenge is not to start from static notions of culture and a priori categories that are likely to be Western rather than objective (see also Pinxten, 1997b, 1999).

Ladd suggests continuing along Mindess's line in exploring "deaf cultural features" and working to "identify commonalities which could inform the development of a central 'core' of cultural identity, similar to those being attempted for the 'Black Atlantic' and for Jewish culture" (p. 406). It is questionable whether a return to an essence is an adequate answer to deal with both deafness and intrinsic human diversity—as the previous literature review illustrates, deaf people and human beings are intrinsically diverse clusters of identity (see also De Clerck & Pinxten, 2011a). Instead, comparitive research, specifically research on non-Western sign languages, deaf cultural practices, and deaf indigenous knowledge, is needed to critically complement the knowledge we have gained so far and may lead toward a posteriori universals. For the theoretical foundation of this epistemological stance, I refer to the earlier discussion of objectivism and relativism.

In documenting deaf communities and deaf people, researchers have analyzed the intertwining of axes of difference in the lives of deaf women (e.g., Brueggemann & Burch, 2006), black deaf people (e.g., Williamsen, 2002; James & Woll, 2004), deaf gay and lesbian people (e.g., Breivik, 2005), and other deaf minorities. For example,

Narajian (2006) interviewed 10 college-educated deaf women in Rochester, New York, and Boston, Massachusetts, on their mothering practices. The empirical sociological study analyzed the intersection of ability and gender in the interviewees' life stories. The study illuminates the role of language in maternal thinking: how women who identify as culturally deaf discuss with their husbands how to communicate with their children, employing a wide range of communication methods: ASL, Signing Exact English, and/or oral methods. The mothers actively made efforts to "normalize" their experiences: The concept of disability was challenged, and when the women were asked whether they preferred their children to be deaf or hearing, they tended to emphasize a preference for "healthy" children with whom they could establish a bond. Whereas their work as mothers was similar to the work of hearing mothers, they also needed to negotiate their deaf identities in mainstream society. They viewed themselves as members of a linguistic and cultural minority group who were not intrinsically different from other people. They also did not want their children to interpret for them. Political decisions on the language(s) they taught their children and used at home were tied to relations to the deaf community and/or the hearing world and helped create room for their families and themselves in both worlds. They strived for their children to be accepted and for themselves to be legitimate mothers in both worlds:

> The contradiction that existed in this aspect of maternal thought was present for these women in a particular way. They had to teach their children the art of going back and forth between these two worlds and to be proud of Deaf culture as a part of their family and balance that within the context of a larger hearing society. (p. 117)

James and Woll (2004) illuminate the influence of educational contexts, language use, social attitudes, and the family context on black deaf people's identity development and life experiences in the United Kingdom. The study finds that "black deaf" is not a unitary notion: Black deaf people create and move between complex identity positions within and beyond the deaf community. Positive experiences of communication in the home context led to positive attitudes toward deafness. Feelings of loneliness and exclusion, poor communication with family members (the use of nonstandard varieties of English, creole English, or other languages is an influential factor), limited participation in the cultural environment, the use of British Sign Language (BSL), and Deaf pride all fostered identification with the deaf community. Informants who had good family relations and were supported in their educational and career trajectories tended to identify with the deaf community. Factors that fostered black community membership were experiences of racism within the deaf community and larger society, positive family experiences, and black pride. Although educational trends moved toward cultural pluralism in the 1970s and 1980s, informants were not able to acquire information related to their own cultural backgrounds at school. Information related to the deaf community and deaf culture was available through interactions with other deaf children; however, racism and stereotyping created a need for information about black culture and black role models. Ambivalent and varied feelings toward the deaf community were noticed, including both pride and exclusion because of racism within the deaf community. Research participants who grew up in an all-black environment abroad developed a strong sense of identity and took leadership roles within the black deaf community and the wider deaf community. Research participants who grew up in the UK but traveled abroad self-identified as both black and black deaf and supported deaf leaders. Research participants who had not traveled expressed a less developed sense of racial identity. People who identified as black deaf experienced black culture as a part of their heritage and deaf culture as an adopted culture; they had access to black hearing communication and communicated primarily in spoken English. People who identified as deaf black primarily identified as deaf because of their access to sign language in the deaf community and had a strong sense of identity and equality. Some informants resisted being identified as black or as deaf. The researchers conclude: "The informants rarely achieved an equal balance in their feelings toward their bicultural identities. They negotiated and renegotiated their identities in different situations" (James & Woll, 2004, p. 157).

These studies illuminate the contextualization and complexity of identity constructions and call for intersectionality as research method and theoretical tool (Crenshaw, 1991; Thorvalsdottir, 2007). In the literature review in the preceding paragraphs, essentialist notions of deaf identity come to the fore as particular constructions of deaf identity situated in a specific social and cultural context and period of time (see De Clerck, 2009a). Essentialized notions of deaf identity are reproduced, while practices of moving between different contexts show multiple identities and conflicts between different identity constructions. Baumann (1999) conceptualizes this process as a *double discursive competence*: "People know when to reify one of their identities, and they know when to question their own reifications" (p. 139). While a unitary notion of deaf identity has been useful in processes of deaf empowerment and emancipation, particularly in a (Western and globalized) context of politicized identities, research studies have also revealed that this construction of deaf identity may be exclusive and oppressive in both Western and non-Western contexts. While it is important to recognize deaf people's shared experiences and the empowering potential of notions of global deafhood, it is also necessary to take the theory-ladenness, situatedness, and partiality of deaf experiences into account (see also Collins, 1990).

Obasi (2008) notices that scholars in black studies and gender studies, in line with postmodern antiessentialism, have recognized the diversity in black, female, and disability identities and criticized the universalizing forms of representation that have failed to take this diversity into account. Reflecting on the development of deaf studies, situated in comparison to gender studies and black studies, and taking into account the relatively young development of the field, Obasi (2008, p. 456) raises the question on whether it is the right time to de-essentialize deaf identities:

> What also needs to be remembered, however, is the historical significance of the development of racial and feminist theories, a significant part of which were developed as a product of resistance to oppressive theories about women and Black people. The subsequent critiques of these generic theories have developed over time, but are critiques that have evolved at a time when the theorizing around these identities is secure enough to withstand such challenge and to resist the threat of nihilism in outcome. The question lies open as to whether Deaf identity or identities are in equally safeguard position.

Ladd (2003) also warns about relativism in a time in which minority groups are moving toward emancipation and are able to represent themselves politically. With the concept of Deafhood, he aims to create "an academic space . . . which recognizes the existence of 'counternarratives' in themselves, a pole around which resistance thinking can even be organized" (Ladd, 2003, p. 81). Simultaneously, he also responds to the "dangers of essentialism": "I hope, then, that in succeeding years others may be able to develop readings which refine and 'de-essentialize' this one, as far as that is necessary" (p. 81).

The naturalized stance in this chapter is a response to this hope, both from analytical and normative points of view. It is a major challenge in the light of the "new era of participation and collaboration" and questions of (1) how to deal with intrinsic human diversity, including deafness, in educational and societal contexts in an increasingly globalized and urbanized world and (2) how to foster human flourishing (Nussbaum, 2006), that is, helping all people to live up to their potential.

This naturalized stance benefits from an anthropological conceptualization of human beings as learners in a particular social, political, economic, and cultural context, which is based on the theories of Vygotsky (1978) and Cole (1996) (De Clerck & Pinxten, 2011a, b). Identities are shaped and constructed in relation to the social and cultural resources that are available and in interaction with peers and other people (for an application to deaf identity as a learning process, see De Clerck, 2009b). Appiah (2005) conceptualizes an ethical self as a dialogical self:

> As we come to maturity, the identities we make, our individualities, are interpretive responses to our talents and disabilities, and the changing social, semantic, and material contexts we enter at birth; and we develop our identities dialectically with our capacities and circumstances, because they are in part the product of what our identities lead us to. (p. 163)

In contrast to these authors, I argue that nihilism is not the only alternative for essentialism. While human beings are genetically relatively homogenous, all human beings are individually different. As a result of these small differences, over ages, human beings have developed various strategies for survival, which differ with the natural and historical context in which individuals were living. From generation to generation, human beings have learned how to become human, and in this learning process there has been room for interpretation. These differences can be acknowledged without turning difference into a dogmatic norm that considers all variation as "deviance" (Pinxten, 2007).

Nobel Prize–winner Amartya Sen (2006) notices that in times of mobilization of cultural and religious identity, the perception of people as members of only one particular group promotes violence. A dominant group or communal identity may become a destiny that can only be discovered through self-actualization. Whereas there is social capital in a sense of community, there is also a risk of exclusion. The solution is in the recognition of "competing affiliations":

> We have to draw on the understanding that the force of a bellicose identity can be challenged by the power of *competing* identities. These can, of course, include the broad commonalities of our shared humanity, but also many other identities that

> everyone simultaneously has. . . . Along with the recognition of the plurality of our identity and their diverse affiliations, there is a critically important need to see the role of *choice* in determining the cogency and relevance of particular identities which are inescapable diverse. (Sen, 2008, p. 4)

> The freedom to determine our loyalties and priorities between the different groups to all of which we may belong is a peculiarly important liberty which we have reason to recognize, value, and defend. (Sen, 2008, p. 5)

If one takes into account research on multiple deaf identities, practices of deaf children and adults of diverse backgrounds in diverse contexts, and both the mobilizing force of unitary constructions of deaf identity and potential of these constructions to be exclusive, then Sen's question as to how educational and societal contexts can create the circumstances in which people will be able to reason about identity constructions and have the freedom to make choices is also a question that must be faced by the fields of deaf education and deaf studies:

> Is multiculturalism nothing other than the tolerance of diversity of cultures? Does it make a difference who chooses the cultural practices, whether they are imposed in the name of "the culture of the community" or whether they are freely chosen by persons with adequate opportunity to learn and reason about alternatives? What facilities do members of different communities have, in schools as well as in the society at large, to learn about the faiths—and nonfaiths—of different people in the world and to understand how to reason about choices that human beings must, if only implicitly, make? (Sen, 2006, p. 152)

Notions of deaf culture and deaf identity have been able to create room for the lives of deaf people; the challenge is now for these concepts to be employed as complex and dynamic notions that create room for and are created by diverse and contextualized practices of deaf people and that also have emancipatory potential. Deaf people are also women, children, people of color, Hindus, workers, people who are living in Third World countries, and so forth. Consequently, deaf people's flourishing will only be possible in a shared orientation toward the flourishing of all people.

CONCLUSION

> The place to test the success of an educational system is not in the schoolroom nor in conversation over the social teacup, but out where men toil and earn their daily bread.
>
> —Schuyler Long (cited in Andersson, 1991, p. 99)

Deaf epistemologies have put value neutrality and objectivity in science into question. The diverse lives and experiences of deaf people should be the methodological basis for research. Criticizing audism in the practice of science, scholars who practice deaf epistemologies have looked at old *problems* from different angles and contributed to a more appropriate science (see also Nader, 2006). I argue for multiple perspectives in the evaluation of research (see also Campbell, 1989) and a reflexive stance on dynamics of (linguistic and cultural) power relations in the academy (Bourdieu, 1990, 1998).

Deaf studies has become institutionalized predominantly in Western countries, and, as anthropological and sociological studies indicate, a critical perspective toward cultural bias in notions of deaf identity, deaf culture, deaf empowerment, and deaf education is needed.

The naturalized epistemological stance discussed in the present chapter calls for cross-cultural comparative research, which may provide a basis for a posteriori universals and for a study of deaf (indigenous) knowledge and practices that can contribute to this project. The deaf studies debate on essentialism can be conceptualized as an epistemological one, challenged by the naturalized stance expressed in the present chapter. Essentialized notions of deaf identity should be situated as particular constructions of multiple identities in a time and place. Taking into account "structural violence" around the globe (Farmer, 2010) among axes of difference, intrinsic diversity in clusters of identity, an orientation toward human flourishing (Nussbaum, 2006), the approaches of Sen (2006) and Appiah (2005) are inspirational for dealing with the complex notion of identity in deaf educational contexts. As an alternative to politicized notions of identity, Sen emphasizes the role of reason and choice in identity formation; Appiah emphasizes that identity formation is an interactive and situated learning process.

Deaf scholars, particularly scholars from deaf minorities, are still underrepresented in the field. Developing different lines in metatheorization is vital to the future of deaf studies and the lives of deaf people. Joint intercultural and interdisciplinary research projects between deaf and hearing scholars will foster methodological reflection and exploration.

A democratic, pluralistic society should encourage individuals and groups to acquire the power to live according to their own views. Deaf people, individually and in association, should be able to organize education according to their own solutions (Andersson, 1991). These include multilingualism (Reagan & Osborn, 2002; Skutnabb-Kangas, 2008) and multiple deaf epistemologies. In a diverse world with equal languages, cultures, and human beings (Skutnabb-Kangas, 1990), multiple literacies change standard views on reading achievement in favor of valuation of deaf people's contextualized and sign language literacy (Brueggemann, 1995, 2004) and a notion of education that looks further than the classroom to include (indigenous) deaf ways of learning (e.g., De Clerck, 2007).

While recognizing that different factors may explain the educational "failure" of deaf students documented in research, true bilingual education for deaf students in ideal conditions is still scarce (Skutnabb-Kangas, 1990, 2008). To provide deaf people with the best circumstances and chances to live up to their potential, diverse forms of knowledge, scientific and indigenous, may be needed (see also Nader, 2006). The wisdom and experiences that deaf people have gained from life may be the best source for evaluating efforts toward this end.

With respect to further theorizing and research, I recommend the following:

- The study of deaf (indigenous) knowledge and practices, both in Western and non-Western contexts, and cross-cultural comparative research.
- Further research on challenges in deaf education in an increasingly globalized and urbanized world; praxis and practices of multilingualism, interculturalism,

multiple literacies, multiple deaf identities, and multiple (deaf) epistemologies in educational contexts.

- Critically complementing the current research base by research in non-Western contexts for further metatheorizing; this is vital to the lives of deaf people around the world and to the future of the field.
- Further reflection on the different lines of metatheorizing on deaf epistemologies.

NOTES

1. In alignment with the naturalized epistemological stance of this chapter, which is oriented toward describing a diversity of human practices, a d/D distinction is not made. Breivik and colleagues reflect upon the (confusing) use of those terms and this distinction, which is in a constant stage of flux within the deaf community (Breivik, Haualand, & Solvang, 2002, p. v). Both spoken and signed practices can be described; this chapter predominantly concentrates on deaf cultural practices in deaf communities around the world. A normative and emancipatory view encourages people to develop their own perspectives. This also means that opportunities should be provided for deaf children to grow up in educational contexts with visual learning, sign language, and contact with deaf adults.
2. I thank Markku Jokinen for discussions of the parallels between the "new era" and "global deaf renaissance themes."
3. I have relied on the literature on feminist epistemologies (e.g., Code, 2006; Collins, 1990; Davis, Evans, & Lorber, 2006; Duran, 1998; Tanesini, 1999). Feminist theorizing has evolved across a large number of publications containing a diverse range of views. Consequently, I am not able to able to cover all the theoretical issues. Code (2006) points out that metatheorizing was put on the feminist agenda rather late. Theories often refer to Sandra Harding's (1980) distinction of three epistemological strands in feminist theorizing: feminist empiricism, feminist standpoint theories, and feminist postmodernism. Harding's classification has been criticized: Distinctions among these lines of inquiry cannot always be clearly drawn, theories cannot always be classified as such, and researchers often employ more than one line of thought at the same time. Despite this, the classification is useful for insight into deaf epistemologies, and the three lines of inquiry might provide inspiration for further metatheorizing in the field of deaf studies. Black and indigenous African/African-centered epistemologies (Asante, 2003; Dei, 2010; Higgs, 2008, 2010) are also inspiring.
4. I am aware that terms such as *indigenous knowledge* and *local knowledge* have different denotations and connotations (see also Sillitoe, 1998). However, in-depth discussion is beyond the scope of the present chapter.
5. Studies have expanded this line of thought, for example, in the exploration of visual rhetoric, ASL literacy/signacy, and the cinematographic characteristics of sign language (e.g., Brueggemann, 1995, 2004; Paul, 2006).
6. Although I do follow Andersson's comparative perspective, I disagree on the positivistic orientation of cross-cultural comparative research in Andersson (1981). Instead, I argue for in-depth empirical, situated, cultural comparison in line with Geertz (1983) and Pinxten (1997b; 2006). I was inspired by my international deaf friends during my three-year stay at Gallaudet University. The emancipation of deaf people in our home countries throughout the world was a favorite topic of discussion and reflection. I consider the strong international bond and solidarity among deaf people and our use of sign language to be one of the most vital aspects of my life. However—and this experience has been confirmed in my encounters with deaf people during travel on different continents—it is crucial to recognize differences. For example, I did not grow up in a country that takes bilingual–bicultural education for deaf people for granted, nor was I born in sub-Saharan Africa, unable to marry because my boyfriend lacked educational opportunities and was unemployed.

7. Ladd (2003) argued that the notion of *insider* does not take into account the academic background of deaf researchers and other differences with nonacademic deaf people, such as growing up mainstreamed and having English as a first language. Drawing upon subaltern studies, Ladd developed the notion of "subaltern elite researcher."

   Another perspective that is useful in explaining differences related to the academic training of deaf researchers and other differences in background is Collins's (1990) concept of "outsider-within," which refers to the position of people who belong to a community but occupy a relatively marginal position. I note that apart from factors mentioned by Ladd (education and mainstreaming), I experienced age and gender as differentiating categories, as well as my cultural (European/white) background. Deaf researchers may relate to the experience of black women in academia who "remain outsiders within, individuals whose marginality provides a different angle of vision on the theories put forth by . . . intellectual communities" (Collins, 1991, p. 12).
8. I use the term *deaf knowledge(s)* to refer to deaf people's ways of knowing. Erting and colleagues (2006) covered this meaning with the term *Deaf indigenous knowledge*; however, in the present chapter, the term *deaf indigenous knowledge(s)* refers to non-Western deaf knowledges. The term *Deaf indigenous knowledge* in Storbeck and Magongwa (2006) may include both meanings—this was not clear to me.

REFERENCES

Aldridge, D. P., & James, E. L. (Eds.). (2007). *Africana studies: Philosophical perspectives and theoretical paradigms*. Pullman: Washington State University Press.

Andersson, Y. (1981). *A cross-cultural comparative study: Deafness* (Unpublished doctoral dissertation). University of Maryland, College Park.

Andersson, Y. (1990). The Deaf world as a linguistic minority. In S. Prillwitz & T. Vollhaber (Eds.), *Sign language research and application* (pp. 155–161). Hamburg, Germany: Signum.

Andersson, Y. (1991, March). *Some sociological implications of Deaf studies*. Paper presented at the National Deaf Studies Conference, Dallas, TX.

Andersson, Y. (1994). Comment on Turner. *Sign Language Studies, 83*, 127–131.

Appadurai, A. (2003). *Modernity at large: Cultural dimensions of globalization*. Minneapolis: University of Minnesota Press.

Appiah, K. (2005). *The ethics of identity*. Princeton, NJ: Princeton University Press.

Asante, M. K. (2003). *Afrocentricity: The theory of social change*. Chicago, IL: African American Images.

Ashcroft, B., Griffiths, G., & Tiffin, H. (Eds.). (1995). *The postcolonial studies reader*. New York: Routledge.

Bahan, B. (1994). Comment on Turner: View from the Deaf world. *Sign Language Studies, 83*, 241–249.

Baker, C., & Battison, R. (Eds.). (1980). *Sign language and the Deaf community*. Silver Spring, MD: National Association of the Deaf.

Banks, J. A. (1994). *Multiethic education: Theory and practice* (3rd ed.). Boston: Allyn & Bacon.

Barcham, L. (1998). The international dimension. In S. Gregory, P. Knight, W. McCracken, S. Powers, & L. Watson (Eds.), *Issues in deaf education* (pp. 245–254). London: David Fulton.

Baumann, G. (1999). *The riddle of multiculturalism: Rethinking national, ethnic, and religious identities*. New York: Routledge.

Bourdieu, P. (1990). *The logic of practice*. Cambridge, UK: Polity Press.

Bourdieu, P. (1998). *Practical reason*. Cambridge, UK: Polity Press.

Bourdieu, P., & Wacquant, L. (1992). *An invitation to reflexive sociology*. Cambridge, UK: Polity Press.

Braidotti, R. (2003). Becoming woman: Or sexual difference revisited. *Theory, culture, and society, 20*(3), 43–65.

Branson, M., & Miller, D. (1998). Achieving human rights: Educating deaf immigrant students from non-English-speaking families in Australia. In A. Weisel (Ed.), *Issues unresolved: New perspectives on language and deaf education* (pp. 88–100). Washington, DC: Gallaudet University Press.

Branson, M., & Miller, D. (2004). The cultural construction of linguistic incompetence through schooling: Deaf education and the transformation of the linguistic environment in Bali, Indonesia. *Sign Language Studies, 5*, 6–38.

Breivik, J. (2005). *Deaf identities in the making: Local lives, transnational connections.* Washington, DC: Gallaudet University Press.

Breivik, J., Haualand, H., & Solvang, P. (2002). *Rome—A temporary deaf city! Deaflympics 2001* (Working Paper No. 2-2003). Bergen, Norway: Stein Rokken Center for Deaf Studies, University of Bergen. Retrieved October 12, 2005, from http://www.ub.uib.no/elpub/rookkan/N/N02-02.pdf

Brueggemann, B. (1995). The coming out of Deaf culture and American Sign Language: An exploration into visual rhetoric and literacy. *Rhetoric Review, 13*(2), 409–420.

Brueggemann, B. (Ed.). (2004). *Literacy and deaf people: Cultural and contextual perspectives.* Washington, DC: Gallaudet University Press.

Brueggemann, B., & Burch, S. (2006). (Eds.). *Women and deafness: Double visions.* Washington, DC: Gallaudet University Press.

Campbell, D. (1989). *Methodology and epistemology for social sciences.* Chicago: University of Chicago Press.

Code, L. (2006). Women knowing/knowing women: Critical-creative interventions in the politics of knowledge. In K. Davis, M. Evans, & J. Lorber (Eds.), *Handbook of gender and women's studies* (pp. 146–167). Thousand Oaks, CA: Sage.

Cole, M. (1996). *Cultural psychology.* Cambridge, MA: Harvard University Press.

Collins, P. H. (1990). *Black feminist thought: Knowledge, consciousness, and the politics of empowerment.* London: Women's Press.

Crenshaw, K. (1991). Mapping the margins: Intersectionality, identity politics, and violence against women of color. *Stanford Law Review, 43*(6), 1241–1299.

Crombie, A. (1994). *Styles of scientific thinking in the European tradition.* London: Redwood Books.

Daniels, H., Cole, M., & Wertsch, J. (2007). *The Cambridge campanion to Vygotsky.* Cambridge, UK: Cambridge University Press.

Davis, K., Evans, M., & Lorber, J. (2006). *Handbook of gender and women's studies.* Thousand Oaks, CA: Sage.

Davis, L. J. (2007, January 12). Deafness and the riddle of identity. *Chronicle Review, 53*(19), B6. Retrieved July 8, 2008, from http://chronicle.com.proxy.cc.uic.edu

De Clerck, G. (2007). Meeting global deaf peers and visiting ideal deaf places: Deaf ways of education leading to empowerment, an exploratory case study. *American Annals of the Deaf, 152*(4), 5–15.

De Clerck, G. (2009a). Identiteitsdynamieken in Vlaamse dove rolmodellen: Een verkenning van tendenzen in emancipatieprocessen in dovengemeenschappen en parallellen met etnische minderheden in Europa [Identity dynamics in Flemish deaf role models: An exploration of trends in emancipation processes in deaf communities and parallels with ethnic minorities in Europe]. *Volkskunde, 110*(2), 117–136.

De Clerck, G. (2009b). "I don't worry because I have my education": International deaf people moving toward emancipation. *Medische Antropologie, 21*(1), 131–158.

De Clerck, G., & Pinxten, R. (2011a). Dealing with intrinsic diversity: Deaf culture as "a concept from the wild." Manuscript in preparation.

De Clerck, G., & Pinxten, R. (2011b). *Capabilities and learning processes.* Manuscript in preparation.

Dei, G. (2010). *Teaching Africa: Toward a transgressive pedagogy.* New York: Springer.

Duran, J. (1998). *Philosophies of science/feminist theories.* Boulder, CO: Westview.

Elzinga, A., & Jamison, A. (1981). *Cultural components in the scientific attitude to nature: Eastern and Western modes?* (Discussion Paper 149). Göteborg, Sweden: Götenborg University Press.

Erting, C. (1976). Introduction. In C. Erting, R. C. Johnson, D. L. Smith, & B. D. Snider (Eds.), *The Deaf way: Perspectives from the International Conference on Deaf Culture* (pp. xxiii–xxxi). Washington, DC: Gallaudet University Press.

Erting, C. (1978). Language policy and Deaf ethnicity in the United States. *Sign Language Studies, 19*, 139–152.

Erting, C., Bailes, C., Erting, L., Thumann-Prezioso, C., & Kuntze, M. (2006). Signs of literacy: Naturalistic inquiry into ASL/English bilingualism at home and at school. In H. Goodstein (Ed.), *The Deaf Way II reader: Perspectives from the Second International Conference on Deaf Culture* (pp. 88–99). Washington, DC: Gallaudet University Press.

Erting, C., Johnson, R. C., Smith, D. L., & Snider, B. D. (Eds.). (1994). *The Deaf way: Perspectives from the International Conference on Deaf Culture.* Washington, DC: Gallaudet University Press.

Erting, C., Thumann-Prezioso, C., & Benedict, B. (2000). Bilingualism in a deaf family. In P. Spencer, C. Erting, & M. Marschark (Eds.), *The deaf child in the family and at school* (pp. 41–54). Mahwah, NJ: Erlbaum.

Fabian, J. (1990). *Power and performance: Ethnographic explorations through proverbial wisdom and theater in Shaba, Zaire.* Madison, WI: University of Wisconsin Press.

Farmer, P. (2010). An anthropology of structural violence. In H. Saussy (Ed.), *Partner to the poor: A Paul Farmer reader* (pp. 350–375). Berkeley: University of California Press.

Feyerabend, P. (1965). Problems of empiricism. In R. Colodny (Ed.), *Beyond the edge of certainty* (pp. 145–260). Englewood Cliffs, NJ: Prentice Hall.

Fisher, R., & Lane, H. (Eds.). (2003). *Looking back: A reader on the history of Deaf communities and their sign languages.* Hamburg, Germany: Signum.

Geertz, C. (1973). *The interpretation of culture.* New York: Basic Books.

Geertz, C. (1983). *Local knowledge: Further essays in interpretive anthropology.* New York: Basic Books.

Geertz, C. (1995). *After the fact: Two countries, four decades, one anthropologist.* Cambridge, MA: Harvard University Press.

Goodstein, H. (2006). *The Deaf Way II reader: Perspectives from the Second International Conference on Deaf Culture.* Washington, DC: Gallaudet University Press.

Groce, N. E. (1995). *Everyone here spoke sign language: Hereditary deafness on Martha's Vineyard.* Cambridge, MA: Harvard University Press.

Hannerz, U. (2003). Macro-scenarios: Anthropology and the debate over contemporary and future worlds. *Social Anthropology, 11*, 169–187.

Hanson, N. R. (1958). *Patterns of discovery.* Cambridge, UK: Cambridge University Press.

Harding, S. (1980). *The science question in feminism.* Ithaca, NY: Cornell University Press.

Haualand, H., & Allen, C. (2009). *Deaf people and human rights.* Helsinki, Finland: World Federation of the Deaf and Swedish Federation of the Deaf. Retrieved from http://wfdeaf.org/projects.html

Haualand, H., Gronningsaeter, A., & Hansen, I. (2003). Uniting divided worlds: Identity, family, and education in the life projects of deaf and hard of hearing young people. *Disability Studies Quarterly, 23*, 75–88.

Higgins, P. (1980). *Outsiders in a hearing world: A sociology of deafness.* Beverly Hills, CA: Sage.

Higgs, P. (2008). Towards an indigenous African educational discourse: A philosophical reflection. *International Review of Education, 54*, 445–458.

Higgs, P. (2010). Towards an indigenous African epistemology of community in education research. *Procedia: Social and Behavioral Sciences, 2*, 2414–2421.

Hofstede, G. (1991). *Allemaal andersdenkenden* [All different-minded]. Amsterdam, the Netherlands: Contact.

Humphries, T. (2007). Talking culture and culture talking. In D. Bauman (Ed.), *Open your eyes: Deaf studies talking* (pp. 35–41). Minneapolis, MN: University of Minnesota Press.

Jamieson, J. R., & Moores, D.F. (2011). Partners in education. In D. F. Moores (Ed.), *Partners in education: Issues and trends from the 21st International Congress on the Education of the Deaf* (pp. 20–28). Washington, DC: Gallaudet University Press.

James, M., & Woll, B. (2004). Black deaf or deaf black? Being black and deaf in Britain. In A. Pavlenko & A. Blackledge (Eds.), *Negotiation of identities in multilingual contexts* (pp. 125–160). Clevedon, UK: Multilingual Matters.

Jankowski, K. A. (1997). *Deaf empowerment: Emergence, struggle, and rhetoric*. Washington, DC: Gallaudet University Press.

Johnson, R. E. (1994). Sign language and the concept of deafness in a traditional Yucatec Mayan village. In C. Erting, R. C. Johnson, D. L. Smith, & B. D. Snider (Eds.), *The Deaf way: Perspectives from the International Conference on Deaf Culture* (pp. 102–109). Washington, DC: Gallaudet University Press.

Johnson, R. E., & Erting, C. (1989). Ethnicity and socialization in a classroom for deaf children. In C. Lucas & C. Valli (Eds.), *Sociolinguistics of the Deaf community* (pp. 41–83). San Diego, CA: Academic Press.

Johnston, T. (1994). Comment on Turner. *Sign Language Studies, 83*, 133–138.

Kuhn, T. S. (1962). *The structure of scientific revolutions*. Chicago, IL: University of Chicago Press.

Kyle, J. (1990). The Deaf community: Culture, custom, and tradition. In S. Prillwitz & T. Vollhaber (Eds.), *Sign language research and application* (pp. 175–185). Hamburg, Germany: Signum.

Ladd, P. (2003). *Understanding Deaf culture: In search of Deafhood*. Clevedon, UK: Multilingual Matters.

Lane, H. (1984). *When the mind hears*. New York, NY: Random House.

Lane, H. (1999). *The mask of benevolence: Disabling the Deaf community*. San Diego, CA: DawnSignPress.

Lane, H. (2005). Ethnicity, ethics, and the Deaf-world. *Journal of Deaf Studies and Deaf Education, 10*(3), 291–301.

Le Master, B. (2003). School language and shifts in Irish Deaf identity. In L. Monaghan, C. Schmaling, K. Nakamura, & G. Turner (Eds.), *Many ways to be deaf: International variation in Deaf communities* (pp. 153–172). Washington, DC: Gallaudet University Press.

Markowicz, H., & Woodward, J. (1982). Language and the maintenance of ethnic boundaries in the Deaf community. In J. Woodward (Ed.), *How you gonna get to heaven if you can't talk with Jesus: On depathologizing deafness* (pp. 3–10). Silver Spring, MD: T. J. Publishers.

Massey, D., & Jess, P. (Eds.). (1995). *A place in the world: Places, cultures, and globalization*. New York, NY: Oxford University Press.

Mindess, A. (1999). *Reading between the signs: Intercultural communication for sign language interpreters*. Yarmouth, ME: Intercultural Press.

Monaghan, L. (1994). Comment on Turner. *Sign Language Studies, 83*, 139–144.

Monaghan, L. (2003). A world's-eye view: Deaf cultures in a global perspective. In L. Monaghan, C. Schmaling, K. Nakamura, & G. Turner (Eds.), *Many ways to be deaf: International variation in Deaf communities* (pp. 1–24). Washington, DC: Gallaudet University Press.

Monaghan, L., Schmaling, C., Nakamura, K., & Turner, G. (Eds.). (2003). *Many ways to be deaf: International variation in Deaf communities*. Washington, DC: Gallaudet University Press.

Moores, D. (2010). Epistemologies, deafness, learning, and teaching. *American Annals of the Deaf, 154*(5), 447–455.

Moores, D., & Paul, P. (2010). Perspectives on deaf epistemologies. *American Annals of the Deaf, 154*(5), 493–500.

Nader, L. (2006). *Naked science: Anthropological inquiry into boundaries, power, and knowledge*. London, UK: Routledge.

Nakamura, K. (2005). *Deaf in Japan: Signing and the politics of identity*. Ithaca, NY: Cornell University Press.

Narajian, C. (2006). Deaf mothers, maternal thinking, and intersections of gender and ability. *Scandinavian Journal of Disability Research, 8*(2–3), 100–119.

Needham, J. (1965). *Science and civilization in China*. Cambridge, UK: Cambridge University Press.

Nussbaum, M. (2006). *Frontiers of justice: Disability, nationality, species membership.* Cambridge, MA: Harvard University Press.

Obasi, C. (2008). Seeing the Deaf in "Deafness." *Journal of Deaf Studies and Deaf Education, 13*(4), 455–465.

Padden, C. (1980). The Deaf community and the culture of deaf people. In C. Baker & R. Battison (Eds.), *Sign language and the Deaf community* (pp. 89–103). Silver Spring, MD: National Association of the Deaf.

Padden, C. (1996a). Early bilingual lives of deaf children. In I. Parasnis (Ed.), *Cultural and language diversity and the Deaf experience* (pp. 99–116). New York, NY: Cambridge University Press.

Padden, C. (1996b). From the cultural to the bicultural: The modern Deaf community. In I. Parasnis (Ed.), *Cultural and language diversity and the Deaf experience* (pp. 79–97). New York, NY: Cambridge University Press.

Padden, C., & Humphries, T. (1988). *Deaf in America: Voices from a culture.* Cambridge, MA: Harvard University Press.

Padden, C., & Humphries, T. (2005). *Inside Deaf culture.* Cambridge, MA: Harvard University Press.

Paul, P. (2006). New literacies, multiple literacies, unlimited literacies: What now, what next, where to? A response to blue Listerine, parochialism, and ASL literacy. *Journal of Deaf Studies and Deaf Education, 11*(3), 382–387.

Perelman, C., & Olbrechts-Tyteca, S. (1957). *La nouvelle rhétorique: Traité de l'argumentation* [The new rhetoric: Treatise on argumentation]. Paris, France: PUF.

Pinxten, R. (1991). Objectivism versus relativism: What are we arguing about? In J. De Wolf et al. (Eds.), *Cognitive relativism and social science* (pp. 181–191). New York: Transaction Press.

Pinxten, R. (1997a). Application in the teaching of mathematics and the sciences. In A. Powel & M. Frankenstein (Eds.), *Ethnomathematics: Challenging Eurocentrism in mathematics education* (pp. 373–401). Albany, NY: State University of New York Press.

Pinxten, R. (1997b). *When the day breaks: Essays in anthropology and philosophy.* Frankfurt, Germany: Peter Lang.

Pinxten, R. (1999). *Culturen sterven langzaam: Over interculturele communicatie* [Cultures die slowly: On intercultural communication]. Antwerp, Belgium: Houtekiet.

Pinxten, R. (2006, September). *The relevance of a noncolonial view on science and knowledge for an open perspective on the world.* Paper presented at the biennial conference of the European Association of Social Anthropologists, Bristol, UK.

Pinxten, R. (2007). *De strepen van de zebra* [The stripes of the zebra]. Antwerp, Belgium: Houtekiet.

Pinxten, R., & De Munter, K. (2006). *De culturele eeuw* [The cultural century]. Antwerp, Belgium: Houtekiet.

Pinxten, R., & Note, N. (2005). A naturalistic and critical view of social sciences and the humanities. In D. Aerts, B. D'Hooge, & N. Note (Eds.), *Worldviews, science, and us: Redemarcating knowledge and its social and ethical implications* (pp. 93–103). Hackensack, NJ: World Scientific.

Pinxten, R., Verstraete, G., & Longman, C. (Eds.). (2004). *Culture and politics: Identity and conflict in a multicultural world.* New York, NY: Berghahn Books.

Pottier, J., Bicker, A., & Sillitoe, P. (Eds.). (2003). *Negotiating local knowledge: Power and identity in development.* Sterling, VA: Pluto Press.

Reagan, T., & Osborn, T. (2002). *The foreign-language educator in society: Toward a critical pedagogy.* Mahwah, NJ: Erlbaum.

Reilly, C. B. (1995). *A Deaf way of education: Interaction among children in a Thai boarding school* (Unpublished doctoral dissertation). University of Maryland, College Park.

Said, E. (1995). *Orientalism: Western conceptions of the Orient.* London, UK: Penguin Books.

Schmaling, C. (2003). A for apple: The impact of Western education and ASL on the Deaf community in Kano State, northern Nigeria. In L. Monaghan, C. Schmaling, K. Nakamura, & G. Turner (Eds.), *Many ways to be deaf: International variation in Deaf communities* (pp. 302–310). Washington, DC: Gallaudet University Press.

Sen, A. (2006). *Identity and violence: The illusion of destiny.* New York, NY: Norton.

Sillitoe, P. (1998). The development of indigenous knowledge: A new applied anthropology. *Current Anthropology, 39*(2), 223–252.

Simms, L. (2006). Deaf education: Whose "way" is it? In H. Goodstein (Ed.), *The Deaf Way II reader: Perspectives from the Second International Conference on Deaf Culture* (pp. 81–86). Washington, DC: Gallaudet University Press.

Skutnabb-Kangas, T. (1990). *Language, literacy, and minorities.* London, UK: Minority Rights Group.

Skutnabb-Kangas, T. (2008, October). *Linguistic human rights of the deaf: Why, when, and what—and decided by whom? The little matter of crimes against humanity.* Paper presented at the Gallaudet University Forum on Linguistic Human Rights and the Future of Sign Languages, Washington, DC.

Spivak, G. (1995). Can the subaltern speak? In B. Ashcroft, G. Griffiths, & H. Tiffin (Eds.), *The postcolonial studies reader* (pp. 24–28). New York, NY: Routledge.

Stokoe, W. C. (1960). *Sign language structure: An outline of the visual communication systems of the American deaf.* Buffalo, NY: University of Buffalo.

Stokoe, W. C. (1994). Comment on Turner. *Sign Language Studies, 84,* 265–270.

Stokoe, W. C., Casterline, D. C., & Croneberg, C. G. (1965). *A dictionary of American Sign Language on linguistic principles.* Washington, DC: Gallaudet College Press.

Storbeck, C., & Magongwa, I. (2006). Teaching about Deaf culture. In D. Moores & D. S. Martin (Eds.), *Deaf learners: Developments in curriculum and instruction* (pp. 113–126). Washington, DC: Gallaudet University Press.

Suppe, F. (1977). *The structure of scientific theories.* Urbana, IL: University of Illinois Press.

Tanesini, A. (1999). *An introduction to feminist epistemologies.* Oxford, UK: Blackwell.

Thorvalsdottir, T. (2007). *"Equal opportunities for all": Intersectionality as a theoretical tool to move equality policies forward.* Retrieved http://www.issa.nl/members/member_docs/ESJ_files/at_docs/add_pdfs/Intersectionality.pdf

Turner, G. (1994). How is Deaf culture? Another perspective on a fundamental concept. *Sign Language Studies, 83,* 103–121.

Turner, G. (2004). Exploring British experiences of language and Deafhood in hypermodernity. In M. Van Herreweghe & M. Vermeerbergen (Eds.), *To the lexicon and beyond: Sociolinguistics in European Deaf communities* (pp. 248–263). Washington, DC: Gallaudet University Press.

Tyson, L. (1999). *Critical theory today.* New York, NY: Garland.

Van Cleve, J. V., & Crouch, B. A. (1989). *A place of their own: Creating the Deaf community in America.* Washington, DC: Gallaudet University Press.

Vygotsky, L. (1978). *Mind in society: The development of higher psychological processes.* Cambridge, MA: Harvard University Press.

Williamsen, C. E. (2002). *Black deaf students: A model for educational success.* Washington, DC: Gallaudet University Press.

Woodward, J. (Ed.). (1982). *How you gonna get to heaven if you can't talk with Jesus: On depathologizing deafness.* Silver Spring, MD: T. J. Publishers.

World Federation of the Deaf. (2010). *Global Deaf renaissance: Durban 2011: XVI World Congress of the World Federation of the Deaf (third announcement).* Retrieved from http://www.wfdeaf.org/pdf/3rd%20Announcement%20of%20WFD%20Congress%20in%20South%20Africa.pdf

Young, R. (1995). *Colonial desire: Hybridity in theory, culture, and race.* New York, NY: Routledge.

SUGGESTIONS FOR FURTHER READING

Geertz, C. (1973). *The interpretation of culture.* New York, NY: Basic Books.

Geertz, C. (1983). *Local knowledge: Further essays in interpretive anthropology.* New York, NY: Basic Books.

Padden, C., & T. Humphries, *Inside Deaf culture.* Cambridge, MA: Harvard University Press, 2005.

Vygotsky, L. (1978). *Mind in society. The development of higher psychological processes.* Cambridge, MA: Harvard University Press.

Woodward, J. (Ed.). (1982). *How you gonna get to heaven if you can't talk with Jesus: On depathologizing deafness.* Silver Spring, MD: T. J. Publishers.

3

Juggling Two Worlds

Michael M. McKee and Peter C. Hauser

Deaf epistemologies constitute a branch of philosophy that investigates the origin, nature, methods, and limits of knowledge that deaf[1] individuals acquire while living in a society that relies heavily on audition to navigate life. Many deaf individuals struggle to meet the expectations and demands of a hearing society while balancing those of the Deaf society (e.g., Hauser, O'Hearn, McKee, Steider, & Thew, 2010; Leigh, 2009). Juggling two different worlds can be a challenge for deaf individuals. It has an impact on their identity, understanding of the world, and ultimately their episteme—that is, their knowledge of themselves.

Our goal in this chapter is to contribute to the theory of deaf epistemologies, which has implications for educators, health-care providers, government leaders, families, researchers, and deaf individuals. The chapter is designed to not only to educate but also to provide strategies to lessen the awkwardness and divisions that often exist between hearing and Deaf cultures. We hope these strategies will decrease social stressors, information and communication barriers, and health disparities while increasing cultural and linguistic recognition, information exchange, and opportunities for deaf individuals.

Deafness creates beings who are more visually oriented than their auditory-oriented peers; therefore, the two groups' experiences of the world are different. How deaf and hearing individuals interact with deaf individuals shapes how deaf individuals acquire knowledge and how they learn. Aspects of the deaf episteme, not caused by deafness but by being Deaf, can have a positive impact on how deaf individuals learn, resist oppression (*audism*), stay healthy, and navigate the world (see Hauser et al., 2010, for discussion). Yet, the prevailing focus of hearing society continues to be on deafness, rather than *Deafhood*—a concept first introduced by Ladd (2003) that demonstrates how deafness can provide a sense of identity to a deaf individual. Some aspects of Deafhood are beneficial to the health of deaf individuals. Many of these key elements can be learned or incorporated by hearing individuals. To alter the hearing individuals' focus from negative (deafness) to positive (Deafhood), deaf individuals must be willing to reach out to hearing individuals to educate and increase awareness on the differences. Legal and political steps must be considered when this fails to ensure deaf individuals' rights are protected.

Social constructivism is a social theory of knowledge on how social expectations and cultures influence conformity or development of identities through cultural artifacts. Given the importance of social factors on deaf epistemologies, the lens of social constructivism is used to better understand several sections of this chapter.

Hauser and colleagues (2010) explored how deaf individuals develop a sense of Deafhood and deafness through their experiences in a world dominated by an auditory-reliant society steeped in technology. These expectations both intentionally and unintentionally influence how deaf individual perceive themselves as well as their health.

DEAF EPISTEMOLOGIES: DEAFHOOD AND DEAFNESS

How deaf people view themselves differs from how hearing people perceive them. This leads to a number of different "faces" that deaf individuals must use, depending on whether they are with hearing people or with deaf people. The dissociation between these two populations' thinking reflects two distinct types of knowledge, epistemologies and ideologies (Lane, Hoffmeister, & Bahan, 1996; Padden & Humphries, 2005; Reagan, 2002). Changes in hearing status, unlike changes in any of the other four senses, create a whole different world, a different experience of life, and a reality that is only known to those who grow up in that life. This is mostly because of changes in access to language, knowledge, and cultural capital (e.g., Listman, Hauser, & Rogers, in press). The fact that a deaf individual must navigate two divergent worlds plays a key role in the development of the deaf episteme for many deaf individuals.

Contemporary social epistemologists believe how an individual justifies a belief as "true" depends on that individual's situation, surroundings, prior knowledge, and sociocultural influences (Foucault, 1980; Goodman, 2004; Rosen, 2001). Feminist epistemologists add that the individual's body or biology needs to be taken into consideration when discussing the nature of knowledge (Haslanger, 2000). This thought could be extended to even genetic components and differences. Societies give individuals the knowledge of how to live in their bodies, how to show capacities unique to one's sex, and how to experience their bodies. Similarly, the way a society interacts with deaf infants, children, and adults impacts what these deaf individuals learn and know and consequently their attitudes, interests, values, and even health (Hauser et al., 2010).

The biological experience of sensory deprivation and the sociocultural experiences of other's reactions and interactions illustrate the different effects of deafness and Deafhood respectively. Deafhood, introduced by Ladd (2003), was described as something different from what is known as Deaf culture. Ladd suggests it is "not a 'static' medical condition like 'deafness.' . . . instead, it represents a process—the struggle by each Deaf child, Deaf family and Deaf adult to explain to themselves and each other their own existence in the world" (Ladd, 2003, p. 3). Deafhood and deafness have strong yet separate influences on the deaf individual and contribute to the individual's knowledge of themselves and the world.

From the biological viewpoint, deafness alone can change, for example, certain aspects of an individual's visual attention (see Bavelier, Dye, & Hauser, 2006, for a review). Specifically, deafness, not experience with sign language, causes an individual to allocate more attention to the visual periphery and be more sensitive to motion in the periphery. This effect might be due to deaf individuals' intrinsic need for survival, relying on the visual modality more than hearing individuals do. There are other influences that are not effects of deafness but effects of life as being deaf such as having fluency in a visual language (Bellugi, O'Grady, Lillo-Martin, O'Grady, van Hoek, & Corina, 1990; Emmorey & Kosslyn, 1996).

The simple notion of not being able to hear does not completely define the deaf individual nor explain Deafhood. "Deafness" begets unique additional experiences for deaf individuals that go beyond auditory sensory input. Deaf individuals by virtue of their biology live their life in a visual reality, which leads to the acquisition of a knowledge base that is different from hearing individuals (Hauser et al., 2010). By living as visually oriented individuals, the deaf episteme is developed with different knowledge and experiences than the "hearing" episteme because of increased attention to the visual world.

TWO WORLDS, ONE INDIVIDUAL

Deaf people are rarely children of deaf parents. Most deaf individuals grow up in a hearing family and adapt to a hearing-dominated culture before they may seek out others who are similar to them (e.g., other deaf individuals). For some, this is their first exposure to Deaf culture and natural signed languages. Despite the fact that many deaf individuals become acculturated into the Deaf community, their consciousness and reasoning continue to hold many of their former ideals and beliefs commonly held by hearing society. Some of these ideals and beliefs are constructed and viewed through a medical model of disability in which the emphasis is on communicating orally through lipreading and speaking, and minimizing hearing loss by the use of hearing aids and cochlear implants to better integrate deaf individuals into a hearing society (Valentine & Skelton, 2009).

Humphries and Humphries (2010) review DuBois's description of African Americans' identification with "double consciousness—the two souls, two thoughts, two un-reconciled strivings; two warring ideals in one dark body" and how this also applies to deaf individuals (Humphries & Humphries, 2010). Many deaf individuals relate to this experience—two contrasting and vastly different expectations are held by deaf people and by hearing society, that is, hearing people who simply perceive deaf individuals as disabled people who are not able to hear (Humphries, 1996). Striving for some balance of expectations by two different cultures, deaf individuals juggle these two worlds. Some deaf individuals are able to juggle with relative ease while others struggle. Individuals who struggle may grow angry, frustrated, anxious, or even depressed.

The perception that there is a difference based on the body (i.e., the perceived imperfection of deaf bodies) is a concept common to audism, racism, and sexism (Hauser et al., 2010). This negative perception leads to the assumption that deaf bodies are undesired, unwanted, inferior, and in need of repair. To the extent that deaf people do not hear and do not speak, they are seen as less intelligent, less capable, and less human (Bauman, 2004). Embedded within cultural practices and coded into social and cultural institutions, audism often appears in the form of treatments, therapies, and interventions connected to a psychology of deficit (Lane, 1992). The most salient impact of audism today may be the act of questioning one's identity by deaf individuals, even to the point of self-doubt or lowered confidence.

The struggle of deaf people to maintain a sense of identity or confidence in the face of others' definition of them has created uncertainty among deaf people about their own linguistic, cultural, and social identities (Humphries, 2008). The pressures to assimilate in hearing society can give some deaf individuals what Gertz (2008) calls *dysconscious audism,* where they accept the perception that they are inferior. This is similar to the findings of the classical study in the 1930s where African American girls were found to prefer to play with white dolls over black dolls and often thought the white doll "looks nice" while the black doll "looks bad" (Clark & Clark, 1939), which suggests internalized oppression among these African American preschoolers.

Dominant societies and cultural groups exert a lot of pressure on immigrant, refugee, and minority groups to assimilate and acculturate (Berry, 1992). Some groups are able to adapt readily while others struggle. Each group also varies in the degree of successful acculturation versus assimilation. For example, many immigrant Hispanic groups are able to acculturate to varying levels but frequently fail to assimilate fully as a result of cultural and language differences, thereby largely preserving their group's identity (Berry, 2006). Countries such as the United States are becoming a plural society with a mixture of minority groups. This helps to lessen the assimilation and, to a lesser degree, acculturation pressures. Hispanic individuals constitute the largest minority group in the United States, which helps to provide a network of supportive communities, schools, governments, organizations, and businesses (e.g., Yosso, 2005). This allows for this group to develop and support bilingual educational programs in many areas, which helps to further preserve the group's cultural and language roots.

Unfortunately, the ability to avoid assimilation pressures does not occur for many deaf individuals because of a variety of factors. For example, deaf individuals are more likely to be poor, unemployed, and less educated than hearing individuals (e.g., Blanchfield, Feldman, Dunbar, & Gardner, 2001). While it is unclear if rates of poverty, low education, and unemployment are also greater within the Deaf community (no reliable national survey exists) than they are for all deaf individuals, it is widely believed that these rates are as dismal if not worse within the Deaf community (Barnett, 1999; Steinberg, Barnett, Meador, Wiggins, & Zazove, 2006; Zazove, Meador, Reed, Sen, & Gorenflo, 2009). Furthermore, the Deaf community is a relatively small linguistic and cultural minority with a population size likely around 250,000 to 500,000 (Mitchell, Young, Bachleda, & Karchmer, 2006).

With a smaller population consisting of individuals who are likely to be poor, these social factors likely influence businesses, organizations, and even politicians to frequently overlook the Deaf community. This social marginalization of many deaf individuals can lead to a sense of loneliness, frustration, and even depression over the loss of societal power and reduced social standing. This can reinforce the dysconscious audism (Gertz, 2008), which can cause deaf individuals to perceive themselves as inferior as they view others perceiving them as inferior. Hence, their deaf episteme might include some internalized oppression.

Most hearing parents struggle with a lack of information on how to raise their deaf child (Eleweke & Rodda, 2000; Jackson & Turnbull, 2004). They often seek information and assistance from their physicians, audiologists, early intervention program educators, and speech therapists. Few opportunities exist for these parents to talk and learn from Deaf adults, but when the opportunities exist, it reduces their parental stress (Hintermair, 2000). A strong majority of deaf children are currently mainstreamed in hearing schools with little exposure to natural signed language and have few interactions with other deaf children (Hauser & Marschark, 2008). The lack of exposure to Deaf culture, American Sign Language (ASL), and other modes of education that foster deaf children's interactions with deaf role models can have lasting negative psychosocial and educational effects on the deaf child (Bat-Chava, 1993; Hauser, Wills, & Isquith, 2006). Because 95% of deaf individuals are born to hearing parents, the loss of opportunities for deaf children to learn in a deaf educational system emphasizing bilingual and bicultural approaches can further erode and impact the ability of the Deaf community to preserve its culture and language (Hauser et al., 2010).

These effects are largely unintentional, as most hearing parents are hungry for all possible sources of information on how to best raise their deaf child. Information from the Deaf community is largely inaccessible for the majority of these hearing parents because of a number of factors: language barriers, marginalization of many deaf individuals, lack of deaf schools in many areas, lack of visible deaf role models, and the scarcity of culturally competent medical professionals. These barriers must be removed to provide parents with opportunities to make fully informed decisions on assistive technologies, education modes, and language development strategies. It is paramount that educational and health researchers, along with the Deaf community, make every effort to disseminate research findings to the medical and educational community. There continues to be a dearth of awareness of peer-reviewed and unbiased research findings that show positive effects of natural signed language learning on language and educational development in deaf children.

Greater collaborations and impartiality by medical professionals and deaf leaders will increase information exchanges and opportunities for parents to meet other deaf individuals and better decide on educational and linguistic strategies for their deaf children (Eleweke & Rodda, 2000; Jackson & Turnbull, 2004). Deaf children and individuals should be encouraged to socialize with other deaf individuals. This would help them develop resiliency while decreasing internalized negative perceptions (*dysconscious audism*) among deaf individuals (Listman et al., in press). This will also alter the origin, method of acquisition, and nature of deaf individuals' self-knowledge in a positive way.

THE GREAT DEAF EXPECTATION

Assimilation pressures deaf individuals act more like people in hearing society. Examples of this type of reinforcement can occur when deaf individuals successfully learn how to talk and lipread (able to communicate with hearing society) or learn to play music or dance (enjoy the arts of a hearing society). Hearing society also strongly encourages deaf individuals to utilize assistive devices such as hearing aids or cochlear implants to correct or minimize their hearing "disability" (Lane et al., 1996; Padden & Humphries, 2005). Hearing individuals frequently become anxious when there may be communication, language, or even cultural barriers between them and deaf individuals. Some hearing individuals might avoid social opportunities with deaf individuals as a way to avoid any potential embarrassment. As a result, deaf individuals may feel ignored and isolated at social events, conferences, or even work situations.

It is not until a deaf individual appears to be "more hearing than expected" do these social exclusions start to disappear. Yet, despite the efforts of the deaf individuals who actually strive to be more "hearing," lowered expectations by hearing society continue to prevent or impair the ability for full inclusion to the hearing society (Leigh, 2009; Nikolaraizi & Makri, 2004). There are always exceptions to any rule, such as deaf individuals who fully assimilate and are able to successfully interact in a hearing world and acculturated deaf individuals who avoid any attempts to assimilate yet are able to thrive in a hearing society.

It is challenging for many hearing individuals to imagine how a deaf person, unable to hear, can become successful in the hearing world because many have never met a deaf adult or professional (Hintermair, 2000). This leads to a continual reinforcement of lowered social and academic expectations. Deaf students often hear guidance counselors or teachers state that certain careers or even classes are not realistic for them (Harris & Vanzandt, 1997; Thumann-Prezioso, 2005). Many deaf individuals even frequently laugh or scoff about how hearing individuals ask if they are able to drive or have children. Parents of deaf children may even begin to lower their expectations as a way to "protect" their deaf child from possible disappointments. The lowered expectations are difficult to overcome, yet some deaf students are resilient enough to pursue their goals (Leigh, 2009; Listman et al., in press). Unfortunately, some of these students may be surprised to encounter lowered expectations from other deaf individuals who have come to accept this as "reality."

The *crab theory* is a phenomenon in which deaf individuals do not believe or support a deaf person who achieves unexpected educational or career success or overcomes significant barriers. The crab theory in part might be an indirect manifestation of hearing society's lowered expectations, a damaging by-product of dyconscious audism (Gertz, 2008). Deaf individuals ingrained with the lowered expectations pass these effects on to their peers and deaf children. The struggle against lowered expectations is an ongoing aspect for many deaf individuals' epistemes. For many deaf individuals, low expectations become a manner of "conformity," shaping what they know and believe. This is why it is so crucial that deaf role models be exemplified by the Deaf community to promote greater well-being and opportunities for deaf individuals.

The lack of exposure to deaf role models makes it more challenging for deaf children to aspire to aim high with their goals and to be self-confident. We know that being a visually oriented learner in an auditory-oriented world creates barriers (Hauser, Maxwell, Leigh, & Gutman, 2000) that can have a negative impact on deaf and hard of hearing individuals' psychosocial development and well-being (Hauser et al., 2005). Unlike with other minority or cultural groups, many deaf individuals lack family members who experience discrimination (i.e., audism) themselves. For example, African American mothers help their hearing (Logan, Freeman, & McRoy, 1989; Pinderhughes, 1995) and deaf (Borum, 2007; Morris, 1992) children develop resiliency, resistance, and tolerance to racism. It is doubtful that deaf children are able to adequately learn about handling, resisting, or coping with audism from their hearing parents.

The inability to learn resilience from parents or family members places deaf individuals at a great disadvantage. It seems that this effect of audism might reduce confidence or resilience of a deaf individual, making it easier to feel defeated or to give up before achieving goals (Listman et al., in press). This is why it is essential that deaf children be able to learn from other deaf individuals. Thew (2007) found that deaf employees who attended a school for the deaf and work in hearing environments have stronger resilience than students who attended mainstream programs, which this might be because the former group learned how deaf role models work with hearing adults. Young deaf individuals aspiring to be physicians, attorneys, scientists, teachers, and so forth would greatly benefit from the mentorship of other deaf professionals who already may have pioneered the way. In addition to mentorship, deaf students need encouragement and support from their families, friends, and the Deaf community.

The social and communication struggles that deaf individuals endure also provide a shared bond. A deaf individual from the United States fluent in ASL has more in common with a deaf Japanese individual fluent in Japanese Sign Language than a hearing individual from the United States fluent in English would have with a hearing individual from Japan fluent in Japanese. The "deaf struggle" often transcends other cultural, linguistic, and social experiences unrelated to deafness (i.e., racial differences). These commonly shared experiences, social marginalization, low expectations, and audism contributes to the development of the deaf episteme.

THE POWER OF INCIDENTAL LEARNING AND ITS EFFECTS ON HEALTH

Incidental learning can be described as informal or unintentional learning (Marsick & Watkins, 1990) that frequently occur throughout the day outside of formal educational or work-related environments. Communication and language barriers can affect how deaf individuals acquire knowledge through incidental learning opportunities. Accommodations such as interpreting services are usually directed for structured or directed learning situations but rarely are available for incidental learning opportunities. Worse yet, many other sources of information and communication technologies such as the telephone, radio, and television historically isolated deaf individuals from information in mainstream society (Valentine, 2009). The deprivation of incidental learning opportunities and poor access to general information are experiences shared by many deaf individuals. These may have a negative impact on deaf individuals' *physical and mental health* (sexual health, cancer, preventive health, cardiovascular disease, suicide, and anxiety) (Heuttel & Rothstein, 2001; Hindley, McGuigan, & Kitson 1994; Margellos-Anast, Estarziau, & Kaufman 2006; McKee, Barnett, Block, & Pearson, 2011;

McKee, Schlehofer, et al., 2011; Peinkofer, 1994; Tamaskar et al., 2000; Wollin & Elder, 2003; Woodroffe, Gorenflo, Meador, & Zazove, 1998; Zazove et al., 2009) and *academic achievement* (Hauser et al., 2010; Traxler, 2000). Deaf signers are considered to be the non-English-speaking minority group at greatest risk for miscommunication, including in areas such as health care (McEwen & Anton-Culver, 1988).

The struggle to acquire information and make decisions despite information gaps forces deaf individuals to adopt a number of coping strategies (McKee, Schlehofer, et al., 2011; Valentine & Skelton, 2009). The Deaf community is very cohesive, likely out of necessity. It greatly values sharing and disseminating information and acquired knowledge with others. This may be partly in response to the challenges of acquiring information from hearing society in the first place. While many hearing individuals may consider social conversations trivial, these conversations often share useful information desperately needed by deaf individuals. However, this can potentially lead to an overreliance on deaf friends and families for information. If the information is distorted, it can be quickly disseminated within a Deaf community. The lack of ability to verify or correct misperceptions or inaccurate information can be problematic for this community (McKee, Schlehofer, et al., 2011).

Many deaf individuals are familiar with the *dinner table syndrome* (Hauser et al., 2010), in which they watch close family members and friends converse with each other but are unable to decipher what is being said. This has an impact on deaf individuals' access to knowledge, which hinders their education and even their health. For example, the lack of incidental learning at home can have a negative impact on deaf individuals' knowledge of family history and health literacy. Health literacy is the degree to which individuals have the capacity to obtain, process, and understand basic health information and services needed to make appropriate health decisions (Nielsen-Bohlman, Panzer, & Kindig, 2004).

To demonstrate how this process occurs, imagine a typical family holiday gathering with several family members conversing about family events that may have happened over the past few months. An uncle may mention that he needs to be careful with his food choices since his doctor told him that his cholesterol was too high. A grandmother may respond back adding that he needs to be careful since her deceased husband followed a poor diet and eventually succumbed to a heart attack at age 51. While this conversation may appear trivial, it is rich in details that will likely be missed by a deaf family member. The deaf individual is therefore less likely to benefit from aggressive screening procedures or interventions because they cannot provide a full family health history to their physician. The loss of incidental learning opportunities affects individuals' abilities to become aware of their diagnoses, potentially affecting their health outcomes (Hauser et al., 2010).

The challenge of incidental learning in auditory-oriented environments most likely has an impact on deaf individuals' health literacy. In one survey, 40.4% of the deaf individuals were not able to identify one symptom of a heart attack (Margellos-Anast et al., 2006) whereas 90% of hearing adults in another survey were able to identify one (Goff et al., 1998). Communication barriers in the family do not have an impact on only cardiovascular knowledge but other areas of health as well. For example, Swartz (1993) found that 23% of hearing individuals learned about sex primarily from their mother compared to only 2.9% of deaf individuals (Swartz, 1993). This appears to affect the sexual behavior of deaf college students, who take more risks than hearing peers (Joseph, Sawyer, & Desmond, 1996).

Parents and educators typically verbally pre-instruct or immediately warn children of dangers as they grow up, and hearing children and adults learn about risks and dangers by being directly instructed or by passively listening to conversations of others. For example, as children leave the home to either walk to school or enter a school bus, parents and teachers routinely shout out warnings such as "be careful when you cross the road" and "do not talk with strangers." Deaf individuals, through the absence of incidental learning about possible dangers, may inadvertently place themselves in harm's way.

According to the National Center for Injury Prevention and Control, injuries are the leading cause of death for children in the United States, accounting for more than 9,700 deaths (National Center for Injury Prevention and Control, 2007). Mann, Zhou, McKee, and McDermott (2007) found that rates of presentation for injury in emergency room visits by deaf children were more than twice that of hearing children even after adjusting for age, race, sex, and the number of hospital or emergency department encounters for treatment of a non-injury-related condition. Deaf individuals are at risk for injuries from inability to identify or react to environmental hazards, especially those with auditory warnings (e.g., alarms) (Gaebler-Spira & Thornton, 2002). Deaf and hard of hearing adults have approximately twice as many occupational injuries as hearing adults (Zwerling et al., 1998).

Limited research suggests that suicidal thoughts and sexual and relationship abuse are more prevalent among deaf individuals (Critchfield, Morrison, & Quinn, 1987; Dobosh, 2002; Glickman & Gulati, 2003; Kvam, 2004; Merkin & Smith, 1995, Sullivan & Knutson, 2000; Turner, Windfuhr, & Kapur, 2007). Developing healthy relationships is a learned skill that is often shared or patterned after parental relationships. If communication or language barriers exist with their loved ones, this can affect the deaf individual's ability to learn the basic constructs of a healthy relationship. Deaf children and hearing parents are more likely to have insecure relationships or attachments because of communication difficulties (e.g., Lederberg, 1993), which can increase the risk for anxiety and depression. This can lead to poor choices of partners and poor reactions in stressful situations. Relationships (attachments) are generally accepted and viewed as an essential component of healthy emotional development in children and emotional maintenance in adults. Secure relationships and attachment styles are related to an increase in health-enhancing behaviors, and conversely insecure attachment styles are linked with participation in fewer health-enhancing behaviors (e.g., Feeney & Ryan, 1994).

Because the loss of incidental learning opportunities can leave lasting damaging effects on the development and health of deaf individuals, hearing family members and friends must make every effort to incorporate their deaf loved ones in their conversations, no matter how trivial they may appear. Parental demonstrations of affection or even quarrels should not be hidden from deaf children. These examples can lead to a healthier understanding on how to handle relationship conflicts. This can help to reduce the unacceptably high rates of relationship abuse, depression, anxiety, and suicide within the Deaf community. Training of deaf health educators can help correct misunderstandings and misperceptions on health topics held by Deaf community members. Health educational outreach by governments, organizations, and schools should utilize natural signed languages, accessible information strategies (easy-to-understand pictorials), and technology (i.e., vlogs).

THE BIOLOGIC BADGE OF DEAFHOOD AND THE EFFECTS OF DEAF GENETICS

Genetic research, testing, and engineering triggers a wide range of emotions for many people, including deaf people. Some deaf individuals are excited about the newfound opportunity to unlock the mysteries on the etiology of their deafness. In the Deaf community, being genetically deaf is often looked upon with a sense of pride, a biological badge of Deafhood (Mand, Duncan, Gillam, Collins, & Delatycki, 2009). During the mid-2000s, many deaf individuals freely donated and mailed their blood to Gallaudet University to discover if they were genetically deaf. This popular program tested and researched the most common cause of hereditary deafness, genes connexin-26 and -30.

Deaf genetics is becoming an important contributor to the deaf episteme. While not necessary, being aware of the presence of their own deaf genes can provide deaf individuals with a further sense of their deaf identity. Yet, there are deaf individuals who are fearful that this may change with the ever-increasing biomedical research on hereditary deafness. They fear that elimination of deafness is not only feasible but inevitable (Arnos, 2002; Emery, Middleton, & Turner, 2010).

Medical researchers and doctors involved with deafness-related research often focus on the elimination of deafness through the use of medical technologies and genetic engineering even in light of increasing recognition of the importance of cultural, ethnic, linguistic, racial, and even genetic diversity (Padden & Humphries, 2005). This is problematic as it conveys conflicting information and the impression of inferiority to many deaf children and adults. Despite the hereditary causes of congenital deafness, approximately 75–80% of the more than 400 identified deaf genes are recessive, with a smaller proportion being autosomal dominant (20%) and X-lined (2–5%) (Marazita et al., 1993; Grundfast, 1993). This explains why most deaf individuals with hereditary deafness continue to be born to hearing families.

A shift in the etiology of congenital deafness appears to be occurring, making hereditary deafness an even more important topic. According to one study, genetic causes of congenital deafness increased from 50.6% in 1969–1970 to 62.8% in 1988–1989 (Marazita et al., 1993). Congenital deafness caused by infections has decreased dramatically over the past few decades, likely because of near-universal immunization and improved neonatal care, including treatment for congenital infections (Hone & Smith, 2001). Some of the most famous examples of these epidemiological shifts of congenital deafness include the eradication of congenital rubella (associated with the rubella epidemic in the 1960s) and the control of meningitis-caused deafness from *Haemophilus influenza* type B through immunization.

Unlike with other cultural and ethnic groups, the future of deaf children can be adversely affected by hearing society through the use of genocide or genetic engineering. With the improvement of genetic testing and counseling, hearing couples will increasingly be notified about their fetus's "defects," including "deafness," which can lead to population-shifting decisions such as abortion. It is unknown how common this ethical issue occurs, but the technology is currently available.

Deaf individuals have historically experienced adverse outcomes from the medical establishment's effort to repair, correct, or eliminate their deafness. This occurred with eugenics and the sterilization of deaf individuals of reproductive ages in the late 19th and early 20th centuries (including in Nazi Germany). There are active government bills and acts in Italy, Australia, and England that state that deafness is a defective condition amenable to genetic screening, elimination, or correction (Emery et al., 2010). The perceptions held by governments and medical establishments on genetic hereditary deafness may hinder deaf individuals' ability to develop a healthy deaf episteme because the knowledge they receive about themselves is that they are broken and a burden to the society.

The fear about the elimination of the Deaf community is not limited to genetic research but includes other medical research such as cochlear implantation. Cochlear implants, although helpful in correcting some deafness, have been used too indiscriminately (Leigh, 2009). Many parents of deaf children are not fully informed by the medical community of the benefits and risks of cochlear implantation, including alternative treatments or doing nothing. Parents often are not aware of the true limits of cochlear implants and may hope that it is a "cure." They might feel that they do not need to learn how to raise a deaf child because the implant will solve everything.

Many deaf leaders are upset by the pressure for children with cochlear implants to enter oral education systems rather than programs that foster their development as visual-oriented beings and that help them develop fluency in a natural signed language (Bat-Chava, 2000). Many of these programs and professions believe that teaching sign language interferes with speech development—a widely disseminated belief that has no empirical support. In fact, research shows that sign language learning actually improves speech development (Woll, Rinaldi, Woolfe, Herman, & Roy, 2010) and some cognitive functions (Bellugi et al., 1990; Emmorey & Kosslyn, 1996).

Despite the issues with genetic research, it has been and potentially continues to be a valuable contributor to deaf health. There is increasing awareness that certain types of hereditary deafness can increase deaf individuals' risk for adverse health outcomes. Some examples such as Usher syndrome (blindness), Pendred syndrome (thyroid issues), and Jervell and Lang-Nielsen (JLN) syndrome (sudden cardiac arrest) are being researched to discover possible treatments to help reduce or avoid health complications. The key is to ensure that genetic research in hereditary deafness maintains its focus on the acquisition of scientific knowledge and improvement of deaf people's health, not on elimination of deaf people.

The medical establishment views deafness through a medical model, necessitating correction of the pathological condition. Many genetic counselors and health-care providers lack impartiality on these issues, which may affect the ability of hearing parents to acquire information about deaf individuals, sign language, and Deaf culture. Anytime there is a sense of unfamiliarity about their child, parents may respond with fear or uncertainty. Hearing parents with a new deaf child are seeking reassurance and guidance from the educational and medical communities. Unfortunately, many hearing parents with deaf children have little experience with successful and well-adjusted deaf individuals, which can negatively affect their perception on deafness and Deaf culture (Hintermair, 2000; Jackson & Turnbull, 2004).

If the focus on deafness is negative, the parents will feel their child is abnormal or even view their child as a failure (Hauser et al., 2010). Training for genetic counselors and medical providers should cover not only the etiology and treatment of congenital deafness but also the linguistic, cultural, and social diversity within the Deaf community. Greater awareness of the Deaf community is essential to protect the interests of the Deaf community and ensure that the population continues to be active and vibrant.

Strict regulations and the use of ethic boards must be involved with genetic research oversight. Both the National Institutes of Health (NIH), a government agency that sponsors much of the medical research on hereditary deafness, and the Centers for Disease Control (CDC), an agency that establishes public policy regarding medical testing and other issues, have taken steps to address these issues. These agencies provide online guidelines and recommendations that address the appropriate use and the ethical implications of genetic testing for deafness (Arnos, 2002). Medical researchers and doctors should become familiar with these guidelines as well as the cultural and linguistic uniqueness of deaf individuals. Additionally, increasing the use of community-based participatory research in deaf medical research would ensure that the "voices" of the Deaf community will be heard.

A collaboration of the Deaf community and researchers can increase acceptance of newer technology, which can have helpful effects on deaf individuals' health. Funding research organizations should require this collaboration if research is to involve members of the community. Also, more deaf researchers must be trained and recruited to work in this field to provide culturally competent approaches.

Deaf genes can contribute to a sense of uniqueness and a sense of belonging to the Deaf community for many Deaf individuals, a Deafhood biological badge. A focus on deafness not as a deficit but as a difference (e.g., visual orientation vs. auditory orientation) would likely result in better outcomes, including a healthier educational and social environment for deaf individuals (Hauser et al., 2010). The recognition of Deaf people as a cultural and linguistic group needs to be clearly stated in publications, web pages, and other research announcements.

CONCLUSION

By failing to acknowledge the existence of deaf epistemes, important strategies to achieve a healthy educational and social environment for deaf individuals may be ignored or lost. Issues of health disparities, social marginalization, discrimination, eugenics, and poor information access are not unique to the Deaf community. They are issues experienced by minority populations around the world. Much can be learned from other groups on how to strengthen resiliency and generate opportunities for change.

Resolving issues will require the efforts of both deaf and hearing individuals. Most deaf individuals live embedded in a hearing society to some degree, whether it is through living with hearing family members and friends, working at a predominately hearing workplace, learning in a mainstreamed educational classroom, interacting with hearing medical professionals, or following the rules established by a government run by hearing individuals. It is essential that deaf individuals continue to develop ways to promote greater awareness about Deafhood and support the education of hearing individuals on deaf issues.

The Deaf community needs to be more accessible to educate parents and medical professionals on healthy and effective strategies to educate and raise a deaf child. Deaf leaders and professionals should make themselves available to mentor and support deaf children and young adults. Ensuring that the expectations are realistic yet ambitious for deaf individuals, we can encourage greater optimism in the learning environment and increase the educational achievement of deaf children. Greater use of natural signed language educational programs, vlogs, web conferencing, and social media tools would help achieve this. The use of technology can make this feasible for most deaf people, even where there may be a dearth of adequately educated deaf professionals, mentors, and supporters in many areas.

Social networking on the web and the use of social media websites have revolutionized how deaf individuals can interact with others. The Internet has provided an avenue for marginalized deaf individuals to become active in political, organizational, and academic arenas. In some ways, social media and networks have leveled the playing field dramatically by incorporating more visual methods of communication (chat rooms, forums, brief emails, instant messaging, blogs, etc.). This can enable deaf individuals to collectively come together to voice their concerns. The Internet and social media websites provide deaf individuals with multiple attractive advantages: ease of communication through the use of text and images and avoidance of initial stigmatizing or stereotypical comments (Barak & Sadovsky, 2008).

It is crucial to ensure access to information is increased, especially to offset the loss of incidental learning opportunities. Knowledge is power, but the key to this power is provision of information in an attainable form. No matter how trivial conversations may seem, families, educators, and health providers caring for deaf individuals must make diligent efforts to ensure their communication is accessible. Educational and health programs targeting deaf individuals should be funded, developed, and disseminated. With greater awareness and understanding of deaf epistemologies, better collaboration among the different communities—medical, educational, political, business, and social—will value and permit the contributions of each deaf individual to take place more fairly. Audism is real but often unintentional. Many aspects of audism can be removed through teaching and promoting greater understanding of the impact of certain actions.

As Gandhi famously said, "If we wish to create a lasting peace we must begin with the children." Change cannot happen unless we ensure that our deaf children are given the tools to fulfill their potential and are permitted to become valuable contributors to both the hearing and Deaf worlds.

Our recommendations for further research and theorizing include an examination of the following questions:

- How can a deaf individual reduce the assimilation pressures without being socially marginalized from the mainstream society?
- What strategies are effective among other minority populations that should be targeted or utilized by deaf populations?
- How can deaf individuals and the Deaf community become more active gatekeepers in areas such as deaf research, education, and health?

NOTE

1. The term *deaf* (lowercase "d") is used here to refer to all deaf and hard of hearing individuals, regardless of hearing acuity, and *Deaf* is used when referring to the community of deaf signers who communicate with each other frequently and share experiences, beliefs, and values (cultural attributes).

REFERENCES

Arnos, K. (2002). Genetics and deafness: Impacts on the Deaf community. *Sign Language Studies, 2*(2), 150–168.

Barak, A., & Sadovsky, A. (2008). Internet use and personal empowerment of hearing impaired adolescents. *Computers in Human Behavior, 24*, 1802–1815.

Barnett, S. (1999). Clinical and cultural issues in caring for deaf people. *Family Medicine, 31*(1), 17–22.

Bat-Chava, Y. (1993). Antecedents of self-esteem in deaf people: A meta-analytic review. *Rehabilitation Psychology, 38*, 221–234.

Bat-Chava, Y. (2000). Diversity of deaf identities. *American Annals of the Deaf, 145*, 420–428.

Bauman, D. (2004). Audism: Exploring the metaphysics of oppression. *Journal of Deaf Studies and Education, 9*, 239–246.

Bavelier, D., Dye, M. W. G., & Hauser, P. (2006). Do deaf individuals see better? *Trends in Cognitive Science, 10*, 512–518.

Bellugi, U., O'Grady, L., Lillo-Martin, D., O'Grady, M., van Hoek, K., & Corina, D. (1990). *Enhancement of spatial cognition in deaf children.* New York, NY: Springer.

Berry, J. (1992). Acculturation and adaptation in a new society. *International Migration, 30*, 69–85.

Berry, J. W. (2006). Acculturative stress. In P. T. P. Wong & L. C. J. Wong (Eds.), *Handbook of multicultural perspectives on stress and coping* (pp. 287–298). New York, NY: Springer.

Blanchfield, B., Feldman, J., Dunbar, J., & Gardner, E. (2001). The severely to profoundly hearing-impaired population in the United States: Prevalence estimates and demographics. *Journal of American Academy of Audiology, 12*(4), 183–189.

Borum, V. (2007). African American mothers with deaf children: A womanist conceptual framework. *Families in Society, 99*, 595–604.

Clark, K., & Clark, M. (1939). The development of consciousness of self and the emergence of racial identification in negro preschool children. *Journal of Social Psychology, 10*, 591–599.

Critchfield, A., Morrison, F., & Quinn, W. (1987). Suicide intervention with hearing impaired adolescents. In G. B. Anderson & D. Watson (Eds.), *Innovations in the habilitation and rehabilitation of Deaf adolescents: Selected proceedings of the Second National Conference on the Habilitation and Rehabilitation of Deaf Adolescents* (pp. 187–203). Little Rock, AR: American Deafness and Rehabilitation Association.

Dobosh, P. (2002). *The use of the Trauma Symptom Inventory with deaf individuals who have experienced sexual abuse and assault* (Unpublished doctoral dissertation). Washington, DC: Gallaudet University.

Eleweke, C., & Rodda, M. (2000). *Enhancing inclusive education in developing countries.* Paper presented at the 2000 International Special Education Congress.

Emery, S., Middleton, A., & Turner, G. (2010). Whose deaf genes are they anyway? The Deaf community's challenge to legislation on embryo selection. *Sign Language Studies, 10*(2), 155–169.

Emmorey, K., & Kosslyn, S. (1996). Enhanced image-generation abilities in deaf signers: A right-hemispheric effect. *Brain and Cognition, 32,* 28–44.

Feeney, J., & Ryan, S. (1994). Attachment style and affect regulations: Relationships with health behavior and family experiences of illnss in a student sample. *Health Psychology, 13,* 334–345.

Foucault, M. (1980). *Power/knowledge.* New York, NY: Pantheon.

Gaebler-Spira, D., & Thornton, L. (2002). Injury prevention for children with disabilities. *Physical Medical Rehabilitation Clinics North America, 13*(4), 891–906.

Gertz, G. (2008). Dysconscious audism: A theoretical proposition. In H. D. L. Bauman (Ed.), *Open your eyes: Deaf studies talking* (pp. 219–234). Minneapolis, MN: University of Minnesota Press.

Glickman, N., & Gulati, S. (2003). *Mental health care of deaf people: A culturally affirmative approach.* Mahwah, NJ: Lawrence Erlbaum Associates.

Goff, D., Sellers, D., McGovern, P., et al. (1998). Knowledge of heart attack symptoms in a population survey in the United States: The REACT trial. *Archives of Internal Medicine, 158*(21), 2329–2338.

Goodman, A. (2004). Group knowledge versus group rationality: Two approaches to social epistemology. *Episteme, 1,* 11–22.

Grundfast, K. (1993). Hereditary hearing impairment in children. *Advanced Otolaryngology and Head and Neck Surgery, 7,* 29–43.

Harris, L., & Vanzandt, C. (1997). Counseling needs of students who are deaf and hard of hearing. *School Counselor, 44*(4), 271–280.

Haslanger, S. (2000). Gender and race: (What) are they? (What) do we want them to be? *Nous, 34,* 31–55.

Hauser, P. C., & Marschark, M. (2008). What we know and what we don't know about cognition and deaf learners. In M. Marschark & P. Hauser (Eds.), *Deaf cognition: Foundations and outcomes* (pp. 439–458). New York: Oxford University Press.

Hauser, P., Maxwell, D., Leigh, I., & Gutman, V. (2000). Internship accessibility issues: No cause for complacency. *Professional Psychology: Research and Practice, 31,* 569–574.

Hauser, P., O'Hearn, A., McKee, M., Steider, A., & Thew, D. (2010). Deaf epistemiology: Deafhood and deafness. *American Annals of the Deaf, 154*(5), 486–492.

Hauser, P., Wills, K., & Isquith, P. (2006). Hard of hearing, deafness, and being deaf. In J. E. Farmer, J. Donders, & S. Warschausky (Eds.), *Neurodevelopmental disabilities: Clinical research and practice* (pp. 119–131). New York, NY: Guilford Publications.

Heuttel, K., & Rothstein, W. (2001). HIV/AIDS knowledge and information sources among deaf and hearing college students. *American Annals of the Deaf, 146*(3), 280–286.

Hindley, P. H. P., McGuigan, S., & Kitson, N. (1994). Psychiatric disorder in deaf and hearing impaired children and young people: A prevalence study. *Journal of Psychiatry and Psychology, 35,* 917–934.

Hintermair, M. (2000). Children who are hearing impaired with additional disabilities and related aspects of parental stress. *Exceptional Children, 66,* 327–332.

Hone, S., & Smith, R. (2001). Genetics of hearing impairment. *Seminars in Neonatology, 6,* 531–541.

Humphries, T. (1996). Of deaf-mutes, the strange, and the modern deaf self. In N. Glickman & M. Harvey (Eds.), *Culturally affirmative psychotherapy with deaf persons* (pp. 99–114). Mahwah, NJ: Lawrence Erlbaum.

Humphries, T. (2008). *Audism.* Unpublished manuscript, University of California, San Diego.

Humphries, T., & Humphries, J. (2010). Deaf in the time of the cochlea. *Journal of Deaf Studies and Deaf Education, 16*(2), 153–163.

Jackson, C., & Turnbull, A. (2004). Impact of deafness on family life: A review of the literature. *Topics in Early Childhood Special Education, 24*(1), 15–29.

Joseph, J., Sawyer, R., & Desmond, S. (1996). Sexual knowledge, behavior, and sources of information among deaf and hard of hearing college students. *American Annals of the Deaf, 140*, 338–345.

Kvam, M. (2004). Sexual abuse of deaf children: A retrospective analysis of the prevalence and characteristics of childhood sexual abuse among deaf adults in Norway. *Child Abuse and Neglect, 3*, 241–251.

Ladd, P. (2003). *Understanding deaf culture: In search of Deafhood.* Bristol, UK: Multilingual Matters.

Lane, H. (1992). *The mask of benevolence: Disabling the deaf community.* New York, NY: Alfred A. Knopf.

Lane, H., Hoffmeister, R., & Bahan, B. (1996). *A journey into the Deaf-World.* San Diego, CA: DawnsignPress.

Lederberg, A. (1993). The impact of deafness on mother–child and peer relationships. In M. Marschark & M. D. Clark (Eds.), *Psychological perspectives on deafness* (pp. 93–119). Hillsdale, NY: Erlbaum.

Leigh, I. (2009). *A lens on deaf identities.* New York, NY: Oxford University Press.

Listman, J. D., Rogers, K. D., & Hauser, P. C. (in press). Rethinking deaf adolescents' resilience: Why cultural capital matters. In D. Zand & K. Pierce (Eds.), *Risk and resilience: Adaptation in the context of being deaf.* New York, NY: Springer.

Logan, S., Freeman, E., & McRoy, R. (1989). *Social work practice with black families: A culturally specific perspective.* Norwood, NJ: Longman.

Mand, C., Duncan, R., Gillam, L., Collins, V., & Delatycki, M. (2009). Genetic selection for deafness: The views of hearing children of deaf adults. *Journal of Medical Ethics, 35*, 722–728.

Mann, J., Zhou, L., McKee, M., & McDermott, S. (2007). Children with hearing loss and increased risk of injury. *Annals of Family Medicine, 5*, 528–533.

Marazita, M., Ploughman, L., Rawlings, B., et al. (1993). Genetic epidemiological studies of early-onset deafness in the U.S. school-age population. *American Journal MedGenet, 46*, 486–491.

Margellos-Anast, H., Estarziau, M., & Kaufman, G. (2006). Cardiovascular disease knowledge among culturally Deaf patients in Chicago. *Preventive Medicine, 42*(3), 235–239.

Marsick, V., & Watkins, K. (1990). *Informal and incidental learning in the workplace.* London, UK: Routledge.

McEwen, E., & Anton-Culver, H. (1988). The medical communication of deaf patients. *Journal of Family Practice, 26*(3), 289–291.

McKee, M., Barnett, S., Block, R., & Pearson, T. (2011). Impact of communication on preventive services among deaf American Sign Language users. *American Journal of Preventive Medicine*, in press.

McKee, M., Schlehofer, D., Cuculick, J., Starr, M., Smith, S., & Chin, N. (2011). Perceptions of cardiovascular health in an underserved community of deaf adults using American Sign Language. *Disability and Health*, in press.

Merkin, L., & Smith, M. J. (1995). A community-based model providing services for deaf and deaf-blind victims of sexual assault and domestic violence. *Sexuality and Disability, 13*, 97–106.

Mitchell, R., Young, T., Bachleda, B., & Karchmer, M. (2006). How many people use ASL in the United States? Why estimates need updating. *Sign Language Studies, 6*, 306–335.

Morris, J. (1992). Personal power in black mothers of handicapped sons. *AFFILIA, 7*, 72–92.

National Association of the Deaf. (2010). *When is captioning required?* Retrieved December 11, 2010, from http://www.nad.org/issues/technology/captioning/when-required

National Center for Injury Prevention and Control. (2007). WISQARS leading causes of death reports. Retrieved December 21, 2010, from http://webappa.cdc.gov/sasweb/ncipc/leadcaus10.html

Nielsen-Bohlman, L., Panzer, A., & Kindig, D. (Eds.). (2004). *Health literacy: A prescription to end confusion.* Washington, DC: National Academies Press.

Nikolaraizi, M., & Makri, M. (2004). Deaf and hearing individuals' beliefs about the capabilities of deaf people. *American Annals of the Deaf, 149*(5), 404–414.

Padden, C., & Humphries, T. (2005). *Inside deaf culture.* Cambridge, MA: Harvard University Press.

Peinkofer, J. (1994). HIV education for the deaf, a vulnerable minority. *Public Health Report, 109*(3), 390–396.

Pinderhughes, E. (1995). Empowering diverse populations: Family practice in the 21st century. *Families in Society, 76,* 131–140.

Reagan, T. (2002). *Language, education, and ideology: Mapping the linguistic landscape of U.S. schools.* Westport, CT: Praeger.

Roberts, I., & Norton, R. (1995). Sensory deficit and the risk of pedestrian injury. *Injury Prevention, 1*(1), 12–14.

Rosen, G. (2001). Norminalism, naturalism, philosophical relativism. *Philosophical Perspectives, 15,* 69–91.

Steinberg, A., Barnett, S., Meador, H., Wiggins, E., & Zazove, P. (2006). Health care system accessibility. *Journal of General Internal Medicine, 21*(3), 260–266.

Sullivan, P., & Knutson, J. (2000). Maltreatment and disabilities: A population-based epidemiological study. *Child Abuse and Neglect, 24,* 1257–1273.

Swartz, D. (1993). A comparative study of sex knowledge among hearing and deaf college freshmen. *Journal of Sexuality and Disability, 11,* 129–147.

Tamaskar, P., Malia, T., Stern, C., Gorenflo, D., Meador, H., & Zazove, P. (2000). Preventive attitudes and beliefs of deaf and hard-of-hearing individuals. *Archives of Family Medicine, 9*(6), 518–525.

Thew, D. (2007). *School to work transition for deaf and hard of hearing: Acculturation stress and resilience.* Paper presented at the 2007 Convention of the American Psychological Association.

Thumann-Prezioso, C. (2005). Deaf parents' perspective on deaf education. *Sign Language Studies, 5,* 425–440.

Traxler, C. (2000). Measuring up to performance standards in reading and mathematics: Achievement of selected deaf and hard-of-hearing students in the national norming of the 9th edition Stanford Achievement Test. *Journal of Deaf Studies and Education, 5,* 337–348.

Turner, O., Windfuhr, K., & Kapur, N. (2007). Suicide in deaf populations: A literature review. *Annals of General Psychiatry, 6,* 26.

Valentine, G., & Skelton, T. (2009). "An umbilical cord to the world": The role of the Internet in D/deaf people's information and communication practices. *Information, Communication, and Society, 12*(1), 44–65.

Woll, B., Rinaldi, P., Woolfe, T., Herman, R., & Roy, P. (2010). *Positive support: A UK study of deaf children and their families.* Paper presented at the Theoretical Issues in Sign Language Research Conference, Purdue University, Indiana.

Wollin, J., & Elder, R. (2003). Mammograms and Pap smears for Australian deaf women. *Cancer Nursing, 26*(5), 405–409.

Woodroffe, T., Gorenflo, D. W., Meador, H. E., & Zazove, P. (1998). Knowledge and attitudes about AIDS among deaf and hard of hearing persons. *AIDS Care, 10*(3), 377–386.

Yosso, T. J. (2005). Whose culture has captial? A critical race theory discussion of community cultural wealth. *Race, Ethnicity, and Education, 8,* 69–91.

Zazove, P., Meador, H., Reed, B., Sen, A., & Gorenflo, D. (2009). Cancer prevention knowledge of people with profound hearing loss. *Journal of General Internal Medicine, 24*(3), 320–326.

Zwerling, C., Sprince, N., Davis, C., Whitten, P., Wallace, R., & Heeringa, S. (1998). Occupational injuries among older workers with disabilities: A prospective cohort study of the Health and Retirement Survey, 1992 to 1994. *American Journal of Public Health, 88*(11), 1691–1695.

SUGGESTIONS FOR FURTHER READING

Berry, J. W. (2006). Acculturative stress. In P. T. P. Wong & L. C. J. Wong (Eds.), *Handbook of multicultural perspectives on stress and coping* (pp. 287–298). New York, NY: Springer.

Ladd, P. (2003). *Understanding Deaf culture: In search of Deafhood.* Bristol, UK: Multilingual Matters.

Leigh, I. (2009). *A lens on deaf identities.* New York, NY: Oxford University Press.

Valentine, G., & Skelton, T. (2009). "An umbilical cord to the world": The role of the Internet in D/deaf people's information and communication practices. *Information, Communication, and Society, 12*(1), 44–65.

Yosso, T. J. (2005). Whose culture has captial? A critical race theory discussion of community cultural wealth. *Race, Ethnicity, and Education, 8,* 69–91.

4

Diversity and Deaf Identity: Implications for Personal Epistemologies in Deaf Education

Ila Parasnis

In this chapter, the term *diversity* refers to sociocultural differences among people. The terms *race/ethnicity* and *racial/ethnic* refer to diversity related to race and ethnicity; the slash does not make the terms *race* and *ethnicity* interchangeable but is used for the sake of brevity. The term *deaf people* refers to people with significant hearing loss and includes those who are American Sign Language (ASL) signers, users of other sign languages and modalities, hard of hearing people, and those with cochlear implants or hearing aids. The term *deaf education* refers to the education of deaf and hard of hearing students, including those who are culturally Deaf (e.g., Padden & Humphries, 1988) and those who view their experience of being hard of hearing as part of their self-identities (e.g., Brueggemann, 1999). The term *Deaf community* refers to a sociocultural group of deaf and hard of hearing people who value the use of a sign language and accept their deafness as a positive difference and not a disability. Deaf people who accept this community affiliation generally regard themselves as having a Deaf identity. More in-depth discussion of the concepts of Deaf community and Deaf identity will follow later.

My perspective in this discussion is shaped by my training as a cognitive psychologist specializing in visual perception, my extensive experience as a researcher in deaf education who uses both quantitative and qualitative methods to study visual cognition and diversity in deaf education (e.g., Parasnis, 1998; 2004; Parasnis, Samar, & Fischer, 2005), and the personal epistemological beliefs I have developed as a hearing, multilingual, Indian American woman, which include recognition of individual differences and sociocultural and linguistic differences among learners as fundamental steps for creating an effective teaching–learning environment.

I thank Vincent J. Samar, Dominique LePoutre, Anjali Parasnis-Samar, and Francois Grosjean for their feedback on the earlier version of this manuscript.

PERSONAL EPISTEMOLOGIES AND DEAF EDUCATION

In the traditional view of epistemology, knowledge and justified beliefs are essentially linked to objective truth as the goal of our cognitive practices, and the existence of objective norms of rationality is presupposed (Steup, 2010). However, many scholars in sociology, psychology, cultural anthropology, and literary theory have advocated the constructivist view that knowledge and justified beliefs are socially constructed and that there is no unified theory of knowledge or set of objective methods for creating knowledge. Put simply, there is growing recognition that who studies what, why, when, and how significantly influences how knowledge is constructed and interpreted. In the field of general education scholars who accept the constructivist view have vigorously discussed the implied multiplicity of epistemological beliefs among individuals and how that may influence the teaching–learning process (see Hofer, 2001; Hofer & Pintrich, 1997, 2002; Pallas, 2001; Schraw, 2001; Schraw & Olafson, 2002; Schraw & Sinatra, 2004). In deaf education in particular, however, it is rare to see an explicit discussion of multiple epistemologies. Yet, it is obvious that professionals from different disciplines such as education, psychology, sociology, linguistics, speech, and audiology have relied on different domain-specific epistemologies in addition to their own personal epistemologies to create and interpret the current common knowledge about deafness and Deaf people. The present volume and the special issue of the *American Annals of the Deaf* edited by Paul (2010) are notable early initiatives to examine the assumptions underlying this knowledge and the future role of epistemological diversity in deaf education.

Historically, theory and practice in the field of deaf education has been driven by the traditional epistemological belief that deafness is a physical disability, a belief seen as value-neutral and objective (Paul & Moores, 2010). More recently, nontraditional epistemological beliefs, centered on the sociocultural model of deafness and informed by the subjective experiences and perspectives of deaf people as members of a linguistic minority culture (e.g., Lane, Hoffmeister, & Bahan, 1996; Padden & Humphries, 1988; Parasnis, 1996), have been gaining acceptance from professionals in deaf education. Within published writings on the sociocultural model of deafness, the concept of diversity is often used to refer to the experience of deaf people as a cultural minority group embedded in a larger hearing society. This conceptualization of the Deaf community as a minority community has opened the way for educators to legitimately propose new, socioculturally informed perspectives on theory and practice within deaf education. Ironically, however, this description of diversity based on the experiences of white American Deaf ASL users has created a perception of Deaf culture as a monolithic overarching trait of all deaf people and has suppressed recognition of the demographic diversity of individuals within the Deaf community itself (see Fernandes & Myers, 2010).

Nevertheless, it seems self-evident that intracommunity demographic diversity related to race, ethnicity, language, gender, sexuality, class, and nationality influences the life experiences of deaf people and, in turn, interacts with their experiences with deafness to shape their self-identities and group identities. Deaf identity development has been discussed as a process by which a deaf person acknowledges and accepts his or her experience with deafness (e.g., Holcomb, 1997; Ladd, 2003). However, recognizing that the multiplicity of experiences of different subgroups of deaf people is relevant to constructing epistemological beliefs, it becomes apparent that conceptualizing Deaf identity only on an experience-with-deafness dimension is an overly restrictive focus on the unifying (but not all-encompassing) elements of experience that deaf people may share solely because of their deafness. Admittedly, those unifying elements are important factors in the emergence of Deaf identity, but there is little reason to believe, and certainly little or no objective research to support, the idea that multiple dimensions of racial, ethnic, linguistic, and social diversity are not potent and interactive factors that may shape unique forms of complex Deaf identities and lead to diverse personal epistemologies within the Deaf community.

INTERSECTIONALITY, PERSONAL EPISTEMOLOGIES, AND DEAF IDENTITY

The construct of intersectionality provides a useful framework for understanding the way in which multiple dimensions of diversity within the Deaf community may create complex Deaf identities and lead to multiple personal epistemologies within that community. Discussed in feminist studies, ethnic studies, and queer studies, the concept of intersectionality refers to the complex relationships among multiple dimensions of social experience or multiple categories of socially constructed knowledge such as race, class, gender, or sexuality (see McCall, 2005; Nash, 2008). As Nash (2008) describes, "Intersectionality emerged in the late 1980s and early 1990s from critical race studies, a scholarly movement born in the legal academy committed to problematizing law's purported colour-blindness, neutrality, and objectivity" (p. 2). The concept of intersectionality was proposed originally by Crenshaw to underscore the multidimensionality of marginalized subjects' lived experiences (Crenshaw, 1989). She points out the importance of speaking against internal exclusions and marginalizations to challenge institutions to hear the silenced voices. In supporting the importance of the intersectionality construct, McCall (2005) acknowledges that methodological approaches to studying intersectionality are challenging and notes the complexity that arises when the subject of analysis expands to include multiple dimensions of social life and categories of analysis. Although the construct of intersectionality has to strengthen its explanatory power, it offers important insights that "identity is complex, that subjectivity is messy, and that personhood is inextricably bound with vectors of power" (Nash, 2008, p. 13). In addressing the intersectionality of race, class, and gender, Andersen and Collins (1995) state that they "are interlocking categories of experience that affect all aspects of human life; they simultaneously structure the experience of all people in the society" (p. xi). Following this reasoning, the idea that all members of a society are affected by the diversity within the society, whether they belong to majority or minority cultures, implies that the diversity within the Deaf community affects *all* members of its subgroups, regardless of their race, as they struggle to create and maintain a Deaf group identity that is both diverse and inclusive at the same time.

Within the general education literature, it is recognized that intersectionality among many socially constructed dimensions creates multidimensional identities and multiple perspectives on knowledge and ways of knowing (Jones & McEwen, 2000; Sellers, Smith, Shelton, Rowley, & Chavous, 1998). As Jones and McEwen point out, multiple dimensions of intersecting identities have different salience for an individual at any given time or in a given context and this complexity of identity construction must be taken into account in conceptualizing the identities of individuals from marginalized groups.

The construct of intersectionality as a complex process affecting identity development and epistemological beliefs has implications for training teachers regarding the role of their personal epistemologies and their students' personal epistemologies in the educational process. Many scholars have made a case for studying the personal epistemologies of educators and learners in addition to domain-specific epistemologies to understand how they influence the educational process (Hofer, 2001; Hofer & Pintrich, 1997; Pallas, 2001; Schraw, 2001). As Hofer states, "The research on personal epistemology . . . addresses students' thinking and beliefs about knowledge and knowing, and typically includes some or all of the following elements: beliefs about the definition of knowledge, how knowledge is constructed, how knowledge is evaluated, where knowledge resides, and how knowing occurs. Although the term 'personal epistemology' has limitations, it is a possible umbrella term for those research programs that address individual conceptions of knowledge and knowing" (p. 355). Schraw and Sinatra (2004) discuss research that demonstrates that beliefs about knowledge interact with individual difference variables such as socioeconomic status, ethnicity, gender, personal interest, or academic major. Furthermore, Schraw (2001), Schraw and Olafson (2002), and Hofer (2001) have shown that teachers' personal epistemological beliefs influence students' personal epistemological beliefs and that the development of sophisticated epistemological beliefs is related to greater academic achievement in students. Schraw and Sinatra (2004) suggest that teacher-training programs need to provide teachers with the opportunity to reflect on their own personal epistemologies and to understand how their beliefs and those of their students come into play in teaching–learning environments.

Pallas (2001) has also stressed the importance of including the study of epistemological diversity in teacher-training programs. He points out that how epistemological perspectives in a field (or in the study of a particular subject) have evolved over time, sometimes in relation to or even in opposition to one another, needs to be studied to understand the common knowledge base. He argues that teacher-training programs should include teaching students how to develop a critical, self-reflective stance that acknowledges multiple perspectives and beliefs, a critical component for preparing students to become teachers and educational researchers.

The construct of intersectionality may play a heuristic role in the self-reflective process by facilitating the understanding that the personal epistemologies of teachers and students do not emerge as disconnected and idiosyncratic ways of knowing but rather are social constructions out of their individual experiences as members of subgroups nested within larger groups. Although educational implications of personal epistemologies have only recently begun to be studied (Brownlee, Schraw, &

Berthelsen, 2011; Hofer & Pintrich, 2002), the current literature supports the idea that there is a significant relationship between sociocultural factors related to identity development and personal epistemology development.

Understanding how the diversity of the experience of deaf people influences their identity development and epistemological development is critical for creating an effective educational environment. Deaf identity can be conceptualized as a dynamic identity that is multidimensional and influenced by psychological, situational, and relational variables. It changes over time and in different contexts. This view discussed by Parasnis (2000, 2004) and Foster and Kinuthia (2003) is not prevalent in the current literature on Deaf culture or deaf education but is essential for developing a perspective that incorporates the personal and domain-specific diverse epistemologies.

LENSES USED TO STUDY DEAF IDENTITY AND THEIR LIMITED VIEWS

Deaf Identity and Focus on the Experience-with-Deafness Dimension

Theoretical discussions in Deaf studies have largely focused on a deaf individual's sociocultural developmental experience with deafness as the single salient dimension that creates that individual's personal and group identity. This salient dimension of experience-with-deafness is expressed by the constructs of Deaf cultural identity (Padden & Humphries, 1988, 2005), Deaf-World (Lane, 2005; Lane, Hoffmeister, & Bahan, 1996), Deafnicity (Eckert, 2010), and Deafhood (Ladd, 2003). This literature has generally attempted to establish the construct of the Deaf self as distinct from the hearing self and of the Deaf community as a cultural entity distinct from the hearing culture. The frame for these constructs is similar to the frame of ethnic multiculturalism and shows how the Deaf people's ways of reflecting on their otherness due to deafness are similar to the ways racial/ethnic minority groups in America reflect on their otherness due to race/ethnicity. They show that knowledge generated by the insiders from the Deaf community is qualitatively different from knowledge generated by outsiders from the hearing society (see Humphreys, 2008).

By defining the construct of a core Deaf group with a common experience-with-deafness dimension binding it together, these authors have advanced the academic and political acceptance of the existence of a culture-based distinction between the perspectives of Deaf and hearing communities. Nevertheless, these analyses of Deaf culture generally ignore how a salient experience-with-deafness dimension may intersect with other biological or socially constructed dimensions such as race/ethnicity, gender, sexuality, and class to create a more general, multidimensional construct of Deaf identity or Deaf community.

Deaf Identity and the Sociocultural Diversity

The sociocultural diversity of the Deaf community is obliquely acknowledged by some scholars such as Padden (1996), who talks about the "ethnic geography" of the Deaf community, and by organizations such as the National Association of the Deaf, which states that the diversity within the Deaf community is one of its core values.

Humphries (1993) states that "unfortunately most of the research into the lives and language of deaf people has tended to be unspecific in reference to particular communities or classes of Deaf people, leaving us to assume that most descriptions of Deaf culture and ASL in the United States are based on studies of white, middle class Americans of indeterminate local community. It is also clear that inquiry in general including inquiry into how best to educate Deaf people has not focused very well on issues of ethnicity among American Deaf people" (p. 10).

Christiansen and Delgado (1993), Christiansen (2000), and other scholars (e.g., Anderson & Grace, 1993; Cohen, 1997) have discussed how the diverse experiences of deaf people, particularly those from underprivileged minority communities, must be acknowledged to provide effective education. However, in these discussions racial/ethnic-minority deaf people are often conceptualized as having several subgroup identities within the Deaf community (Woll & Ladd, 2003). The issue of how sociocultural diversity impacts the very construct of Deaf identity is not generally addressed. Viewing the effects of race, gender, class, and so on as separate additive factors in their influence on identity formation is missing the complex connections and interactions among these dynamically changing, socially constructed categories that are likely to interact in complex ways with experience with deafness.

More than 20 years ago, Cohen, Fischgrund, and Redding (1990) pointed out that a black deaf person is neither a black person who is deaf nor a deaf person who is black, but someone with his/her own persona (i.e., a black deaf person). Their insight about incorporating such understanding about Deaf identity has not been followed in subsequent theory or practice in deaf education.

Experiential evidence collected directly from diverse Deaf community members could play a central role in defining the construct of a multidimensional Deaf identity, but at present, very few studies are available with diverse deaf people as primary sources of information (Anderson & Grace, 1991; Anderson & Miller, 2005; Aramburo, 1989; Brooks, 1996; Dively, 2001; Foster & Kinuthia, 2003). These studies show that racial/ethnic minority deaf people are aware of their Deaf identity, racial/ethnic identity, and their perceived minority status within the Deaf community. For example, Anderson and Miller state that one common experience that deaf people of color have is dealing with stereotypes, cultural conflicts, or discrimination.

The intersectionality of race/ethnicity, gender, and sexuality differences in the construction of Deaf identity has begun to receive some attention in the Deaf studies discourse on Deaf identity. Several scholars have articulated the feeling of being "othered" when considering different dimensions of Deaf identity. Dunn (2008) reflects on how he feels as a black deaf person when he goes to Deaf clubs with his white friends. The most recurring comment is, "I am so happy to see you here. I hope you can bring more of your people to come here next time" (p. 241). Dunn states, "It's as if I am a foreigner and the people here are unsure as to how to respond to my presence at their establishment" (p. 242). Kelly (2008), reflecting on the experience of Deaf women, states, "In spite of its attention to the issues of marginalization and oppression by the dominant hearing culture, the field of deaf studies has yet to include the study of the deaf female experience" (p. 259). Bienvenu (2008) wonders, "What about Deaf Lesbians/Gay men? Are we welcomed to take our place at the table of the

Deaf community? We do not know for sure, but I'd think, no. Deaf identity is highly valued. To clearly assert one's L/G identity might be to jeopardize one's Deaf identity" (p. 264). More in-depth studies with diverse deaf people are needed to explore how different dimensions such as race/ethnicity, gender, sexuality, and class intersect with the experience-with-deafness dimension to create an emergent complex Deaf identity.

Deaf Identity Viewed in Political Context

Historically, the pressing political need to elevate the American Deaf community to minority culture status has served to reinforce the dominance of the experience-with-deafness dimension over intracommunity diversity issues related to race, ethnicity, language, class, and nationality. The two successful protests at Gallaudet in 1988 and 2006 against the board of trustees' choice of its president demonstrated that the socio-cultural experience of deafness can unify people of different races and ethnicities in a common minority-culture cause. In fact, sociopolitical discourses of Deaf power and Deaf Way generally rely on showing unity among deaf people who differ in race, ethnicity, class, gender, and sexuality when the goal is to persuade hearing society that being Deaf is culturally transformative, not equivalent to being culturally Hearing with a functional sensory limitation. However, after achieving the initial political goal of societal recognition of the Deaf community's distinctiveness, subsequent study of the relevance of intersections of the experience-with-deafness dimension with other salient dimensions of diversity will be necessary to advance new political goals that respect the full complexity of Deaf identity in American society and its epistemological relevance to contemporary deaf education. While this research agenda may tear at the old-guard monolith of Deaf identity, it will ultimately support the political agenda of equal access to education and knowledge for deaf children with diverse multidimensional identities, inevitably including children on the periphery of the Deaf core as currently conceived.

Deaf Identity Viewed in the Context of Minority Identity Development

Several authors (Glickman, 1996; Holcomb, 1997) have discussed how the stages of Deaf identity development are similar to the stages of racial identity development in African Americans that Cross (1991) envisioned. Racial identity development is seen as related to self-esteem (Cross, 1991). The Deaf Identity Development Scale (Fischer & McWhirter, 2001; Glickman, 1996) and the Deaf Acculturation Scale (Maxwell-McCaw & Zea, 2011) have been developed to determine how deaf and hard of hearing people move from a culturally hearing to a culturally Deaf or bicultural identity based on how they perceive their experience with deafness. However, these scales do not account for the currently unknown influence of multidimensional diversity factors on the development of these stages.

Bat-Chava (1993, 2000) has shown that self-esteem is greater among those who have a culturally Deaf or bicultural identity, and Nikolaraizi and Hadjikakou (2006) have shown the positive role of educational experience in developing such identities. However, the complexities of race and other diversity dynamics may modulate the role of identity in developing self-esteem, and hence these and other findings from studies that do not take fundamental dimensions of diversity into account cannot be assumed to generalize to subcultural groups within the Deaf community.

Deaf Identity Viewed in a Bilingualism–Biculturalism Context

Another way identity development in deaf people has been traditionally studied is by comparing it to bilingual–bicultural identity development in hearing people. Grosjean (1996, 2010) has eloquently argued that Deaf ASL signers have bilingual–bicultural life experiences like many hearing bilingual–bicultural people. Grosjean's (1996) definition of a bilingual person recognizes that such a person may use two or more languages in daily life, and his definition of a bicultural person recognizes that a person may negotiate two or more cultures, but he defines bilingualism in deaf people as involving the sign language used by the Deaf community and the spoken language used by the hearing majority (Grosjean, 2010, p. 141). Bilingual or multilingual experiences of the racial/ethnic minority subgroup members in a given Deaf community are not fully addressed, although he acknowledges the diversity within the Deaf community (p. 139). His work addresses the psychological and psycholinguistic issues related to bilingualism–biculturalism but only addresses peripherally the sociocultural issues related to power and oppression that influence a racial/ethnic minority Deaf culture member's experience in moving between cultures or in using different languages. Such discussion is needed in the field to fully represent cultural and language diversity of deaf people.

Grosjean (2001), Lane, Hoffmeister, and Bahan (1996), and recently Cummins (2009) specifically discuss access to ASL for deaf children as a human rights issue. However, many American deaf children from minority culture backgrounds have access to different spoken languages and/or different sign languages at home. By overlooking this fact, these authors fail to adequately specify the scope and complexity of the actual human rights issue involved in the way society and the educational system may restrict language access for deaf children in general. Taken literally, addressing this human rights issue by providing access to only ASL and spoken English in the multicultural American context may simply substitute one human rights violation for another.

In general, the issue of the rights of culturally and linguistically diverse deaf students is not adequately addressed by the general emphasis on an ASL–English bilingual–bicultural identity development model or by the "bi–bi" program's emphasis on ASL–English language learning. The emphasis on ASL–English bilingualism may not help racial/ethnic minority children in their education because they may not have adequate exposure to English in their daily life and may use other spoken or signed languages at home. Delgado (2001) has discussed how teaching ASL to Hispanic deaf children sometimes creates problems in their ability to communicate with their families and how teachers who only speak English do not recognize the quality of children's language skills in Spanish.

Parsons and Jordan (1994) have discussed how bilingual special education policies and school practices do not address the needs of deaf minority children from families of non-English speakers (NES). Natapoff (1995) has argued that the intersectionality of deafness and NES children's cultural and language origins must be taken into account in how to view a NES deaf child's identity and how to provide educational access. She points out that deafness and NES status are not unitary traits to be dealt with pedagogically in isolation and states, "Intersectionality theory . . . forbids this sort of reductionism holding that such important aspects of complex identities cannot be neatly separated and prioritized in this way. In fact, such reductionism is in itself a form of discrimination because it fails to define equality in the complex terms demanded by NES identity" (p. 276). These considerations support the idea that the multicultural, multilingual experiences of Deaf community members of all social classes need to be studied to develop how Deaf identities are developed.

Deaf Identity Viewed in Global Context

There is a growing interest in learning about deaf people across national boundaries with the notion that Deaf identity can be a transnational global identity. The evidence from autobiographical information (e.g., Vasistha, 2006), cultural anthropological studies (e.g., Nakamura, 2006), and international perspectives on deaf education (e.g., Moores & Miller, 2009) has shown some similarity in the struggle deaf people have in constructing Deaf identities as distinct from hearing identities. However, as De Clerck (2010) and Nakamura (2006) caution, the construction of Deaf identity in each country is related to local sociocultural, political, educational, and social policy constructions and hence differs among countries.

These cultural anthropologists' observations underscore the problems in building a construct of Deaf identity that is globally universal. The construct of a multidimensional model of Deaf identity can be applied universally, but the multidimensional identities themselves are not universal. This distinction needs to be kept in mind as we learn about Deaf identities in different nations and communities. To clarify, Deaf people everywhere are potentially susceptible to the formative effects of the same underlying biological and sociocultural dimensions on their identity development, but the relevant underlying dimensions are not always present in the environment of specific countries and communities and are therefore not always selected by the identity development process to influence their emergent identity patterns. Hence, deaf people from different nations can have culturally conflicting identities, just like hearing people can, and still have a multidimensional Deaf identity in all cases.

DIVERSITY OF DEAF IDENTITY, PERSONAL EPISTEMOLOGIES, AND DEAF EDUCATION

Accepting the notion that complex Deaf identity emerges from the intersection and interaction of multiple dimensions has some important implications for understanding the scope and complexities of personal epistemologies in deaf education. The first implication is that studying how interpersonal diversity among deaf people, their diverse language and communication preferences, their diverse cultural and religious backgrounds, their gender, class, sexuality differences, and so on influences their identity development is essential for understanding the development of their personal epistemologies. Furthermore, these personal epistemologies cannot be understood simply as the sum of epistemological beliefs that come out of independent component experiences with deafness, gender, race/ethnicity, and so on. The second implication is that building effective epistemological frameworks to guide deaf education is unlikely to succeed by simply attempting to transfer to deaf people what is already known about the effect of race or gender or class separately, or even jointly, on identity development and epistemological beliefs in the general hearing population. Third, evidence from diverse members of the Deaf community needs to be examined to understand how multiple dimensions of identity intersect and how the complex interactions between these dimensions influence Deaf identity development. Fourth, those who are involved in such study need to understand and acknowledge their own personal epistemological and domain-specific beliefs when interpreting the evidence. Finally, this perspective motivates a commitment to change teacher-training programs and educational policies and practices to support multidimensional Deaf identity development as an integral part of deaf education.

DIVERSITY OF DEAF STUDENTS AND EDUCATORS AND PERSONAL EPISTEMOLOGIES

To understand how diversity and personal epistemologies influence deaf education, the sociocultural factors that influence development of personal and domain-specific epistemologies of students as well as teachers need to be studied because education is a dynamic interactive process engaging students and teachers. Acknowledging that diversity of deaf students and their educators needs to move from a peripheral to a central issue is the necessary first step to create a significant shift in thinking about deaf education and epistemologies in deaf education.

There is demographic evidence to suggest that deaf students and their educators are diverse in their sociocultural experiences. Research shows that the deaf student population is becoming increasingly diverse and the educational achievements of racial/ethnic minority deaf students continue to be lower than those of white students (Kluwin, 1994; Myers et al., 2010). A recent Gallaudet Research Institute Survey conducted in 2007–8 (GRI, 2008) showed that of the 36,710 deaf and hard of hearing school children in the United States, 46.4% are white, 28.8% are Hispanic/Latino, 15% are black/African American, 3.8% are Asian or Pacific Islander, and 0.7% are American Indian or Alaska natives. English is a home language for 82.5%, Spanish for 21.9%, and ASL for 3.8%. About 75% of deaf and hard of hearing children are enrolled in regular school settings. Speech is used as the primary communication mode to teach for 50% of the students, and speech with sign is used for 34.9% of the students. Most (71%) come from families where family members do not regularly sign, and about 77% have parents who both are hearing. For the entire deaf population (including people both in and out of school), it is estimated that 95% of deaf and hard of hearing people are born to hearing parents (Mitchell & Karschmer, 2004) and the majority of Deaf community members are exposed to the Deaf community and ASL when they go to school (Johnson & Erting, 1989).

These statistics show clearly that the typical deaf student cannot be conceptualized as a fluent ASL signer attending a residential school program. This obvious fact is worth emphasizing because much of the literature has focused on understanding the experience of Deaf ASL signers to build the construct of Deaf identity, and this literature is routinely used in teacher-training programs to convey to teachers a canonical understanding of the experience of deaf people. In point of fact, the nonrepresentative community sample that this literature is based on makes it inadequate to build a complex multidimensional construct of Deaf identity. Planning the education of deaf students based on the information about Deaf ASL signers alone would tend to marginalize the majority of deaf students in the educational process.

Less diversity exists among educators of deaf people in their race, hearing status, and gender than among their students, with the majority being white, hearing, and female (Andrews & Jordan, 1993; Simms, Rusher, Andrews, & Coryell, 2008). In their survey of 6,043 professionals in 349 deaf education programs, Andrews and Jordan reported that the majority of teachers of the deaf were white and hearing (75.5). Simms et al. (2008), based on a survey conducted in 2004 of 3,227 professionals in 313 deaf education programs, found that these percentages have not changed much: There were 69.9% who were classified as white and hearing. Deaf teachers of the deaf remained a small group: 15.6% in 1993 (Andrew & Jordan, 1993) and 22.1% in 2004 (Simms et al., 2008). Deaf teachers of the deaf who were not white were only 1.2% in 1993 and 2.5% in 2004. The majority of teachers were female (78.4% in 1993 and 80.3 in 2004). Most states do not require proficiency in sign language for certification of teachers of the deaf, and even those educators who become fluent signers generally learn ASL as adult second-language learners.

A substantial difference thus exists between the typical sociocultural and linguistic experiences of teachers and deaf students. These sociocultural and linguistic differences undoubtedly influence the structure of personal epistemologies and the interpersonal dynamics among teachers and students. However, these differences have not been examined to see what impact they have on deaf education.

Racial/ethnic minority educators of deaf people and racial/ethnic minority deaf students have suggested that the diversity of deaf educators needs to be increased to provide role models for deaf students of color and to create a campus climate that promotes pluralism and inclusiveness (Parasnis & Fischer, 2005; Parasnis et al., 2005). However, just increasing the number of diverse educators to serve as role models is not sufficient to address the issue of providing education that is sensitive to the needs of diverse students. Their diverse identities alone do not make teachers effective role models. Teachers need to be trained in understanding diversity and multiculturalism and engage in self-reflection about sociocultural diversity to become effective role models. In addition, they need to understand how their personal epistemologies have been influenced by sociocultural diversity and how these personal epistemologies have been shaped by their attitudes toward deaf students and their perceptions of the ways deaf students learn. Research is needed to show how the personal epistemologies of teachers develop and how they influence the teaching–learning process, and such research will empower teachers to be more effective role models for deaf students in the classroom.

CENTERING DIVERSITY AND MULTICULTURALISM IN DEAF EDUCATION

In discussing the general American education system, proponents of multicultural education, antiracist education, and feminism have noted that knowledge has been primarily constructed and transmitted based on the experiences and perspectives of white, Judeo-Christian, heterosexual, male, native English speakers and has marginalized the experiences and perspectives of many racial/ethnic minorities, women, and people with different sexual orientations. Such marginalization diminishes the educational experience of minorities who are not able to relate their own socioculturally based experiences and perspectives to the established traditional knowledge being taught in schools. The American deaf education system follows the general tradition in American education and is subject to the same criticism. Additionally, American deaf education, like general education, continues to view a typical American student as hearing and able-bodied (Bauman, 2008; Davis, 2007, 2008). Deafness and disabilities are viewed as *modifying* the general construct of an American student, not *transforming* that general construct. Furthermore, it typically ignores or de-emphasizes the racial, cultural, and linguistic diversity among educators and children and the role that this diversity plays in the construction and transmission of knowledge.

In deaf education, diversity and multiculturalism are often acknowledged as important goals, but the implementation of diversity and multiculturalism training in deaf education needs to go beyond providing information about different cultures and various standard demographic statistics about student census categories. The availability of multicultural events on campus or providing a few specific professional development activities for accommodating diverse students is not sufficient to fulfill the goals of promoting diversity and multiculturalism because they do not directly address how the dynamics of race, class, gender, and other sociocultural dimensions influences the development of an individual's identity and personal epistemology and how it shapes the educational experiences.

A more aggressive and effective agenda is needed that would include opportunities for in-depth exposure of students in teacher-training programs to assumption-challenging experiences, for example, a multicultural curriculum that examines the dominant culture of whiteness in America and discusses what whiteness and white privilege means (see Nakayama & Martin, 1999; Steinberg, 2009). Asher (2007) discusses how a multicultural teacher-training program that fosters critical, self-reflective ways of teaching can promote equity and democratic ways of being. She suggests that teachers should engage, rather than deny or repress, differences that emerge at the dynamic, context-specific intersections of race, culture, gender, and sexuality when they engage in self-reflection.

Teacher-training programs need to offer courses that critically review diversity and multiculturalism in American society and courses that connect these reviews to concepts regarding the development of epistemological beliefs. Such courses would help teachers understand their own identities and epistemological beliefs and understand the genuine educational implications of epistemological diversity in the classroom.

Commitment to studying diversity and multiculturalism can lead to examining how sociocultural differences influence teaching and learning, how stereotypes and prejudice influence human interactions, and how the established knowledge base and traditional methods of teaching and learning are inadequate to accommodate multiple identities and ways of knowing and often leave minorities feeling disenfranchised. Teachers should be formally engaged in self-reflection and in discussions with representatives of diverse racial, ethnic, linguistic, class, gender, sexuality, and religious groups to understand how stereotypes, stereotype threat, and prejudice influence social behavior and educational performance.

Self-reflections and discussion about self-identity and group identity development, which in turn influence epistemological development, can occur through a variety of ways including the use of web blogs and vlogs. Electronic media can be used effectively to document testimonial evidence, autobiographical reflections, group discussion, and historical information and to establish and maintain contact across diverse groups, all of which can make identity discourse more inclusive.

Centering the concepts of diversity and multiculturalism in these ways within deaf education will lead naturally to focused critique of curricular and educational practices and of the common knowledge base, who creates and interprets it, and who teaches it, leading in turn to more effective epistemological approaches to the multicultural community of deaf learners.

CONCLUSION

A review of current literature in deaf education reveals that the construct of experience-with-deafness as a unifying dimension has captured primary attention in our construction of knowledge about Deaf identity and Deaf community while other personal dimensions that involve diverse experience related to race/ethnicity, gender, class, and sexuality, all of which affect identity development, have been underplayed or ignored. Moving beyond this overly restrictive focus on experience-with-deafness as the single salient dimension of identity development will allow educators and scholars to create a valid construct of Deaf identity as a complex multidimensional identity built on the intersectional experience of deafness and other dimensions of identity. Self reflections, personal testimonial evidence, and theorizing by Deaf and hearing scholars in Deaf studies are culturally sensitive approaches that have begun to build knowledge about the Deaf community and Deaf identity, but much work needs to be done to represent the full scale of sociocultural experiences of the American Deaf community, its language use, its self-defining criteria for membership, and the potency of its members' multidimensional experiences in forming group and individual identities.

Developing the knowledge constructs of Deaf identity and Deaf community is necessary to understand how diverse deaf people develop personal epistemologies. How these personal epistemologies influence deaf students' educational experiences needs to be considered to develop epistemological frameworks to inform deaf educational policies and practices. Teacher-training programs should incorporate teaching about diversity and multiculturalism as well as epistemological diversity so that teachers understand how sociocultural diversity influences the epistemologies of deaf people.

With respect to further theorizing and research, there are several areas to explore. Redefining Deaf identity as a complex intersectionality of diverse dimensions prompts new questions about the role of multiple perspectives in the creation and sharing of a common knowledge base within the teaching–learning environment. How do personal epistemologies among deaf students develop out of complex multidimensional Deaf identities? How do personal epistemologies and domain-specific epistemologies of deaf students interact with the personal epistemologies and domain-specific epistemologies of the teachers in a teaching–learning environment? These questions need to be investigated.

The recognition that Deaf identity may be shaped by the intersectionality of multiple dimensions of diversity begs the question of what is the scope of those dimensions. While dimensions such as race, gender, class, and sexuality are obvious candidates that intersect with the experience-with-deafness dimension, there are many other physical, sensory, cognitive, cultural, religious, and linguistic dimensions of diversity that contribute to Deaf identity development. Research that discovers the full range of dimensions relevant to the emergence of multidimensional Deaf identity is needed.

The attitudes of the American Deaf community regarding how deaf people define themselves vis-à-vis the many dimensions of diversity also need to be studied. What are the self-affirmed markers of Deaf identity? How does the Deaf community maintain social cohesiveness within and across racial and ethnic boundaries and gender, sexuality, and class differences? More research needs to be done to understand Deaf community members' language preferences and language use in distinct communication environments. How do diverse Deaf people differ in the way they code switch? How do they negotiate communication in different domains and with different groups? How do the sociocutural issues related to power and oppression influence a racial/ethnic minority Deaf person's choice to use different languages?

Major changes in educational policies, curriculum design, and campus climate have to occur in addition to teacher-training program changes to make issues related to diversity and multiculturalism become an integral part of deaf education. An educational framework that shows how to bring about this change needs to be developed. Theoretical arguments and research that articulate the relationship between identity development and personal epistemological development, interactions between personal epistemologies and domain-specific epistemologies, and how diverse epistemological beliefs influence the teaching–learning process will help improve deaf education and make it relevant to living in today's global society.

REFERENCES

Andersen, M. N., & Collins, P. H. (1995). *Race, class, and gender: An anthology* (2nd ed.). Belmont, CA: Wadsworth.

Anderson, G., & Grace, C. (1991). Black deaf adolescents: A diverse and underserved population. *Volta Review, 93*, 73–86.

Anderson, G., & Miller, K. (2005). Appreciating diversity through stories about the lives of deaf color. *American Annals of the Deaf, 149*, 375–383.
Andrews, J., & Jordan, D. L. (1993). Minority and minority professionals: How many and where are they? *American Annals of the Deaf, 138*, 388–396.
Aramburo, A. B. (1989). Sociolinguistic aspect of the black deaf community. In C. Lucas (Ed.), *The sociolinguistics of the deaf community* (pp. 103–119). New York, NY: Academic Press.
Asher, N. (2007). Made in the (multicultural) U.S.A.: Unpacking tensions of race, culture, gender, and sexuality in education. *Educational Researcher, 36*(2), 65–73.
Bat-Chava, Y. (1993). Antecedents of self-esteem in deaf people: A meta-analytic review. *Rehabilitation Psychology, 38*, 221–234.
Bat-Chava, Y. (2000). Diversity of deaf identities. *American Annals of the Deaf, 145*, 420–428.
Bauman, H.-D. (Ed.). (2008). *Open your eyes: Deaf studies talking.* Minneapolis, MN: University of Minnesota Press.
Bienvenu, M. J. (2008). Queer as deaf: Intersections. In H.-D. Bauman (Ed.), *Open your eyes: Deaf studies talking* (pp. 251–263). Minneapolis, MN: University of Minnesota Press.
Brooks, D. (1996). In I. Parasnis (Ed.), *Cultural and language diversity and the deaf experience.* NewYork, NY: Cambridge University Press.
Brownlee, J., Schraw, G., & Berthelsen, D. (Eds.). (2011). *Personal epistemology and teacher education.* New York, NY: Routledge.
Brueggemann, B. (1999). *Lend me your ear: Rhetorical constructions of deafness.* Washington, DC: Gallaudet University Press.
Christensen, K. (Ed.) (2000). *Deaf plus: A multicultural perspective.* San Diego, CA: DawnSignPress.
Christensen, K., & Delgado, G. L. (Eds.). (1993). *Multicultural issues in deafness.* White Plains, NY: Longman.
Crenshaw, K. (1989). Demarginalizing the intersection of race and sex: A black feminist critique of antidiscrimination doctrine, feminist theory, and antiracist politics. *University of Chicago Legal Forum*, 139.
Cohen, O. P. (1993). Educational needs of African American and Hispanic deaf children and youth. In K. Christensen & G. L. Delgado (Eds.), *Multicultural issues in deafness* (pp. 45–68). White Plains, NY: Longman.
Cohen, O. P. (1997). Giving all children a chance: Advantages of an antiracist approach to education of deaf children. *American Annals of the Deaf, 142*, 80–82.
Cohen, O. P., Fischgrund, J., & Redding, R. (1990). Deaf children from ethnic, linguistic, and racial minority backgrounds: An overview. *American Annals of the Deaf, 135*, 67–73.
Cross, W. E. (1991). *Shades of black: Diversity in African American identity.* Philadelphia, PA: Temple University Press.
Cummins, J. (2009). Pedagogies of choice: Challenging coercive relations of power in classrooms and communities. *International Journal of Bilingual Education and Bilingualism, 12*, 261–271.
Davis, L. (2007). Deafness and the riddle of identity. *Chronicle of Higher Education, 53*(19), 1.
Davis, L. (2008). Postdeafness. In H.-D. Bauman (Ed.), *Open your eyes: Deaf studies talking* (pp. 314–326). Minneapolis, MN: University of Minnesota Press.
De Clerck, G. (2010). Deaf epistemologies as a critique and alternative to the practice of science: An anthropological perspective. *American Annals of the Deaf, 154*, 435–446.
Delgado, G. (2001). *Hispanic/Latino deaf students in our school.* Knoxville, TN: Postsecondary Education Consortium, University of Tennessee.
Dively, V. L. (2001). Contemporary native deaf experience: Overdue smoke rising. In L. Bragg (Ed.), *Deaf world: A historical reader and primary sourcebook* (pp. 390–405). New York, NY: New York University Press.
Dunn, L. (2008). The burden of racism and audism. In H.-D. Bauman (Ed.), *Open your eyes: Deaf studies talking* (pp. 264–276). Minneapolis, MN: University of Minnesota Press.

Eckert, R. C. (2010). Toward a theory of deaf ethnos: Deafnicity D/deaf (Ho´maemon. Homo´glosson. Homo´threskon). *Journal of Deaf Studies and Deaf Education, 15,* 317–333.

Fernandes, J. K., & Myers, S. S. (2010). Inclusive deaf studies: Barriers and pathways. *Journal of Deaf Studies and Deaf Education, 15,* 17–29.

Fisher, L. C., & McWhirter, J. J. (2001). The Deaf Identity Development scale: A revision and validation. *Journal of Counseling Psychology, 48,* 355–358.

Foster, S. (2001). Examining the fit between deafness and disability. In B. Altman and S. Barnartt (Eds.), *Research in Social Science and Disability: Vol. 2. Exploring theories and expanding methodologies: Where we are and where we need to go* (pp. 101–123). Oxford, UK: Elsevier Science.

Foster, S., & Kinuthia, W. (2003). Deaf persons of Asian American, Hispanic American, and African American backgrounds: A study of intraindividual diversity and identity. *Journal of Deaf Studies and Deaf Education, 8,* 271–290.

Gallaudet Research Institute. (2008). *Regional and national summary report of data from the 2007–8 Annual Survey of Deaf and Hard of Hearing Children and Youth.* Washington, DC: Gallaudet Research Institute, Gallaudet University.

Glickman, N. D. (1996). The development of culturally deaf identities. In N. S. Glickman & M. A. Harvey (Eds.), *Culturally affirmative psychotherapy with deaf persons* (pp. 115–153). Mahwah, NJ: Lawrence Erlbaum.

Grosjean, F. (1996). Living with two languages and two cultures. In I. Parasnis (Ed.), *Cultural and language diversity and the deaf experience* (pp. 20–37). New York, NY: Cambridge University Press.

Grosjean, F. (2001). The right of the deaf child to grow up bilingual. *Sign Language Studies 1*(2), 110–114.

Grosjean, F. (2010). Bilingualism, biculturalism, and deafness. *International Journal of Bilingual Education and Bilingualism, 13,* 133–145.

Hofer, B. K. (2001). Personal epistemology research: Implications for learning and teaching. *Educational Psychology Review, 13,* 353–383.

Hofer, B. K., & Pintrich, P. R. (1997). The development of epistemological theories: Beliefs about knowledge and knowing and their relation to learning. *Review of Educational Research, 67,* 88–140.

Hofer, B., & Pintrich, P. R. (2002). *Personal epistemology.* New York, NY: Lawrence Erlbaum.

Holcomb, T. K. (1997). Development of deaf bicultural identity. *American Annals of the Deaf, 142,* 89–93.

Humphries, T. (1993). Deaf culture and cultures. In K. Christensen & G. L. Delgado (Eds.), *Multicultural issues in deafness* (pp. 3–15). White Plains, NY: Longman.

Humphries, T. (2008). Talking culture and culture talking. In H.-D. Bauman (Ed.), *Open your eyes: Deaf studies talking* (pp. 35–41). Minneapolis, MN: University of Minnesota Press.

Johnson, R. E., & Erting, C. (1989). Ethnicity and socialization in a classroom for deaf children. In C. Lucas (Ed.), *The sociolinguistics of the Deaf community* (pp. 41–83). New York, NY: Academic Press.

Jones, S., & McEwen, M. (2000). A conceptual model of multiple dimensions of identity. *Journal of College Student Development, 41,* 405–414.

Kannapell, B. (1993). *Language choice–identity choice.* Burtonsville, MD: Linstock Press.

Kelly, A. B. (2008). Where is deaf herstory? In H.-D. Bauman (Ed.), *Open your eyes: Deaf studies talking* (pp. 251–263). Minneapolis, MN: University of Minnesota Press.

Kluwin, T. (1994). The interaction of race, gender, and social class in the education of deaf students. *American Annals of the Deaf, 139,* 465–471.

Ladd, P. (2003). *Understanding deaf culture: In search of deafhood.* Clevedon, UK: Multilingual Matters.

Lane, H. (1992). *The mask of benevolence: Disabling the deaf community.* New York, NY: Alfred A. Knopf.

Lane, H. (2005). Ethnicity, ethics, and the Deaf-world. *Journal of Deaf Studies and Deaf Education, 10,* 291–310.

Lane, H., Hoffmeister, R., & Bahan, B. (1996). *A journey into the Deaf-world.* San Diego, CA: DawnSignPress.

Leigh, I. (2008). Who am I? Deaf identity issues. In K. Lindgren, D. DeLuca, & D. J. Napoli (Eds.), *Signs and voices: Deaf culture, identity, language, and arts* (pp. 21–29). Washington, DC: Gallaudet University Press.

Maxwell-McCaw, D., & Zea, M. C. (2011). The deaf acculturation scale (DAS): Development and validation of a 58-item measure. *Journal of Deaf Studies and Deaf Education, 16,* 325–342.

McCall, L. (2005). The complexity of intersectionality. *Signs, 30*(3), 1771–1800.

Mitchell, R., & Karschmer, M. (2004). Chasing the mythical ten percent: Parental hearing status of Deaf and hard of hearing students in the United States. *Sign Language Studies, 4,* 138–163.

Moores, D., & Miller, M. (2009). *Deaf people around the world: Educational and social perspectives.* Washington, DC: Gallaudet University Press.

Myers, C., Clark, M. D., Musyoka, M. M., Anderson, M. L., Gilbert, G. L., Agyen, S., & Hauser, P. (2010). Black deaf individuals' reading skills: Influence of ASL, culture, family characteristics, reading experience, and education. *American Annals of the Deaf, 155,* 449–457.

Nakamura, K. (2006). *Deaf in Japan: Signing and the politics of identity.* Ithaca, NY: Cornell University Press.

Nakayama, T. K., & Martin, J. N. (Eds.). (1999). *Whiteness: The communication of social identity.* Thousand Oaks, CA: Sage.

Nash, J. (2008). Rethinking intersectionality. *Feminist Review, 89,* 1–15.

Natapoff, A. (1995). Anatomy of a debate: Intersectionality and equality for deaf children from non-English-speaking homes. *Journal of Law and Education, 24,* 271–278.

Nikolaraizi, M., & Hadjikakou, K. (2006). The role of educational experiences in the development of deaf identity. *Journal of Deaf Studies and Deaf Education, 11,* 477–492.

Padden, C. (1980). The deaf community and the culture of deaf people. In C. Baker & R. Battison (Eds.), *Sign language and the deaf community: Essays in honor of William C. Stokoe* (pp. 89–103). Silver Spring, MD: National Association of the Deaf.

Padden, C. (1996). From the cultural to the bicultural. In I. Parasnis (Ed.), *Cultural and language diversity and the deaf experience* (pp. 79–98). New York, NY: Cambridge University Press.

Padden, C., & Humphries, T. (1988). *Deaf in America: Voices from a culture.* Cambridge, MA: Harvard University Press.

Padden, C., & Humphries, T. (2005). *Inside Deaf culture.* Cambridge, MA: Harvard University Press.

Pallas, A. (2001). Preparing education doctoral students for epistemological diversity. *Educational Researcher, 30*(5), 6–11.

Parasnis, I. (1996). On interpreting the Deaf experience within the context of cultural and language diversity. In *Cultural and language diversity and the Deaf experience* (pp. 3–19). New York, NY: Cambridge University Press.

Parasnis, I. (Ed.). (1996). *Cultural and language diversity and the deaf experience.* New York, NY: Cambridge University Press.

Parasnis, I. (1997). Cultural identity and diversity in deaf education. *American Annals of the Deaf, 142,* 72–79.

Parasnis, I. (1998). Cognitive diversity in deaf people: Implications for communication and education. *Scandinavian Journal of Audiology, 27*(Suppl. 49), 109–115.

Parasnis, I. (2000, July). Deaf ethnic-minority students: Diversity and identity. *Proceedings of the 19th International Conference on Education of the Deaf,* Sydney, Australia.

Parasnis, I. (2004). Diversity and identity: Implications for deaf education. In S. Brodaric-Joncic & V. Ivasovic (Eds.), *Sign language, deaf culture, and bilingual education* (pp. 101–110). Zagreb, Croatia: Faculty of Education and Rehabilitation Sciences, University of Zagreb.

Parasnis, I., & Fischer, S. D. (2005). Perceptions of diverse educators regarding ethnic-minority deaf college students, role models, and diversity. *American Annals of the Deaf, 150*, 341–349.

Parasnis, I., Samar, V. J., & Fischer, S. D. (2005). Deaf students' attitudes toward ethnic diversity, campus climate, and role models. *American Annals of the Deaf, 150*, 47–58.

Parillo, V. N. (2011). *Understanding race and ethnic relations* (4th ed.). New York, NY: Prentice Hall.

Parsons, L., & Jordan, T. (1994). When educational reform results in educational discrimination: A case in point. *Journal of Law and Education, 23*, 211–231.

Paul, P. (Ed.). (2010). Deaf epistemologies [Special issue]. *American Annals of the Deaf, 154*, 417–496.

Paul, P., & Moores, D. (2010). Introduction: Toward an understanding of epistemology and deafness. *American Annals of the Deaf, 154*, 421–427.

Preston, P. (1996). *Mother father deaf: Living between sound and silence*. Cambridge, MA: Harvard University Press.

Schraw, G. (2001). Current themes and future directions in epistemological research: A commentary. *Educational Psychology Review, 13*, 451–464.

Schraw, G., & Olafson, L. (2002). Teachers' epistemological world views and educational practices. *Issues in Education: Contributions from Educational Psychology, 8*, 99–148.

Schraw, G., & Sinatra, G. (2004). Epistemological development and its impact on cognition in academic domains. *Contemporary Educational Psychology, 29*, 95–102.

Sellers, R. M., Smith, M. A., Shelton, J. N., Rowley, S. A. J., & Chavous, T. M. (1998). Multidimensional model of racial identity: A reconceptualization of African American racial identity. *Personality and Social Psychology Review, 2*, 18–39.

Simms, L., Rusher, M., Andrew, J. F., & Coryell, J. (2008). Apartheid in deaf education: Examining workforce diversity. *American Annals of the Deaf, 153*, 384–395.

Steinberg, S. (Ed.). (2009). *Diversity and multiculturalism: A reader*. New York, NY: Peter Lang.

Steup, M. (2010, Spring). Epistemology. In E. Zalta (Ed.), *The Stanford encyclopedia of philosophy*. Retrieved January 12, 2010 from http://plato.stanford.edu/archives/spr2010/entries/epistemology.

Tatum, B. (2003). *"Why are all the black kids sitting together in the cafeteria?" and other conversations about race*. New York, NY: Basic Books.

Vasistha, M. (2006). *Deaf in Delhi: A memoir*. Washington, DC: Gallaudet University Press.

Woll, B., & Ladd, P. (2003). Deaf communities. In M. Marschark & P. E. Spencer (Eds.), *Oxford handbook of deaf studies, language, and education* (pp. 151–163). New York, NY: Oxford University Press.

SUGGESTIONS FOR FURTHER READING

Brownlee, J., Schraw, G., & Berthelsen, D. (2011). *Personal epistemology and teacher education*. New York, NY: Routledge.

Hofer, B., & Pintrich, P. R. (2002). *Personal epistemology*. New York, NY: Lawrence Erlbaum.

Nakamura, K. (2006). *Deaf in Japan: Signing and the politics of identity*. Ithaca, NY: Cornell University Press.

Padden, C., & Humphries, T. (2005). *Inside Deaf culture*. Cambridge, MA: Harvard University Press.

Parillo, V. N. (2011). *Understanding race and ethnic relations* (4th ed.). New York, NY: Prentice Hall.

Steinberg, S. (Ed.). (2009). *Diversity and multiculturalism: A reader*. New York, NY: Peter Lang.

Tatum, B. (2003). *"Why are all the black kids sitting together in the cafeteria?" and other conversations about race*. New York, NY: Basic Books.

5

Valuing Deaf Indigenous Knowledge in Research Through Partnership: The Cameroonian Deaf Community and the Challenge of "Serious" Scholarship

Goedele A. M. De Clerck

Science is a practice developed by human beings in a particular context and a particular time. It can describe diverse perspectives and practices, including deaf knowledge and deaf worldviews. As long as science is a master narrative and deaf knowledge continues to be excluded from science, the concept of deaf epistemologies is necessary.

Parallel to developments in science, master narratives have also developed in deaf studies and deaf education. In Chapter 2, I argued for a descriptive project of cross-cultural comparison as an alternative to a top-down approach. The question of

---

This project has been supported by a postdoctoral research grant and travel grants from the Research Foundation–Flanders. I give special thanks to Dr. Donald F. Moores and Dr. Peter V. Paul for their encouragements and constructive feedback during the writing of this chapter. I also thank Dr. Rik Pinxten for his generous support of my work. I wholeheartedly thank the deaf people of Cameroon for participating in the present study, the Cameroon National Association of the Deaf for supporting the research, and Cameroonian deaf leaders for their cooperation in the study. The staff at the University of Buea, where I was a visiting scholar, has been very supportive, including Dr. Gratien Atindogbe, Mr. Patrick Shey, Dr. Moses Einstein, Dr. Euphrasiah Yuh, Dr. Therese Tchombe, and Dr. Victor Ngoh. Thanks go to Dr. Bame Nsamenang for informing me about his inspiring research. I also thank the World Federation of the Deaf (WFD) and the WFD Human Rights trainers Megan Youngs and Ablavi Dziku for their collaboration and for the opportunities to participate in and observe the training in Cameroon and to present a workshop. I also express gratitude to the Buea School for the Deaf—its generous support, especially in the first stages of this research, has helped make this project possible. I thank Ivo Ngade for sharing his Cameroonian experiences views, and research, and Sam Lutalo-Kiingi for inspiring discussions on deaf community development and empowerment in sub-Saharan Africa.

how deaf indigenous knowledge can be valued during this ongoing research process, that is, a question on adequate research methods, is illustrated by discussion of the development of the research methodology of an exploratory case study on emancipation processes in the Cameroonian deaf community, which, in line with performance ethnography (Fabian, 1990) has been largely developed during the fieldwork. In a joint venture of negotiation and control (Pinxten, 2006), the Cameroonian deaf community has been involved in all stages of the research process, and research findings have been shared and reflected upon.

This interdisciplinary project involves deaf studies, deaf education, (sign) linguistics, anthropology, and critical pedagogy. In alignment with the organization of the Cameroonian deaf community, including Cameroonian deaf leaders as epistemic authorities, a community-based and participatory approach (Higgs, 2008, 2010) has been developed. A methodological stance of intersectionality has been beneficial in the research process: Intertwining axes of oppression (based, for example, on one's status as African, black, deaf, or female or on one's educational or class background) have been analyzed and taken into account (Farmer, 2010a; Thorvaldsdottir, 2007). A bottom-up approach seemed beneficial for the description of Cameroonian deaf knowledge and philosophy of life. The moral concept of "being serious" is employed in the Cameroonian deaf community to guide deaf Cameroonians toward "being succesful." This research project was placed in the local semantic framework of "development": Support for the development of the Cameroonian deaf community was a necessary condition for deaf Cameroonians to participate in the present study. To meet this challenge of enabling "serious" scholarship, it seemed useful to pursue development of "pragmatic solidarity" (Farmer, 2010c, p. 450) with an interactive partnership of the deaf community, nongovernmental organizations (NGOs), and academia.

An interview in Spring 2010 with a Cameroonian deaf man in his early twenties is illustrative of the structural limitations young deaf people experience in Cameroon and of the emancipation process that has begun.[1] The interview itself was remarkable: I did not ask any question for more than an hour; the man had his story ready. Earlier, in a meeting with the local deaf community, I had introduced myself, my research study, and the methods and topics of the interview and provided members of the deaf community with the opportunity to participate in the study. The man had put his name on the list of people who wanted to be interviewed, and I had invited him by a text message. No need to re-explain the goals and ethical conditions of the study! The man remembered everything and was eager to start with his life story. I started the video recorder and he signed for more than an hour on all the topics I had intended to cover. He explained how he had to argue to be allowed to stay in school after the death of his father:

> When I was 9 years old, my father died. My family supported us. My mom considered our situation and told me, "You have to stop going to school." I was very angry: "No, I must learn how to write!" My mom said, "Ah, but we don't have money, that's a problem." I said, "No, I want to learn how to write!" I asked my sister for money, but she wouldn't pay. My mom said, "I can't afford to pay school." Then we

went to the director and he said, "Well, try to pay." He allowed us to pay a cheaper school fee, and we could manage.

The topic of education—the key to better life chances—and this young man's efforts on his own behalf to gain access to it are central in his life story. The interview had a clear purpose for him, and in telling his life story, he worked toward a concrete question that is currently jeopardizing his efforts to improve himself: "The teacher doesn't sign well. He/she doesn't know how to teach. I need to pass my FSLC [First School Leaving Certificate, a primary education national exam]. But how do I learn English?" The young man was very concerned about his future, and he knew that this structural problem needed to be solved if he was to have better life chances. Hoping to pass his exam this time and waiting to move on with his life, he had already started in a secondary deaf education program. When I met him a year later, I learned that he had failed the exam again and was still experiencing the same barriers but still had the same hope. He had also retained the strength to be critical and ask for structural solutions to his problem.

There is some ambiguity in his question. On the one hand, it is rhetorical in relation to the Cameroonian context—as my informant philosophically said, "Maybe, in 2020, Cameroon will develop. But if not . . . if not, then we have to work hard and set up a business." On the other hand, the question also appeals to me as a white female deaf scholar. As a visitor with a project, I am placed in a history: a history of globalization and inequality, a history of corruption of government and local leadership, a history of broken promises of white people, a history of deaf Cameroonians who moved to Europe and the United States and did not come back. "And now you are here." I swallowed and nodded: "Yes, I am here." I was here for fundamental research. Though genuinely necessary and probably helpful in some way, opportunities for supporting deaf community development are limited within the project. The young man's analysis was less surprising than confrontational: "And then white people come, and they say that it is not easy to find funding, but they have a computer, a photo camera, all those things." In his analysis and conclusion of his experiences, he moved between a sense of hopelessness (will you be the same?) and a sense of hope, in a clear call for what Paul Farmer (2010c) has called "pragmatic solidarity" (p. 450): making room for research that contributes to social justice and equality. This call for pragmatic solidarity for the Cameroonian deaf community is a necessary condition for supporting this research.

COMMUNITY-BASED RESEARCH: VALUING AFRICAN AND DEAF EPISTEMOLOGIES

The sense of moving between hope and hopelessness expressed in the interviews is a common feeling among Cameroonians, both deaf and hearing. In modern Africa, the "optimism of postwar movements of decolonization and the building of 'new nations'" have disappeared "as everyday life in Africa is increasingly marked by a gap between people's dreams of a better life and their actual disconnection from the structures on which the materialization of this dreams depends" (Geschiere, Pels, & Meyer, 2008, p. 2). The Republic of Cameroon has a history of German, French, and British colonization. It is officially bilingual (French and English), with more than 200 ethnic groups and languages. Paul Biya, the president, has been able to stay in power for almost 30 years. Known for a lack of transparency in both its governance and its commercial life, Cameroon has been listed as one of the world's most corrupt countries (Ceuppens & Geschiere, 2005). Yet despite these problems, and regardless of political tensions in neighboring countries such as Côte d'Ivoire, Cameroon has been politically stable. The United Nations Human Development (UNDP) index, "a composite measure of three basic dimensions of human development: health, education and income" (Human Development Reports, 2010), provides a broader indication of well-being than statistics based solely on economic growth. The 2010 UNDP index lists a life expectancy of 51.7 years, an average of 5.9 years of schooling, and a gross national income per capita of US$7.70. With an index of 0.460 in 2010 (compared to 0.354 in 1980), Cameroon is doing better than the index of the sub-Saharan African region (0.389 in 2010, compared to 0.293 in 1980); however, it is listed as a "low human development country" (ranking 131st out of 169 countries in the world) (Human Development Reports, 2010).

The Cameroonian economy is predominantly agricultural; bananas, cocoa, coffee, timber, tobacco, and cotton are major export products. Cameroonians are still suffering from the economic shock that resulted from the decline in the prices of oil, coffee, and cocoa in the 1980s. In spite of structural reforms undertaken by the government, economic stagnation persists (World Bank, 2010). The global economic downturn has seriously affected the lives of Cameroonians: Expenses for education and housing have increased, whereas incomes and opportunities for employment have decreased. There is an ongoing brain drain, and with an average age of only 18 years (only 3.7% of the population is above 65), the Cameroonian labor force consists in large part of adolescents who are looking for opportunities abroad (World Population Prospects as cited in Fleischer, 2007).

In 2009, 58% of the population lived in urban areas (UNICEF, 2009). The poverty rate in rural areas, more than 55% of households, is much greater than in cities, where it is just 12% (World Bank, 2010). Increased poverty, unemployment, and the attraction of modernity have driven young people to the cities (Nsamenang, 1992). These social transitions, in combination with increased suffering and sickness, have bred strong feelings of uncertainty: Community-based safety nets are collapsing. These social transitions are also related to a moral crisis: Modern education, which was introduced in colonial times, has marginalized indigenous knowledge; community elders are losing authority and respect because they are not able to provide answers to questions about the changed world in which young people today are living; the failing state is also losing authority. More and more people are finding alternative explanations for unfortunate life conditions in witchcraft (Fisiy, 1998; Johnson-Hanks, 2007; Nsamenang, 1992).

The Cameroonian deaf community came into my life when I met Aloysius N'jok Bibum at Gallaudet University. He is a deaf Gallaudet alumnus from Cameroon who returned to his country to establish the Buea School for the Deaf with his wife, Margaret Bibum. During my visit to the school in 2007, I was impressed with its educational ambitions. I learned that the Buea School for the Deaf was the second deaf school in Cameroon to start a secondary education program. All deaf schools in Cameroon are private, and many parents cannot afford school fees. Consequently, there are many deaf children in Cameroon who do not have access to education. Most deaf schools only offer primary education, after which deaf students leave school or are mainstreamed. There are no programs for interpreting training, or interpreting services, in Cameroon. Some deaf schools offer some form of tutoring after school, but often students give up. The limited educational opportunities for deaf people in Cameroon made me wonder about the lives of deaf adults.

I was introduced to a gathering of deaf people in the seaport city of Douala on a Sunday afternoon. What followed was a more or less formal meeting in which deaf leaders and deaf community members expressed their anger, frustration, and concerns about their lives. A vicious circle of little or no education, illiteracy, unemployment, and the inability to pay a dowry and/or gain family consent to marry a deaf spouse has left these people with few prospects for the future.[2] They had seen little change in Cameroonian society over the past 10 to 15 years, and they felt abandoned by the government and the Cameroon National Association of the Deaf (CANAD).

Their stories and their raw and energetic anger inspired me to work on Cameroonian deaf lives as part of a 3-year cross-cultural comparative study of emancipation processes in deaf communities in Sweden, Flanders, and Cameroon. For the Cameroonian case study, I collaborate with the University of Buea, where I am affiliated as a visiting scholar during fieldwork periods. In an initial 1-month exploratory visit in October 2009, I introduced my study to CANAD and the Cameroonian deaf community. Data from informal interviews and participant observation during this stay enabled me to gain insight into native terminology and common themes in the life stories of Cameroonian deaf people and to develop a contextualized list of questions for ethnographic in-depth interviews (Spradley, 1997). This is the first study on this topic in Cameroon; therefore, the research is exploratory and employs a bottom-up approach (Stebbins, 2001; Yin, 1994).[3] Tailoring the study to the collective identification and organization of the Cameroonian deaf community, from an interdisciplinary stance of African and deaf epistemologies, I have employed a community-based research process (Dei, 2010; Higgs, 2008, 2010). The creative development of the research method during the fieldwork, in interaction with the Cameroonian deaf community, is an example of performance ethnography (Fabian, 1990). The case study includes multiple sources of data (participant observation, ethnographic interviews, document study, and discussion groups).

During a 3-month stay from March to June 2010 and a 1-month stay from February to March 2011, I interviewed 59 deaf Cameroonians of different backgrounds (in regard to gender, religion, ethnicity, age, schooling, class, onset of deafness, and language) from five regions in Cameroon. Research participants were recruited through presentations and discussions of the research studies and discussions in local deaf community meetings organized by deaf leaders in the Central, Littoral, North-West, and South-West regions.[4] (Cameroon is divided into 10 regions; they are the country's primary administrative divisions.) The research followed the ethical guidelines of the American Anthropological Association. All interviews were individual, private, and conducted in Cameroon Sign Language (CSL). Because I am deaf and already had knowledge of American Sign Language (ASL), which has heavily influenced CSL, I was able to gain fluency in CSL fairly quickly.

The study was limited to deaf communities in cities in the Central, Littoral, North-West, and South-West regions; I am not aware of any other research on the development of the Cameroonian deaf community in the country's other six regions. Because of financial constraints and other restrictions on travel opportunities, the CANAD and individual Cameroonian deaf adults also have limited information on the other regions.[5]

During my first stay, I noticed that the concept of research was new to the Cameroonian deaf community, as well as the method of ethnographic interviewing. Research on the emancipation topic was associated with the work of NGOs. Therefore, I tried to find creative ways to communicate my research concept. Based on data collected during my first month of fieldwork, I asked Eyonga Beltus, a Cameroonian deaf artist, to make drawings of key moments and experiences in deaf people's lives, such as becoming deaf, communication within the family, going to a deaf school, learning sign language (instead of the gestural communication and home signs that are used in villages and with families), helping parents at the farm, and getting married (see Figures 1 and 2). Deaf community members could identify with the drawings and recognize the topics. The drawings also helped to "break the ice" and make people more comfortable and less shy when meeting a deaf scholar. Another tool that I used

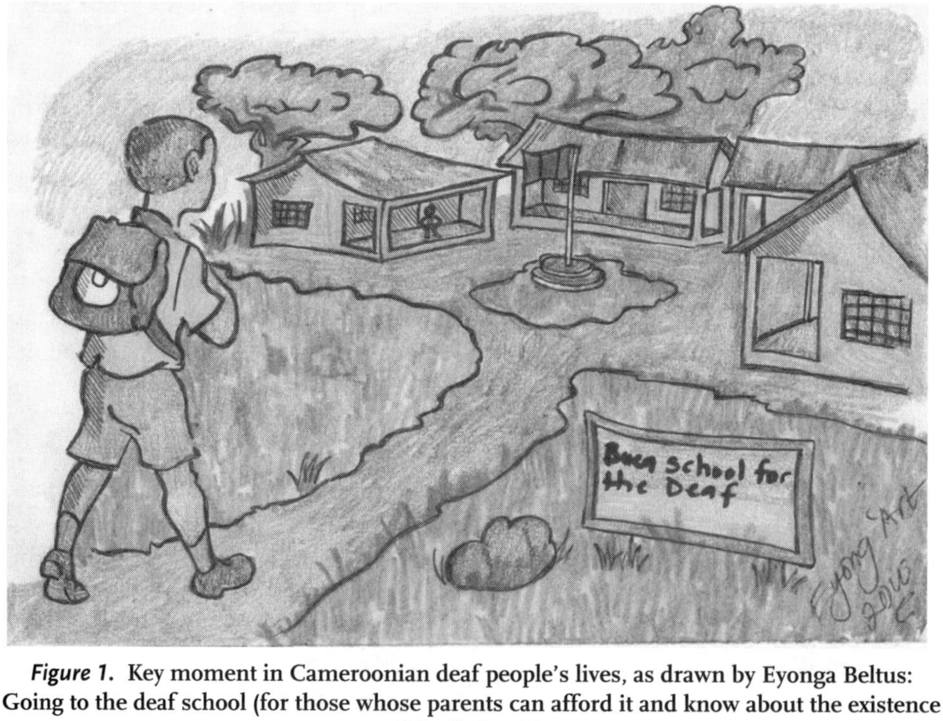

Figure 1. Key moment in Cameroonian deaf people's lives, as drawn by Eyonga Beltus: Going to the deaf school (for those whose parents can afford it and know about the existence of deaf schools).

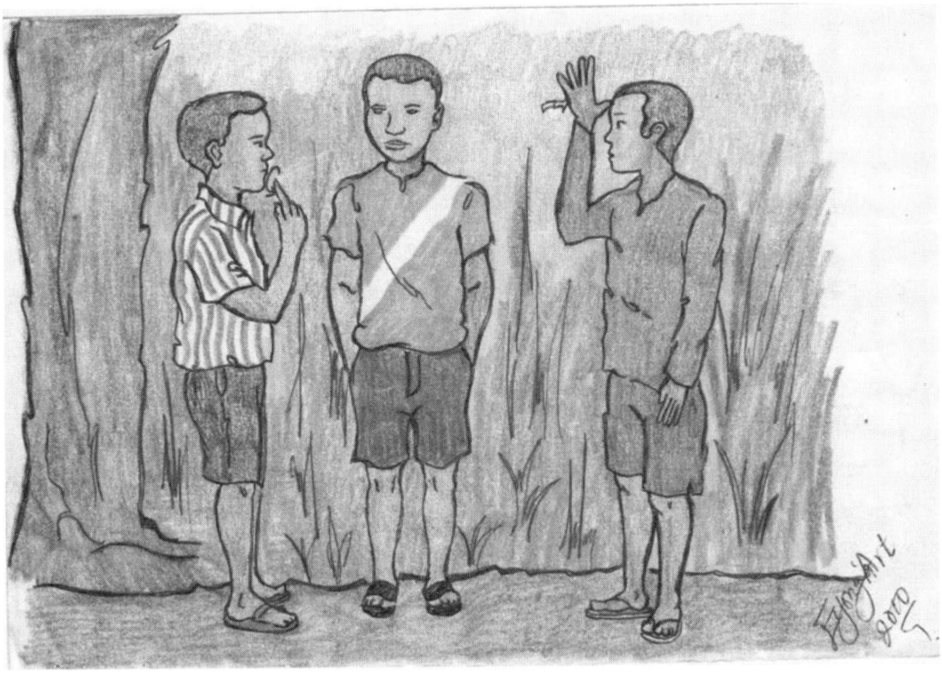

Figure 2. **Key moments in Cameroonian deaf people's lives, as drawn by Eyonga Beltus: Learning sign language at the deaf school, replacing home signs and gestures. The signs shown in the picture are WHO? FATHER.**

in these meetings is Ruth Morgan's 2008 book *DEAF ME NORMAL*, a collection of life stories of deaf people in South Africa. The deaf participants in the meetings were very enthusiastic about this work. For most of them, it was the first time they had ever seen a book about deaf people. Some information, such as the existence of deaf families, was received with surprise and wonder. The idea of a book about the Cameroonian deaf community was received as a signal of hope: It can inform the Cameroonian government ("you are white, you can do that"), and, even more important for most people, the outside world could learn about deaf people in Cameroon. Even if they themselves might not be able to go out of the country, at least their stories could.

I tried to be sensitive to indigenous African epistemologies and to respect "*the double role* of individuals in African societies"; that is, elders and other "epistemic authorities" (Kaphagawani & Malherbe, 1998, p. 214) "should not only be perceived as important informants, but also as research colleagues with critical perspectives on educational practices" (Higgs, 2010, p. 2418; see also Dei, 2010). Deaf leaders introduced me to Cameroonian deaf collective life and advised me on both the organization of research topics and the interpretation of the research findings. They were very generous in their support of my study, in organizing local deaf community meetings, and in helping me to contact and meet adults who wanted to be interviewed.

The Cameroonian deaf community was involved in all stages of the research process. Grounded analysis has led to tentative generalizations and theory development (Stebbins, 2001). Preliminary research findings were discussed individually with some deaf leaders and key informants during my first periods of fieldwork. During my visit of February–March 2011, I had the opportunity to observe the World Federation of the Deaf (WFD) Deaf Human Rights and Capacity Building Training Project in western and central Africa for national and regional deaf board members in the national capital, Yaoundé, and to present and discuss the preliminary research findings presented in the present chapter with the participants in the training. During that stay, I also received feedback from discussions with the broader community in local meetings in Douala and the nearby city of Kumba.

PICTURE OF A YOUNG DEAF COMMUNITY

As in many other countries in Africa and elsewhere, the development of the deaf community in Cameroon is tied to the foundation of deaf schools. The history of formal deaf education in Cameroon is a recent one; this is in alignment with the history of special education in Cameroon. Although missionaries provided care for people with disabilities in precolonial and colonial times, schools were established only after the independence of Cameroon in 1960 (see also Yuh & Shey, 2008). In 1972, French missionaries founded the first deaf school in Cameroon in Yaoundé. The school employed an oral philosophy. Narratives of deaf adults in Yaoundé reveal the emergence of signed communication among deaf children on the playground in the early years of the school, which differed from the gestures used in home and village environment. (Gestural communication accompanying speech is widely used in sub-Saharan Africa; see, e.g., Dalle-Nazébi, 2009, and Sorin-Barreteau, 1996.) In 1979, American missionary Andrew Foster established the second deaf school, in Kumba, in the Anglophone area of Cameroon. The missionary was the first African American to obtain a bachelor's degree from Gallaudet University. Noticing that formal deaf education was almost nonexistent in Africa, Foster had started his work by founding a deaf school in Ghana in 1956. Altogether, he would establish 31 deaf schools in western and central Africa, which is why he is called "the father of deaf education in Africa" (Kamei, 2006). He is well remembered and highly respected by the Cameroonian deaf community. Foster also founded the Christian Mission of the Deaf and deaf gospel churches in those regions before he died in 1987.

ASL was used as a language of communication and instruction in these schools and churches, which ensured a strong ASL influence on deaf communications in western and central African countries. In a teacher-training center for deaf Africans in Ibadan, Nigeria, established by Foster, 161 deaf adults from 19 African countries received training. Kamei (2006) writes that in this training institute ASL was "changed" to teach French and fit in the francophone African context; a dictionary was published on this, titled *Langage des Signes du Sourds Africain Francophone* (sign language of deaf francophone Africans) (Tamomo 1994, in Kamei, 2006). A francophone deaf trainee from Cameroon, who graduated from the training in 1986, confirmed that he was trained in French. However, he brought a different English dictionary from the training, probably because he was prepared to work in the anglophone Ephata Institute for the Deaf in Kumba. The book, which is titled *Sign Language Lessons for the Deaf: Handbook for*

Teachers of the Deaf (Silas, n. d.), contains a collection of signs that reveal a form of an English signed system rather than ASL. This use of this communication system would be in alignment of Total Communication philosophies at the time in the United States and in Europe. The use of a sign system as a language of instruction was also confirmed by interviews with deaf adults who worked in the school at Foster's time, most of whom were trained in Nigeria and became deaf at a later age. Influence of sign systems (in forms of CSL influenced by ASL and *langue des signes francophone* [LSF]) can also be seen in the use of CSL today.

The establishment of the Kumba School for the Deaf not only introduced ASL but also contributed to the dissemination of ASL throughout Cameroon by means of deaf school students and graduates who socialized with deaf adults in other places, such as Yaoundé. Another source of ASL influence in Yaoundé was a deaf church where a missionary, who had been trained by Foster in Nigeria, used ASL as the language for the church services. In the 1990s, LSF was introduced in deaf schools in some places where French was the primary language (such as Yaoundé and a city in the interior, Bafoussam). The (ideological) motivation was that French could only be taught in LSF and not in the ASL-based sign language that was being used in the adult deaf community. However, the use of LSF and ASL does not simply mirror the spoken-language French–English bilingualism of Cameroon. Most Cameroonian deaf adults in the areas of research use an ASL-influenced variant of CSL. The introduction of LSF has resulted in the first generation of young deaf people using an LSF-influenced variant. The linguistic colonialism manifested by the introduction of ASL and LSF is the result of ideology and politics (in the case of Foster, maybe also of a limited knowledge of sign language linguistics in that period of time). Ideological and political arguments, as well as the influence of dominant spoken languages (French, English, pidgin) and influences of gestures must be taken into account if one is to gain a full understanding of the linguistic mosaic of signed languages in Cameroon and its sociolinguistic context. Linguistic research is needed to determine whether CSL is a national language with regional variations or whether different sign languages are used in Cameroon. Investigation of this issue will help advance recognition of CSL and support the preservation of Cameroonian indigenous signs.

So far I have been unable to find any signing deaf families in Cameroon[6]—as I have noted, Cameroonian deaf people were very surprised when they learned about the existence of deaf families in South Africa from Ruth Morgan's book. There are several cases of deaf siblings in a family. Intergenerational transmission of sign language within deaf families seems to be beginning—some deaf parents are starting to communicate in sign language with their hearing children. Cameroonian deaf people share stories of the marginalization and linguistic and communicative exclusion they experienced before coming into contact with other deaf people: All the deaf people in my study who made the transition from gestures to sign emphasized that they had felt limited before and that sign helped them to "develop."

However, the picture is different from a Western one—some rural contexts seem to be communicatively and socially inclusive, with a commonly used gestural basis that enables in-depth conversation. Liliane Sorin-Barreteau (1996) studied gestural communication among the Mofu-Gudur in Cameroon's North region. Her doctoral study included deaf people's signing. She found that the gestures used by hearing people seem to form the basis for signed communication, which is characterized by an expanded vocabulary and enables faster communication. Further anthropological and linguistic research on gestural communication between hearing and deaf people in Cameroon and sub-Saharan Africa is needed to gain a better understanding of this point of view.[7]

Cameroonian collective life is organized through "deaf gatherings" (CSL sign) in cities on the weekends. In the course of the present study, a "deaf map" was developed identifying deaf schools and places where deaf people gather. Deaf adults meet each other after church on Sunday, in deaf schools, after sports events on weekends, and any time deaf leaders organize meetings. CSL is a border marker distinguishing members of the deaf community from "chickens," that is, deaf people who have grown up in rural areas, have not attended deaf schools, and/or have not been in contact with other deaf adults. (This label is applied because these people's gestural form of communication is said to resemble the flapping of a chicken's wings.) The transition from gestural communication to formal signing in deaf schools or in the adult deaf community is a turning point in deaf people's lives. Deaf people's description of this transition also illustrates the ideologies of Western education, sign language, and religion imported into the country. For example, common iconic gestures in Cameroon to refer to *father* and *mother*, respectively indicating a man's beard and a woman's breasts, have had to be replaced by formal ASL signs (see Figure 2). Gradually, the narrative goes, as deaf Cameroonians' signing "improves" (and the gestures are replaced), they became "successful." Having an education, "signing beautifully," and knowing how to read and write are also perceived as signs of being "smart." This ideology is also reflected in the current organization of deaf leadership in the CANAD and in the Cameroonian deaf community, which is largely represented by deafened people who have more educational background and knowledge of the written and spoken dominant languages.

There is a sense of collective identification among deaf adults in terms of the African notion of an extended family; for example, deaf peers are called "brothers and sisters" in deaf community meetings, and older male leaders are called "papa." For those who have attended deaf schools, this sense of care and responsibility starts at the deaf school with deaf teachers or older deaf students taking care of younger students, but it is broader than that. Local deaf leaders are concerned about the well-being of deaf community members and often visit deaf people to see how they are doing or to act as negotiators in case of family problems. The context of a wider distribution of gestural communication and the lack of access to rehabilitative technology results in a border marking between members of the deaf community and "chickens" that is different from the symbolic marker distinguishing oral and signing deaf people in Western societies. "Chickens" are also considered part of the extended deaf family and welcomed to learn sign language and join the group. Deaf leaders will also take responsibility for "chickens" in case of problems with the larger society.

However, this sense of family is an ambiguous one. In its lack of confidence and collaboration among deaf adults, it differs from the sense of collectivity in Western deaf communities (see, e.g., Ladd, 2003; Mindess, 1999; Padden & Humphries, 1988) and in deaf communities in the Far North region of Cameroon and in Chad (see note 5). The broader moral crisis and collapse of the community safety net is probably also a factor, as well as the absence of deaf elders (and their epistemic authority) who can serve as examples of successful deaf people. Most deaf adults respond that they do not have any friends and need to solve problems on their own. Those who attended a deaf school often recall a feeling of belonging; however, this feeling seems to be overshadowed by the hard realities of adult life. The lack of secondary education and of room for continuous bonding, at an age when maturity and independence is being developed, is another explanatory factor. A reason for the lack of trust among deaf community members may also be found in reported systematic sexual abuse of deaf children and women in deaf schools and in the adult deaf community (particularly in begging groups). Jealousy and gossip in the deaf community are experienced as damaging, for example, when they lead to the loss of a boyfriend or girlfriend or the closing of a business. These problems are a challenge for the Cameroonian deaf family. The training offered as part of the WFD Deaf Human Rights and Capacity Building Training Project in western and central Africa addressed this challenge by emphasizing collaboration and unity.

Another challenge is posed by deaf begging groups. When I ask deaf people whether they socialize with other deaf people or whether they have good friends, the response is mostly negative. Socializing with deaf people is associated with the destructive behavior of groups of deaf beggars in big cities. The beggars operate as part of a transnational (western and central African) deaf criminal group that takes advantage of the limited educational background and marginalized social position of Cameroonian deaf people. Promises of money attract naive, poor, and otherwise marginalized young deaf men and women, who are then exploited in a network of begging, stealing, slavery, and sexual violence and abuse (see also note 5).

EMANCIPATION PROCESSES IN THE CAMEROONIAN DEAF COMMUNITY

"Life is very hard here." "We suffer." The Cameroonian case study is "an anthropology of human suffering" (Farmer, 2010b, p. 137). The social position of deaf people in society is one of dehumanization, exploitation, and exclusion: "Hearing people think that we are animals." Deaf people emphasize that they are seen as people who are not able to "reason" and learn (see also the interview at the beginning of this chapter). Consequently, they are also not involved in decision making and in family meetings and have only limited access to African indigenous education.[8] Domestic labor is part of African indigenous education and usually evolves with the growth of the child, without being exploitative (Nsamenang, 1992). However, deaf adults report having had to work in the household or on the farm "as a slave." The semantic framework of causality that explains deafness and disability in cosmological or magical terms (e.g., as a manifestation of witchcraft) and often casts the entire family in a negative light (see also Mekang, 2007; Nsamenang, 1992; Shey, 2003) when a child is born deaf or becomes deaf is one of the reasons for the exclusion of deaf people. Nsamenang finds in poverty, hunger, ignorance, disease, and exploitation reasons why parents may not be able to meet the needs of their children.

I incorporated the question *How can Cameroon deaf people develop?* into my research because the theme of development is often discussed in deaf community gatherings. The variety of responses I received can be placed on a continuum of self-esteem and of hope. Some deaf adults have internalized negative perceptions of deaf people: "My mind is blank. I know nothing." "I only went to school for 3 years. I'm only a little bit smart." "Hearing people develop. Deaf people are low." "No, there are no successful deaf people in Cameroon." Other deaf people, especially those who are or were enrolled in secondary education, have more positive and hopeful perspectives: "Deaf people are smart. We can do many things." "It's a long way for development, but God is there." "I must show hearing people that I can be successful."

A process of emancipation has begun, particularly in young deaf people with the experience of secondary education. This is illustrated by the interview with the young man at the beginning of this chapter. He disagreed with his mother, who wanted him to stop going to school because of a lack of financial resources. Rancière (1999, 2009) uses the notions of subjectivation and disagreement to refer to this process of protesting against a given social position. This process can only start from the assumption of equality. The young man also noticed that European and American people seem to have money to fly around and have some knowledge about how to organize more educational opportunities for deaf people, but somehow seem to miss the money or the courage to support changes in Cameroon. The concept of critical consciousness articulated by Freire (2005) refers to the process of becoming aware of contrasts in social, political, and economic structures and standing up against oppression. Although there has been no collective action so far in Cameroon, deaf Cameroonians do not "sleep." They discuss and imagine approaching the government by marching or writing letters. The Internet is an inspiring course on developments in other countries; some deaf adults are also inspired by their past educational experiences in Nigeria.

The kind of self-advocacy expressed by the young man in the interview is not exceptional. Because the limited financial resources of households tend to go to hearing children first and deaf schools are private, attendance at a deaf school is often something that has to be fought for (and this is also done by deaf children). Forms of adult education such as literacy, vocational and entrepreneurial training, teacher training, and access to advanced education, are high among the needs of the deaf community. Many deaf adults experience their restricted access to information and opportunities for learning as frustrating and limiting. Although most deaf adults are not aware of it, Cameroon does have an enabling legal framework of antidiscrimination legislation, as well as legislation in alignment with the United Nations Convention on the Rights of Persons With Disabilities. However, these laws are not implemented (Mekang, 2007; Pouagam, 2000; Titjani, 2008; Yuh & Shey, 2008).

Cameroonian deaf people complain that corruption keeps the CANAD and the government asleep. Observation during the training associated with the Human Rights and Capacity Building Training Project in western and central Africa revealed a lack of knowledge on the part of CANAD board members of how to advocate for sign language recognition, interpreting, quality deaf education, teacher training, and other needs. The training emphasized practices of collaboration, information sharing, and transparency in working toward the common goal of development of all deaf Cameroonians. The training inspired the CANAD to take action—in forms that may have an impact in the near future. Another criticism of the CANAD in the deaf community was the lack of information sharing by the board with the larger deaf community.

Before the WFD training, there had been hardly any transnational knowledge transfer of deaf cultural rhetoric or of alternative life trajectories in Cameroon, but concepts of "deaf can" and human rights have started to be distributed. The WFD's training provided the first exposure for most participants and seems to have contributed to raising awareness. The WFD strongly encouraged the transfer of the contents of the training by CANAD board members to the broader Cameroonian deaf community. Because of limited financial resources, unfortunately, this objective cannot be realized within the project. It is the responsibility of the CANAD and the participants in the training, who seem to have taken initiatives in this direction. Sharing knowledge about advocacy and the workings of a deaf association, including how to bring about a new constitution and elections, may be key to the development of a participatory and democratic deaf community.

Although structural changes are needed, transfer of the contents of the WFD training and positive action by the CANAD would meet some of the needs and requests of the Cameroonian deaf community for more information and more advocacy. Deaf adults are eager to learn how to advocate for themselves, but how and where can they learn this? "If I go to America and study and learn how to be active, then I can do all things that hearing people can do. Then I can write more and meet the government." Hopefully, the WFD project can be continued in long-term projects and provide further support to this process.

"(BEING) SERIOUS": DEAF INDIGENOUS EDUCATION AS A SITE OF EMPOWERMENT

Despite little structural support and transnational exposure, indigenous "sites of empowerment" (Dei, 2010, p. 75) can be identified. Deaf leaders, both women and men, are actively employing the concept of *being serious* (expressed by the Cameroon sign SERIOUS; see Figure 3) to keep and bring deaf adults on the right track and to enhance their well-being. African indigenous education is oriented toward becoming a *good person* (Nsamenang, 1992; Reagan, 1996); this translates in practice in deaf indigenous education into an orientation toward being a *serious person*. This is particularly relevant in the light of deaf people's limited access to African indigenous knowledge that is traditionally transmitted in the family. The moral concept stands in opposition to the concept of *playing*, which refers to *bad* or *damaging* behavior, at both the individual and collective levels. For example, deaf adults are encouraged to *take care of the future*. This includes saving money in the bank or through indigenous savings and credit associations known as money-go-rounds (Rowlands, 2009) instead of *eating* or *drinking* money, which is what is done in begging groups (see Figure 4). The concept aims to create a moral network, and it is applied to diverse realms of life, such as employment, education, marriage, sex, family, and leadership.

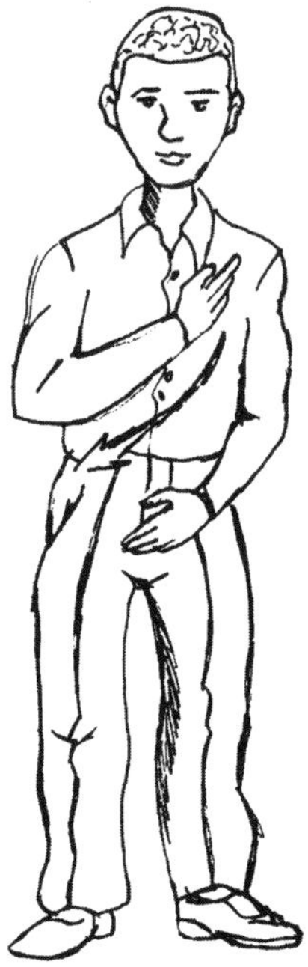

Figure 3. The Cameroon sign SERIOUS, as drawn by Eyonga Beltus.

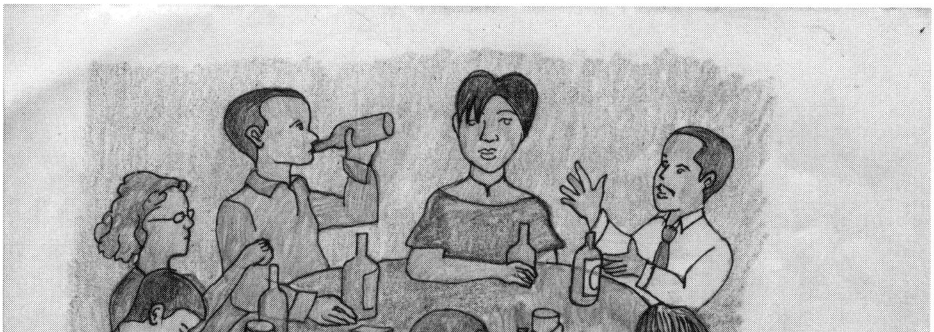

Figure 4. An example of behavior that is "not serious": "drinking" money, as drawn by Eyonga Beltus.

The directors of deaf schools are employing the concept in education to raise deaf children to be *good people*. They keep deaf adults away from their deaf schools so as to not to expose deaf children to bad behavior (i.e., the behavior of begging groups) before the children are mature enough to deal with this. A deaf leader explained how a deaf child can grow into a *serious* person (which illustrates the need of secondary education):

> There are many deaf who are wandering around. Some become beggars and thieves. They are without work; their families are poor and hearing people take advantage of them. What should they do? Because they don't have education, there is no one to follow up. . . . They are responsible for themselves.
>
> I want deaf children to develop first and to follow them until they are grown-ups and have become responsible people. . . . I want deaf to have something to learn when they finish school, so that they can set up a business themselves or join another work and get paid every month. That's better than always having their family help and feed them. Then they can also feed their family. If deaf can continue school until college, then we can follow up with them.

Being serious also means *not wandering around*. In a time of rampant HIV and AIDS,[9] moral crisis, and sexual violence, older deaf women are drawing upon their own life experiences and knowledge related to HIV and AIDS, relationships, marriage, and the unequal position of women in society to advise young deaf women on sexual behavior and morality. This is also related to the concept of what it means to be a *good woman* in Cameroon and to the moral crisis and lack of *serious* men in Cameroon (cf. Johnson-Hanks, 2007). Sexual abuse of young deaf girls is perceived as *damage*, and there is concern about increased teenage pregnancies. Advice from older deaf women sometimes leads to positive awareness and more responsible behavior of young women. Male leaders are also taking responsibility for advising young men—for instance, teaching them about pregnancy and how to use condoms, information that is often unavailable to young and "uneducated" deaf people.

Without explicitly introducing this concept as a deaf indigenous notion, the diverse meanings of the sign SERIOUS were food for a lively discussion during the presentation of the research findings in the deaf community meeting in Douala. The discussion concluded with a feeling of a sense of "ownership" when a leader recognized the concept as a "true" Cameroonian deaf concept, which has potential to inspire the Cameroonian deaf community to work toward the common goal of further development and action and to inspire individual members to take responsibility for their own lives. Whether the concept is actually Cameroonian and is not used by deaf communities in neighboring countries (there is transnational interaction) will need to be revealed by empirical research in the region.

This description of the practices and philosophy of life of the Cameroonian deaf community illustrates the relevance of a plural concept of deaf epistemologies in the light of a Western view of this concept. Miller (2003, cited in Miller, 2010) coined the concept of "culture of common experience" (p. 483) to describe commonalities in deaf people's individual epistemologies before coming into contact with other deaf people. Then they receive culturally situated group epistemologies. This culture "may be a major force in Deaf epistemology" (p. 483); the mixture of the experiences of deaf children growing up in deaf schools and mainstream environments and deaf children of deaf parents in Western societies "creates the continuing epistemology of social and linguistic culture creation, maintenance, and survival—a Deaf epistemology" (p. 484). The Cameroonian case study, which describes the development of a young deaf community, provides a different yet complementary view to this perspective. Apparently, there has not been any intergenerational transmission of sign language and deaf culture within deaf families so far. Deaf people share a sense of linguistic and social marginalization and exclusion— although in a different context of a widely distributed gestural communication and multilingualism and with some form of communicative and social inclusion in some rural areas. Also, the moral net that is being created through informal deaf education of the concept of being serious, which seems to be a vital force for the maintenance and survival of the Cameroonian deaf community, is illustrative of a deaf indigenous worldview.

VALUING DEAF INDIGENOUS KNOWLEDGE IN RESEARCH THROUGH PARTNERSHIP

Reflecting on my own position in my study, I realize that the concept of *researcher* is nonexistent in the semantic framework of the setting. I have been put in the roles of coach/counselor, deaf sister, and missionary: someone who is able to listen, guarantee privacy, not judge, and solve problems. Each person has his or her own question or concern: how to set up a business or build a bigger store, whether I can explain how one gets pregnant, if it is still possible to have children when one is HIV positive, and so on.

New research methods, such as community-based, participatory research that ties research to the knowledge and needs of communities (Dei, 2010; Higgs, 2008, 2010), seem fruitful for deaf communities as well. Cameroonian deaf people's interpretation of the research project in terms of "development" and the working of an NGO can be understood as "sidetracking." De Sardan (2008, p. 40) notes that sidetracking is common in development work, where different logics are in conflict and actors try to obtain their own goals: "Sidetracking is a sign that the actors involved have 'appropriated' the development project."

Discussions of the research findings with the Cameroonian deaf community started from ethical considerations and "principled engagement" (Janes & Corbett, 2009, p. 176), as opposed to "epistemological naiveté" (p. 178), and I encouraged participation, awareness, and local practices by Cameroonian deaf leaders and deaf community members.

Searching for answers to the question *How can deaf people in Cameroon develop?* also challenged me to reflect on my own research process and on deaf studies research in developing countries. Cameroonian deaf people are not asking for research. They are asking for service and solutions to problems (see also Farmer, 2010a, 2010d). This is in alignment with African universities' orientation toward teaching and community service, which is in contrast to the research emphasis common among Western universities

(Neubert, 2008) but consistent with African scholars' advocacy of solution-oriented and contextualized research (Dei, 2010; Higgs, 2008, 2010; Nsamenang, 1992).

Sidetracking in the direction of serious scholarship was a necessary condition for the CANAD and the community to support the study. Partnership with the Cameroonian deaf community, negotiations of the research process and research findings, and movement to "a third position" (beyond mutual bias) have provided some (temporarily valid) answers to this challenge. In this process, I have been guided by the naturalized epistemological stance discussed in the present chapter in areas of anthropology, deaf studies, sign linguistics, and critical pedagogy. For the approach of critical pedagogy, I have found inspiration in Paolo Freire's *Pedagogy of the Oppressed* (2005) and in the presupposition articulated by Rancière (2009) that "all intelligence is equal," not in the sense of IQ but in the sense that all people can make observations, analyze data, make conclusions, and communicate these conclusions to other people (Verstraete & Pinxten, 2009). This approach also aims to be helpful in encouraging leadership in the light of the (ideological) separation of "uneducated"/"illiterate" and "educated"/"literate" deaf people.

In the workshop I provided as part of the WFD training (De Clerck, 2011), I had the opportunity to illustrate how the research put a triangular and interactive model of partnership of NGOs, academics, and deaf community (De Clerck & Lutalo-Kiingi, 2011) into practice that is supportive of the development of the Cameroonian deaf community. In deaf studies and sign language research, there is increased attention to research ethics, the involvement of deaf people in the research process, and the benefits deaf communities gain from research. Among NGOs working with deaf communities, there is increased awareness of human rights and inclusion of deaf people in all stages of project planning and decision making. Deaf studies research benefits from collaboration with NGOs in the implementation of the research findings, and NGOs can integrate developments in research and teaching into their operations (De Clerck & Lutalo-Kiingi, 2011).

Discussing this model and the research process was part of a workshop that was oriented to "giving back" the research findings to the Cameroonian deaf community. Higgs (2010, p. 2420) writes that researchers should "expose indigenous communities to knowledge production and dissemination founded on indigenous cultural and social values." During presentation of the research process, I sometimes employed a dramatic style that is common in sub-Saharan Africa and is also used by the WFD trainers. Exaggerating unwanted behavior is an indirect and unthreatening way of confrontation that has a catalyzing and humorous effect and creates room for negotiation. (This approach is illustrated in the drawings that accompany the present chapter; see, for example, Figure 4, which depicts behavior that is "not serious.") Understanding experiences of exclusion, exploitation, and oppression and recognizing and acknowledging that these experiences may have motivated some of the initial resistance to the research process was crucial: "Oh, what do you think? I am white; maybe I will, like many other people before me, just take the information and leave. Shall I do that?" It was also important to take time for negotiation and discussion of the research process and to search for a basis of confidence and collaboration. I also aimed to work in a dialogical way (Freire, 2005), encouraging questions and interaction and fostering "epistemological curiosity" (Freire, 2005, p. 19). Deaf adults appreciated that the study was documenting and collecting information on Cameroonian deaf history, on the emergence and development of the Cameroonian deaf community and CSL. To promote their sense of ownership of the study, I emphasized that I was documenting and collecting their own knowledge, gathered through multiple sources of data, with the most important ones being private interviews and discussion groups. Deaf adults appreciated the exposure to this deaf indigenous knowledge and felt comfortable completing the information with further discussions of topics of the study. They also appreciated that the study would be published in a book and would be supportive of the advocacy efforts of CANAD. The collaboration with the WFD, the broader framework in which the study was situated, and the WFD's support of the research facilitated this process.

Cameroonian deaf people have explicitly asked for Western knowledge. The knowledge gained so far about sign languages, deaf communities, and deaf education, but also about deaf people's experiences of survival and advocacy, can be useful. There is a lot of confusion in the Cameroonian deaf community and in the Cameroonian government about which sign languages and sign language varieties are being used in Cameroon. There are also misconceptions about the status of sign language in academic circles: Is it an assistive tool, like a wheelchair, or a real language? In an effort to introduce some clarification, my workshop in the WFD training was complemented by a workshop provided by Sam Lutalo-Kiingi (2011), an Ugandan deaf linguist who is completing his PhD on Ugandan Sign Language (USL). The workshop, in combination with awareness of Uganda as a regional leader in regard to deaf interests in sub-Saharan Africa (with constitutional recognition of USL, publication of a USL dictionary, and the presence of deaf staff and a deaf studies diploma course at Kyambogo University in Kampala) seems to have had an impact on the Cameroonian deaf community. CANAD has expressed a strong need for research on CSL (in its regional variations and with involvement of the Cameroonian deaf community) and a strong wish for a CSL dictionary. The University of Buea is taking the initiative to start CSL research.

The recognition of Cameroonian deaf people's multilingual background (most deaf Cameroonians have some knowledge of one or more tribal languages, gestural communication, and sign languages, as well as French or English) has validated the feelings of alienation deaf adults experienced in their childhood when they entered the deaf school. Feelings were quite strong when people reflected on this tabula rasa experience, in which the learning process neither acknowledged nor connected with the local knowledge and communication skills they had acquired before entering the deaf school. This devalued background included indigenous skills and experiences such as working on the farm, cooking, and participating in traditional forms of dance. (These skills are currently included in educational programs of some deaf schools led by deaf directors.) These concerns should be placed in the broader context of the failure of formal deaf education and standardized tests in Cameroon, which has its origins in colonial history and the exclusion of indigenous languages and knowledge (Ngwabine, 2010). Another factor that stimulated discussion was the presence of a deaf leader from the Extreme North region in Cameroon (see note 5). He provided alternative views of deaf indigenous knowledge, transmission of sign language, social inclusion of deaf people, and the existence of strong networks of informal education in both the deaf and mainstream hearing communities. Conditions in the Extreme North region had equipped this man with adequate knowledge to deal with different aspects of life. He did not experience his limited literacy skills as a barrier to being an equal participant in society. His dignity and alternative perspective challenged common ideological notions of the superiority of educated deaf people and sometimes painfully illustrated the inadequacy of formal education.

For deaf educational programs to be successful, there is a need to reflect on an integrative epistemological framework (Dei, 2010; Higgs, 2008, 2010) and on how African (deaf) indigenous knowledge, local languages, and local cultural patterns (Lutalo-Kiingi, 2010) can be incorporated into the teaching of deaf children and deaf adults. Changing societal views of deaf people will be a challenge and a condition for educational success, and this is experienced as such by young deaf people in Cameroon.

Reflecting upon the Cameroonian and African contexts, Nsamenang (1992) argues that new conceptions of family and community are needed, as well as agency-based forms of social service. Nsamenang also emphasizes that development cannot succeed unless basic human rights are ensured (see also Farmer, 2010c, 2010d, 2010e). Clean water, shelter, food for children, access to health care (including treatment of tuberculosis, malaria, and HIV and AIDS): These are all basic needs that must be addressed if deaf people in Cameroon are to flourish.

The capability approach, a theoretical framework developed by Nobel Prize–winner Amartya Sen and by Martha Nussbaum, focuses on the evaluation of quality of life in the effort to achieve social justice (Nussbaum, 2006). Distinguishing between *functioning* (what people actually are and do) and *capabilities* (the range of options and choices that people have and can make), the capability approach makes room for self-determination and the opportunities that people have to live the life they wish to live. Although the Cameroonian case study has been only partially discussed, it illustrates that increased agency of deaf people is a necessary condition for their flourishing.

CONCLUSION

> Throughout the history of social science the debate about what is science and what is scientific knowledge rages. "It is a question as much for North America or Western Europe as for Africa" (Wallerstein, 1988, pp. 332–333). . . . Science is one way of viewing and exploring phenomena, a critical, systematic way of thinking in the fact-finding process.
>
> —Nsamenang, 1992, p. 218

Working toward "epistemological equity" (Dei, 2010, p. 98) implies granting an equal status to deaf (indigenous) knowledge in science. This is a methodological challenge. Discussion of an ethnographic case study on emancipation processes in the Cameroonian deaf community illuminates the development of research methods during fieldwork and through negotiation and involvement of the research participants (Fabian, 1990; Pinxten, 1997).

Valuing the collective organization of the Cameroonian deaf community, taking into account the epistemic authority of deaf leaders, and being sensitive to input from the broader community led to a community-based and participatory approach (Higgs, 2008). Cameroonian deaf people challenged me to develop serious scholarship—that is, scholarship that can support the development of the Cameroonian deaf community.

Meeting this challenge and developing contextualized, and temporarily valid, answers to the question *How can deaf people in Cameroon develop?* requires a "synthesis of multiple knowledge systems" (Dei, 2010, p.104; see also Nsamenang, 1992). This synthesis includes the wisdom developed by deaf communities around the world and the scientific knowledge that has been developed in my field of study; it also takes into account African indigenous knowledge and African deaf knowledge.

A stance of "humility of knowing" and "uncertainty of knowledge" (Dei, 2010, p. 105) with openness for multiple perspectives is called for. Scientific knowledge is partial, situated, and fallible. Scientific knowledge is preferred wherever it is possible and whenever it is relevant (Verstraete & Pinxten, 2009). However, scientific knowledge cannot replace daily knowledge of taking care of a baby, growing cassava, or visual and gestural ways of communication to sell vegetables or shoes on the market. Cameroonian deaf knowledge, philosophy of life, and practice, such as agency through the concept of *being serious,* can be strengthened by scientific research.

Complementing fundamental research with a solution-oriented approach and a practice of partnership of scholars, NGO, and deaf communities (De Clerck & Lutalo-Kiingi, 2011) has been crucial in meeting some of the needs of deaf community development. Several questions merit further attention in scholarship and praxis:

- How can opportunities be fostered for all deaf people to live up to their potential and flourish?
- How can indigenous knowledge, indigenous deaf knowledge, and indigenous languages and sign languages be included in formal education?
- How can local initiatives by deaf leaders be supported? How can local systems of social security be supported?

Describing deaf indigenous practices in a bottom-up research method contributes to a cross-cultural perspective in deaf studies and deaf education. The case study of the Cameroonian deaf community documents the development of a young deaf community and a young sign language: Deaf gatherings, the extended family metaphor, and the notion of being serious are tools that enable deaf Cameroonians both to manage life and to imagine future life. These conceptual tools provide an alternative and complementary view of the notions of deaf community, deaf epistemology, and the global claim in concepts such as "a global deaf renaissance."

NOTES

1. Portions of the case study described in the present chapter were presented at the Deaf Community Leadership Conference at the University of Central Lancashire, United Kingdom, on June 27, 2010; at the Citizenship Platform at Ghent University, Belgium, on October 15, 2010; and in a workshop during the WFD Deaf Human Rights and Capacity Building Training Project in Western and Central Africa, in Yaoundé, on February 26, 2011.

2. Cameroonians currently face considerable obstacles to getting married because of the economical and moral crisis; they nonetheless regard taking a spouse as a key moment in life (Fleisher, 2007) and a prerequisite to full personhood (Nsamenang, 1992). This is also the case for deaf Cameroonians, who experience even more obstacles.
3. A bottom-up approach has been found fruitful in enhancing democratic participation (Pinxten, 2011) and in development contexts (Dei, 2010).
4. Within the limits and time frame of the study, I have not been able to do interviews yet in the western regions of Cameroon, although I have interviewed some deaf people from this region.
5. Interviews (lasting a total of about 10 hours) with a key informant from the Extreme North region in Cameroon revealed different dynamics of deaf community and sign language in the area and throw light on the marginalization of deaf people in the central regions. The interviews indicate the existence of an indigenous sign language, a strong collective sense of deaf community, a transmission of deaf history by deaf elders, and inclusion of deaf people in all aspects of society (see also note 8). This has deaf awareness that has enabled the local deaf community to resist pressures from globalization, dominant sign languages, and normalizing ideologies. A strong tradition of informal learning both among deaf peers and in the broader community has created room for deaf adults to acquire knowledge of the world and take up equal positions in society. I am currently exploring opportunities to include this area in the study.

   A deaf informant from Chad who has been living in Cameroon for a couple of years has provided another comparative view: Social marginalization and the phenomenon of begging are nonexistent in Chad. Reasons are found in the strong collective sense and the social and moral network—both in the broader community and the deaf community. Inclusion of deaf people in the community, apprenticeship, formal and informal education, and the epistemic authority and care of deaf elders and deaf leaders are other factors that come to the fore.
6. A deaf woman told me that her mother and grandmother were both deaf. However, they did not sign, and the concept of "a deaf family" does not exist or have cultural meaning for her. I also know of the existence of deaf siblings, which also does not have the cultural meaning it has in Europe and America, where deaf families tend to have leadership roles in deaf communities.
7. Further research is needed to better understand gestures and sign language in Africa generally.
8. Many deaf adults in my study did not know their ethnic group or only had limited education on the history and culture of their tribe (see also Lutalo-Kiingi, 2010, on the same problem in Uganda). Farm work and domestic work are acquired through visual learning (see also Nsamenang, 1992, on indigenous education in Cameroon).
9. UNAIDS (2008) reports a 5.1% rate of HIV infection among the Cameroonian adult population (i.e., people 15–49 years old), and 60% of the infected individuals are women. In my research study, which is not representative, infection rates seemed to be greater and are particularly high in some regions and among some groups of deaf people. This should be examined further. Research in Kenya found a comparable infection rate (about 7%) among deaf and hearing clients of a HIV test and counseling program (Taegtmeyer et al., 2009). The risk factors for HIV and AIDS among people with disabilities identified by Groce (2004) also apply to the Cameroonian deaf community: poverty, limited access to education, illiteracy, inaccessibility of information and health care, the orphaning of deaf children of people with AIDS, greater risks for sexual violence in combination with limited legal protection and access, and the misuse of alcohol and drugs. Representative research on HIV and AIDS among the Cameroonian deaf population is needed. Some initiatives have been taken by NGOs, and some deaf adults have received training. However, nationwide community-based prevention and counseling programs in CSL, access to health services, and in-depth training of deaf HIV educators and counselors are needed (see Groce, 2004; Taegtmeyer et al., 2009).

REFERENCES

Ceuppens, B., & Geschiere, P. (2005). Autochthony: Local or global? New modes in the struggle over citizenship in Africa and Europe. *Annual Review of Anthropology, 34*, 385–407.

Dalle-Nazébi, S. (2009). Les sourds au Congo-Brazzaville, entre sorcellerie locale et pratiques occidentals. In Gardou (Ed.), *Le handicap au risqué des cultures: Variations anthropologiques [Disability at the risk of cultures: Anthropological variations]*. Paris, France: Erès.

De Clerck, G. (2011, March). *The deaf community in Cameroon: Emancipation processes.* Workshop presented at the WFD Deaf Human Rights and Capacity Building Training Project in Western and Central Africa, Yaoundé, Cameroon.

De Clerck, G., & Lutalo-Kiingi, S. (2011, February). *Partnership of academia, deaf communities, and NGOs in deaf empowerment and development.* Workshop presented at the Supporting Deaf People Conference, online conference, United Kingdom.

De Clerck, G., & Pinxten, R. (2011). Dealing with intrinsic diversity: Deaf culture as "a concept from the wild." Manuscript in preparation.

De Sardan, J. P. O. (2008). Excerpts from anthropology and development. In P. Geschiere, B. Meyer, & P. Pels (Eds.), *Readings in modernity in Africa* (pp. 34–41). Oxford, UK: International African Institute and James Currey.

Dei, G. (2010). *Teaching Africa: Toward a transgressive pedagogy.* New York, NY: Springer.

Fabian, J. (1990). *Power and performance: Ethnographic explorations through proverbial wisdom and theater in Shaba, Zaire.* Madison, WI: University of Wisconsin Press.

Farmer, P. (2010a). An anthropology of structural violence. In H. Saussy (Ed.), *Partner to the poor: A Paul Farmer reader* (pp. 350–375). Berkeley, CA: University of California Press.

Farmer, P. (2010b). From Haiti to Rwanda: AIDS and Accusations. In H. Saussy (Ed.), *Partner to the poor: A Paul Farmer reader* (pp. 136–154). Berkeley, CA: University of California Press.

Farmer, P. (2010c). Making human rights substantial. In H. Saussy (Ed.), *Partner to the poor: A Paul Farmer reader* (pp. 545–559). Berkeley, CA: University of California Press.

Farmer, P. (2010d). Never again? Reflections on human values and human rights. In H. Saussy (Ed.), *Partner to the poor: A Paul Farmer reader* (pp. 487–527). Berkeley, CA: University of California Press.

Farmer, P. (2010e). On suffering and structural violence: Social and economic rights in the global era. In H. Saussy (Ed.), *Partner to the poor: A Paul Farmer reader* (pp. 228–249). Berkeley, CA: University of California Press.

Fisiy, C. (1998). Containing occult practices: Witchcraft trials in Cameroon. *African Studies Review, 41*(3), 143–163.

Fleischer, A. (2007). Family, obligations, and migration: The role of kinship in Cameroon. *Demographic Research, 16*(13), 413–437.

Freire, P. (2005). *Pedagogy of the oppressed.* New York, NY: Continuum.

Geschiere, P., Pels, P., & Meyer, B. (Eds.). (2008). *Readings in modernity in Africa.* Oxford, UK: International African Institute and James Currey.

Groce, N. E. (2004). *HIV/AIDS and Disability—Capturing hidden voices: Global survey on HIV/AIDS and disability.* Retrieved from Yale University/World Bank website on January, 5, 2010: http://globalsurvey.med.yale.edu/capturing_hidden_voices_english.pdf

Higgs, P. (2008). Towards an indigenous African educational discourse: A philosophical reflection. *International Review of Education, 54*, 445–458.

Higgs, P. (2010). Towards an indigenous African epistemology of community in education research. *Procedia: Social and Behavioral Sciences, 2*, 2414–2421.

Human Development Reports. (2010). *Country profile of human development indicators—Cameroon, 2010.* Retrieved April 8, 2011, from http://hdrstats.undp.org/en/countries/profiles/CMR.html

Janes, C. R., & Corbett, K. K. (2009). Anthropology and global health. *Annual Review of Anthropology, 38*, 167–183.

Johnson-Hanks, J. (2007). Women on the market: Marriage, consumption, and the internet in urban Cameroon. *American Ethnologist, 34*(4), 642–658.

Kamei, N. (2006, November). *The birth of Langue des Signes Franco-Africaine: Creole ASL in west and central French-speaking Africa.* Paper presented online at the Languages and Education in Africa Conference (LEA2006), University of Oslo, Oslo, Norway.

Kaphagawani, N. D. N., & Malherbe, J. (1998). African epistemology. In P. H. Coetze & A. J. Roux (Eds.), *Philosophy from Africa* (pp. 210–222). South Africa: Thomson International.

Ladd, P. (2003). *Understanding Deaf culture: In search of Deafhood.* Clevedon, UK: Multilingual Matters.

Lutalo-Kiingi, S. (2010, September). *Bilingual education and deaf studies in East Africa.* Paper presented at the Sign Language in Deaf Education Conference, Kyambogo University, Kampala, Uganda.

Lutalo-Kiingi, S. (2011, March). *Language(s).* Workshop presented at the WFD Deaf Human Rights and Capacity Building Training Project in Western and Central Africa, Yaoundé, Cameroon.

Mekang, N. D. (2007). *Challenges encountered by specialized institutions educating the blind in the North-West and South-West provinces in Cameroon* (Unpublished master's thesis). University of Buea, Cameroon.

Miles, M. (2004). Locating deaf people, gesture, and sign in African histories, 1450s–1950s. *Disability and Society, 19*(5), 531–545.

Miller, M. (2010). Epistemology and people who are deaf: Deaf worldviews, views of the deaf world, or my parents are hearing. *American Annals of the Deaf, 154*(5), 479–485.

Mindess, A. (1999). *Reading between the signs: Intercultural communication for sign language interpreters.* Yarmouth, MA: Intercultural Press.

Moores, D., & Paul, P. (2010). Perspectives on deaf epistemologies. *American Annals of the Deaf, 154*(5), 493–500.

Morgan, R. (Ed). (2008). *DEAF ME NORMAL: Deaf South Africans tell their life stories.* Pretoria, South Africa: Unisa Press.

Neubert, N. (2008). University cooperation between Germany and Africa: Challenges and some lessons learnt. In E. W. Schamp & S. Schmid (Eds.), *Lessons for partnership in higher education* (pp. 93–110). Berlin, Germany: Lit Verlag.

Ngwabine, S. F. (2010). *The impact of standardized tests on diverse cultures in Cameroon* (Unpublished doctoral dissertation). University of Buea, Cameroon.

Nsamenang, B. (1992). *Human development in cultural context: A Third World perspective.* London, UK: Sage.

Nussbaum, M. (2006). *Frontiers of justice: Disability, nationality, species membership.* Cambridge, MA: Harvard University Press.

Padden, C., & Humphries, T. (1988). *Deaf in America: Voices from a culture.* Cambridge, MA: Harvard University Press.

Pinxten, R. (1997). *When the day breaks: Essays in anthropology and philosophy.* New York, NY: Peter Lang.

Pinxten, R. (2006, September). *The relevance of a noncolonial view on science and knowledge for an open perspective on the world.* Paper presented at the biennial conference of the European Association of Social Anthropologists, Bristol, England.

Pinxten, R. (2011). *The plezier van het zoeken. Filosofie tegen de angst* [The pleasure of searching: Philosophy against fear]. Antwerp, Belgium: Houtekiet.

Pouagam, J. (2000). *Disabled: Do you know your rights?* Yaoundé, Cameroon: Établissement La Foire des Foirés.

Rancière, J. (1999). *Disagreement: Politics and philosophy.* Minneapolis, MN: University of Minnesota Press.

Rancière, J. (2009). *The ignorant schoolmaster: Five lessons in intellectual emancipation.* Stanford, CA: Stanford University Press.

Reagan, T. (1996). *Nonwestern educational traditions: Alternative approaches to educational thought and practice.* Mahwah, NJ: Erlbaum.

Rowlands, M (2009). Looking at financial landscapes: A contextual analysis of ROSCAs in Cameroon. In S. Ardener & S. Burman (Eds.), *Money-go-rounds: The importance of rotating savings and credit associations for women* (pp. 111–124). Oxford, UK: Berg.

Schmaling, C. (2003). A for apple: The impact of Western education and ASL on the Deaf community in Kano State, northern Nigeria. In L. Monaghan, C. Schmaling, K. Nakamura, & G. Turner (Eds.), *Many ways to be deaf: International variation in Deaf communities* (pp. 302–310). Washington, DC: Gallaudet University Press.

Sen, A. (2008). *Identity and violence: The illusion of destiny.* New York, NY: Norton.

Shey, P. (2003). *Parents' perspectives on the education of children with disabilities in regular schools in Cameroon* (Unpublished master's thesis). University of Oslo, Norway.

Silas, N. O. (n.d.). *Sign language lessons for the deaf: Handbook for teachers of the deaf.*

Sorin-Barreteau, L. (1996). *La langue gestuelle des Mofu-Gudur au Cameroun* [The gestural language of the Mofu-Gudur of Cameroon] (Unpublished doctoral dissertation). University of Paris V—René Descartes, Paris.

Spradley, J. P. *The ethnographic interview.* New York, NY: Wadsworth, 1997.

Stebbins, R. (2001). *Exploratory research in the social sciences.* Thousand Oaks, CA: Sage.

Taegtmeyer, M., Hightower, A., Opiyo, W., Mwachiro, L., Henderson, K., Angala, P., Ngare, C., & Marum, E. (2009). A peer-led HIV counselling and testing programme for the deaf in Kenya. *Disability and Rehabilitation, 31*(6), 508–514.

Tamomo, S. (1994). *Le Langage des Signes du Sourds Africain Francophone.* Cotonou, Bénin: PEFISS.

Thorvalsdottir, T. (2007). *"Equal opportunities for all": Intersectionality as a theoretical tool to move equality policies forward.* Retrieved on April 8, 2011, from http://www.issa.nl/members/member_docs/ESJ_files/at_docs/add_pdfs/Intersectionality.pdf

UNICEF. (2009). *Cameroon—Statistics.* Retrieved on April 8, 2011, from http://www.unicef.org/infobycountry/cameroon_statistics.html

Titjani, P. (2008). Education for all in Cameroon: What principals need to know and do. *African Journal of Special Education, 1*(1), 105–115.

Verstraete, G., & Pinxten, R. (2009). Een pleidooi om ons denken en handelen te oriënteren [A plea to orient our thinking and acting]. In G. Verstraete & R. Pinxten (Eds.), *Doe het zelf democratie* [Do-it-yourself democracy] (pp. 233–252). Berchem, Belgium: EPO.

World Bank. (2010). *Cameroon: Country brief* Retrieved from http://web.worldbank.org/WBSITE/EXTERNAL/COUNTRIES/AFRICAEXT/CAMEROONEXTN/0,,menuPK:343823~pagePK:141132~piPK:141107~theSitePK:343813,00.html

Yin, R. K. (1994). *Case study research: Design and methods.* Thousand Oaks, CA: Sage.

Yuh, E., & Shey, P. (2008). The education of persons with special needs in Cameroon: A historical perspective. *African Journal of Special Education, 1*(1), 27–31.

SUGGESTIONS FOR FURTHER READING

Nsamenang, B. (1992). *Human development in cultural context: A Third World perspective.* London, UK: Sage.

Pinxten, R. (1997). *When the day breaks: Essays in anthropology and philosophy.* Frankfurt, Germany: Peter Lang.

Polish, L. (2005). *The emergence of the deaf community in Nicaragua: "With sign language you can learn so much."* Washington, DC: Gallaudet University Press.

Reagan, T. (1996). *Non-Western educational traditions: Alternative approaches to educational thought and practice.* Mahwah, NJ: Lawrence Erlbaum.

Reilly, C., & Reilly, N. (2005). *The rising of lotus flowers: The self-education of deaf children in Thai boarding schools.* Washington, DC: Gallaudet University Press.

PART III

HISTORICAL/PSYCHOLOGICAL AND LITERARY PERSPECTIVES

6

Dueling Epistemologies: Between Scylla and Charybdis in the Education of Deaf Learners

Donald F. Moores

In Greek mythology, Scylla and Charybdis were hideous sea monsters occupying two sides of a narrow strait. If a ship sailed too close to Scylla, it might hit the rocks and Scylla would devour the sailors. If the ship sailed too close to Charybdis, it might be sucked into a whirlpool and all would perish. Occasionally, an intrepid leader would navigate the treacherous waters. According to legend, Jason successfully accomplished this with the *Argo*. Odysseus was partially successful; he steered too close to Scylla, who consumed six sailors, but Odysseus and the rest of the crew survived.

Being between Scylla and Charybdis means that one is between two dangers and that moving away from one involves increasing proximity to, and danger from, the other. For me, as an educator of d/Deaf students, Scylla represents the prevailing reality when I first entered the field. (In this chapter, *deaf* refers to individuals with an audiometric hearing loss, and *Deaf* refers to those individuals who have a cultural attachment to a Deaf community or who possess a Deaf identity or Deafhood.) Although there was a vibrant Deaf community, education of d/Deaf students was parochial and repressive. Deaf epistemologies existed, but they were not considered by the decision makers (see Holcomb, this volume). There were no d/Deaf school superintendents and very few administrators at any level. Signing was forbidden, even punished, at least until students were 12 years of age. With few exceptions, the curriculum was weak; little attention was devoted to content areas such as science, social studies, and mathematics. Postsecondary opportunities were essentially constrained to Gallaudet College (now University), and even there d/Deaf students were not allowed into the graduate school.

From my perspective, Charybdis represents the danger of complete assimilation, of going so far as to obviate the actual characteristics of d/Deaf individuals and their unique needs and learning styles. Less than one child in a thousand, d/Deaf children can be swallowed up in the mainstream whirlpool and forced to sink or swim in a curriculum designed for students who learn both auditorially and visually. The responsibility is to educate d/Deaf children to the highest academic levels possible; the goals are similar to those for hearing children but the procedures may vary. I believe this can be accomplished through a judicious mix of standard and special epistemologies. However, I remain aware of the truism that individuals or groups with less power live in environments constrained by those with more power to influence and even dominate their lives.

In considering epistemologies, it is tempting but intellectually misleading to think in dichotomous terms. In the introductory chapter of this text, Peter V. Paul and I present some characteristics of deaf epistemologies and contrast them with the standard epistemology, which may not in actuality have a standard version anymore. Deaf epistemologies, as they relate to education and instruction, typically contain certain beliefs including but not limited to the idea that deaf education has been controlled by hearing educators who harbor a deficit or deficiency model of deafness and who are insensitive to the needs and learning styles of d/Deaf learners. In essence, the argument goes that general theories of instruction and research do not apply to the education of d/Deaf students.

In addition, deaf epistemologies posit that there is no specific psychology of deafness, but there are differences in the ways that d/Deaf and hearing individuals learn; d/Deaf learners are visual learners, and consequently the d/Deaf brain may be organized differently from the hearing brain. Another consistent theme is that a sign language should be the natural language of a d/Deaf child from birth.

A standard epistemology has a more general or universal perspective. It operates under the assumption that there are external knowable realities that can be discovered or developed through the scientific method. Theories can be tested, with the result being closer approximations of truth (Lehrer, 2000).

An epistemology, stripped to its barest essence, is a way of knowing, understanding, structuring, and interacting with the world. It focuses on the nature, uses, and limitations of knowing. Among those who think about such matters, the consensus is that the standard epistemology represents a white male weltanschauung, or view of the world. Its literary canon consists of white males (Shakespeare, Dante, Cervantes, Dostoevsky, Twain, etc.), with analogous representation in art (Da Vinci, Raphael, Rembrandt, Dali, Picasso, Michelangelo), philosophy (Socrates, Plato, Aristotle, Kant, Kierkegaard), music (Bach, Beethoven, Verdi, Rimski-Korsakov), and numerous other fields of endeavor. Such a worldview excludes most of the human race. In the United States, this exclusion applies to women, racial and ethnic minorities, and d/Deaf people, among others who have been marginalized.

If one believes that the standard epistemology is inadequate and misleading, that there is no external, knowable reality, and that knowledge and truth are relative and situational constructs, how do the constructs of gender, race, and deafness situate knowledge and how does the production of knowledge affect women, racial minorities, and d/Deaf individuals? To a large extent, racial minorities, women, and d/Deaf individuals have been excluded from inquiry, portrayed as inferior, and denied access to power; thus, the production of knowledge has not been beneficial to them.

It was inevitable that domination by a minority of the population would be challenged and fundamental changes would be instituted. Significant change has occurred, although more needs to be done. Change can be effected in different ways. One approach is to be integrated into and be accepted by an existing system. This was an effective strategy for d/Deaf leaders in the 1970s and to a lesser extent remains so today. Access to power and decision making by individuals with diverse perspectives can be quite beneficial. Another approach is to declare the system itself repressive and oppressive in a sexist, racist, or audist way and strive to change it in a revolutionary manner or to withdraw from it. An example of this is provided by Paulo Freire's *Pedagogy of the Oppressed* (1970), in which he argued that the purpose of education for poor people was to change education to help them understand the nature of their oppression so that they could then change the system.

The situation for women, racial and ethnic minorities, individuals with disabilities, and gay/lesbian/bisexual/transsexual individuals in the United States has improved over the past 50 years, and the rate of improvement seems to have accelerated. However, there are two caveats: Conditions changed only because of the leadership of people from marginalized groups, and the situation is better but not good. Much more needs to be accomplished.

STANDARD EPISTEMOLOGY, THE SCIENTIFIC METHOD, AND RESEARCH ON EDUCATION OF THE DEAF

As discussed by Paul and Moores in the first chapter of this text, the standard epistemology is based on the assumption that there is an external, knowable reality that is universal—and not situated—and that this external knowable reality can be attained through the scientific method. There are several definitions of the scientific method, but in essence it must consist of theory building and involve observation, experimentation, and hypothesis testing, leading to refinement of theories and hypotheses and ultimately to knowledge. Any legitimate theory must be falsifiable; if it is not true, it must be stated and tested in such a way that application of the scientific method can demonstrate it to be wrong or false. It has been argued (Popper, 1977) that no theory can be completely verified; it can be only disproven or shown to be false.

It is instructive to investigate the effect the scientific method has had on education of d/Deaf children and adolescents. Although there was substantial research on genealogy and vocational status of the d/Deaf in the 19th century and research on cognition and academic achievement in the first part of the 20th century, the studies did not match the criteria for scientific inquiry. The establishment of the Institute for Research on Exceptional Children (IREC) at the University of Illinois in 1953, under the direction of Samuel Kirk, was the first university-based multidisciplinary research center in education of exceptional children (Kirk, 1983) and served as a research model for all aspects of special education, including deafness. Although not explicitly stated, it emphasized adherence to the scientific method—statement of a problem, observation, literature review, hypothesis development, experimentation, analysis and interpretation of data, drawing conclusions, publication, and repeating the process. It should be noted that both editors of this text received their PhD training at the University of Illinois, and I was a member of the IREC; we both still function under the influence of the Illinois research zeitgeist of that time.

The establishment of the Bureau of Education for the Handicapped (BEH) in 1967, the forerunner of the U.S. Office of Special Education Programs (OSEP) in 1974, was a major impetus for the growth of research in special education as a whole and education of d/Deaf children and adolescents in particular. Research funding was provided through the BEH Division of Research, and graduate training was supported through a division of training. However, as difficult as conducting research itself is, conducting practical research leading to change in educational practice is much more complex. James Gallagher (1968), the first director of BEH and a charter member of IREC, postulated five phases of translation of knowledge from research to adoption into educational practice:

1. Research: The discovery or development of new knowledge.
2. Development: Packaging of knowledge into appropriate curricula.
3. Demonstration: Effectiveness must be demonstrated in a school or school-like setting.
4. Implementation: Local school systems test the procedures.
5. Adoption: Acceptance of the new program at the policy level.

Unfortunately, this ideal process for research to application was never fully realized. There are many possible explanations for this. For one, there is often a disconnect between the university researcher and the classroom teacher, whereas successful implementation of the model requires cooperation in every phase. Second, federal support for special education research is focused on the short term, with projects supported at most for three or four years. It is difficult, if not impossible, to establish continuity or move from one phase to another in such a short time. Third, educational and special educational research increasingly has to follow a federal agenda. Much funding now is allocated under requests for proposals (RFPs) or requests for applications (RFAs), in which the federal agency delineates the type of research that will be funded. There is less support for field-initiated studies, in which the researcher has the flexibility to propose a creative line of research.

Finally, current research in education, special education, or education of the d/Deaf has little impact on educational practice. The research-to-adoption paradigm promulgated by Gallagher does not apply in the present reality of American education. Much of the explanation for this may be attributed to the Individuals With Disability Education Improvement Act of 2004 (IDEIA) and the No Child Left Behind (NCLB) Act of 2002. For purposes of clarity, IDEIA has replaced previous legislation entitled Individuals With Disabilities Education Act (IDEA), and the abbreviation *IDEA* commonly is used for the current legislation. I follow the practice and refer to it as IDEA.

For now, the reader should keep in mind that IDEA identified d/Deaf and hard of hearing children as one of the 13 disability categories. Over the years approximately,

12%, or one school-aged child out of eight, has been classified as having a disability under federal regulations. Approximately one child in a thousand of the school-aged population, or 1% of the disabled population, has been diagnosed as deaf or hard of hearing, a small minority of a minority. However, all mandates of IDEA apply to d/Deaf children, regardless of whether they are appropriate. The most obvious is the Least Restrictive Environment (LRE) regulation, which has never been defined in a satisfactory manner. The primary issue is not whether educational placement of d/Deaf children with hearing peers, or any other federal mandate, is advantageous—there are many factors to consider—but that federal regulations with little or no research support stifle flexibility and creativity.

As limiting as IDEA is, it pales in comparison with NCLB, which has a number of laudable goals but also significant weaknesses, which may or may not be rectified in subsequent reauthorizations. NCLB contains 10 goals, including improved academic achievement of disadvantaged youth, preparation of qualified teachers, language instruction for limited-English-speaking students, increased parental choice, education for Native American children, and so forth. Children classified as having a disability, one-eighth of the American school-aged population are not included as a major category (Moores, 2011), an inexcusable omission. Regardless of this error of omission, NCLB regulations apply to all children, including those who are d/Deaf. With very few exceptions, they must be taught through a general education curriculum based on standards of learning developed by individual states and approved by the federal government. They must be tested by state-developed tests with allowance for few accommodations and even fewer modifications. The system is stultifying, and opportunities for applied research are restricted to very constricted areas. The promise of an individualized educational plan, or perhaps multiple epistemologies, under IDEA is overridden by the one-size-fits-all rigidity of NCLB. Practice does not follow research; unfortunately, research must follow established practice. NCLB represents the domination of a standard epistemology, albeit one that is weakly buttressed by research involving the scientific method.

DEAF EPISTEMOLOGIES

Deaf epistemologies present a complex picture, in part because there are relatively few Deaf studies departments, where much of the research and logical debate would take place, and because such departments have been established in academia more recently than the comparable women's studies or African American studies departments. The first Deaf studies department was established at Boston University in 1981 (R. Hoffmeister, personal communication, February 2009), so the field has had a relatively short time span in which to develop a comprehensive body of work. Additionally, hearing educators controlled higher education for d/Deaf students, at least until the Deaf President Now protest at Gallaudet University in 1988 (Gannon, 1989). Therefore, with some notable exceptions, currently there is not a history of inquiry or body of knowledge reflecting Deaf perspectives or epistemologies.

Adherence to any epistemology is not necessarily contingent upon any condition per se, such as hearing status in the present case. A d/Deaf person may or may not agree with any or all of the characteristics of deaf epistemologies, as presented here, and a hearing person might be a strong supporter of deaf epistemologies. Further, everyone has multiple references and points of self-identification. In 1983, Hairston and Smith published a book with a provocative title, *Black and Deaf in America: Are We That Different?* More recently, Kelly (2008) raised the question "Where is Deaf herstory?" in her eponymously titled chapter. If there is a deaf epistemology (or epistemologies), or an American deaf epistemology, that is different from the standard epistemology, is it essentially a white d/Deaf male epistemology and thus an extension to some degree of the standard epistemology? How does this affect d/Deaf women, African Americans, Hispanic Americans, Native Americans, Asian Pacific Americans, gay and lesbian Americans? Among national organizations, there are the National Black Deaf Advocates, National Council of Hispano Deaf and Hard of Hearing, Intertribal Deaf Council, National Asian Deaf Conference, and the Rainbow Coalition. Each organization serves as an advocate for an identified subgroup of d/Deaf Americans.

The danger is that people can identify themselves by increasingly narrow characteristics, beginning with categories such as hearing status, gender, race, ethnicity, religious affiliation (if any), social class, or geography. Because each human being is unique, reductio ad absurdum, there could be seven billion categories. The issue is too complex to address in the allocated space and is better resolved with attention to more detail elsewhere, but the reader should remain cognizant of the complexity of multiple identities.

Most readers of the present chapter probably agree that a Deaf community and a Deaf culture exist, although there may be some varying definitions of these terms. Readers not familiar with these terms and with the concept of Deafhood should refer to the work of Ladd (2003, 2008) and other sources.

To provide a perspective for the present, it is important to consider the status of d/Deaf people from the beginnings of the education of deaf children and adolescents in the United States. Throughout history, d/Deaf leaders have played significant, although frequently unacknowledged, roles and have influenced the development of d/Deaf children even when pure oralism was dominant.

AMERICAN EDUCATION: SALIENT CHARACTERISTICS

As stated earlier, the goal of the present article is not to define deaf culture or deaf epistemologies in depth but rather to take common constructs that have been developed and examine their present and potential relationships to the reality that is American education today.

American education reflects the goals and aspirations of American society in general. American education has gone through periods in which either equity of access or excellence has been emphasized. Since passage of the No Child Left Behind

Act in 2001, both goals have been embraced, at least in theory. The goal is that all children will achieve academic proficiency. In other words, quality of access by itself is no longer acceptable; access has been replaced by academic success as the measuring stick for all children.

In American schools today, in general, diversity is embraced and celebrated. It is built into the curriculum and, although the situation is not ideal, is supported by teachers and staff to greater extent. From my observations, everyone seems much less judgmental. In effect, there seems to be an atmosphere of multiple epistemologies.

There are opposing forces, however, in society and education. As most readers are aware, No Child Left Behind has several ambitious mandates. Each state must develop standards of learning for each grade for academic subjects, with the approval of the federal government. The standards should provide guidance for school districts in curriculum development. Individual states must also develop rigorous standardized tests to assess educational progress of schools, school districts, and states themselves, with the results disaggregated by categories such as gender, racial/ethnic status, second-language learners, poverty indicators, and disability. With very few exceptions, all schoolchildren must participate in this testing, with the goal of 100% demonstrating academic proficiency by 2014.

The sole criterion for success is passing a standardized, state-administered, grade-level test. Although some states are more flexible than others in making accommodations, the test must be in English, not in American Sign Language (ASL) or any spoken language other than English. Despite the growing acceptance of diversity, it is not taken into account in the most important assessments of student progress. The idea of one test given to all students at any particular grade level, regardless of the range of achievement at that level, is a reflection of, or perhaps a distortion of, the standard epistemology. At present, when diversity comes into conflict with uniformity, as represented by the requirements of No Child Left Behind, in American education uniformity wins.

EDUCATION OF THE DEAF IN THE UNITED STATES: THE BEGINNINGS

Although there were previous efforts in Virginia and New York City, what is now the American School for the Deaf was the first permanent school for d/Deaf children in America, founded in Hartford, Connecticut, in 1817. Fortunately for the school, its first principal, Thomas Hopkins Gallaudet, recruited Laurent Clerc, a deaf French instructor, as the first teacher at the school. Clerc was probably the dominant educator of the d/Deaf in the United States for 40 years or more, contributing a deaf presence and influence to the formative years of American deaf education. He remained at the school long after Gallaudet left, and his influence was felt in several ways. First, he adapted the French system of methodical signs to English, relying heavily on the manual alphabet to initialize signs. Some of his invented initialized signs continue to exist 200 years later in American Sign Language (ASL) today, including signs for many colors and for the days of the week, except Sunday. Second, Clerc adapted French systems for teaching grammar, ending up with five basic parts to teach correct grammar (Clerc, 1851).

Third, he not only trained the d/Deaf and hearing teachers at the American School in his sign system and curriculum, he also trained many of the teachers and founders of schools across the country, a number of whom were d/Deaf.

Many schools for d/Deaf children and adolescents in the 19th century were founded by d/Deaf leaders (Gannon, 1981). To a large degree, d/Deaf and hearing educators shared a common vision of d/Deaf individuals, the goals of education, and the answers to three fundamental questions: how to teach d/Deaf students, where to teach d/Deaf students, and what to teach d/Deaf students. Education took place within residential settings, instruction was through manual communication (either a natural sign language or an invented sign system), and the curriculum concentrated on reading, writing, arithmetic, moral training, and vocational preparation (Moores, 2001). There were no apparent separate deaf and hearing epistemologies.

The situation was not ideal. Many hearing school administrators, including Thomas Hopkins Gallaudet, were ordained ministers, and some viewed their calling in a missionary sense (Moores, 2001). All teachers were white. Several schools limited the roles of d/Deaf teachers, and for the first half of the 19th century there were no female teachers, hearing or d/Deaf. Deaf African American children were not allowed in schools for the deaf in the South and parts of the Midwest, and there were no schools at all for deaf African American children in these areas until after the Civil War. There were also conflicts between the advocates of methodical signs and natural signs, including some of the issues that have arisen in recent times over the relative benefits of Signed English systems and ASL. Deaf leaders were on both sides of the methodical signs–natural signs debate (Stedt & Moores, 1990). The debate lost much of its relevance with the rise of oral education, culminating in the Milan Congress in 1880, in which participants condemned both the use of signs alone and signs in coordination with speech and advocated the use of the pure oral method for all d/Deaf students.

Education of the d/Deaf in the United States endured a dark age from 1880 to 1960. Until near the end of that period, all schools used only oral methods for students up to age 12 and for most students throughout all grades. For those schools that allowed signs, d/Deaf teachers were limited to teaching high school or in vocational departments. Deaf leaders were not passive during this period (Boyd & Van Cleve, 2007; Reis, 2007), although the range of their influence was limited. Ladd (2008) argued that there are two approaches to Deafhood: One is to maintain it within the boundaries of an oppressive world, and the second is to enlarge the idea of what Deafhood means. Clearly, the goal from 1880 to 1960 was to maintain the Deaf community in the face of threat and attack. It is no coincidence that the National Association of the Deaf (NAD) was established in 1880, the same year as the Milan Congress, and that since then it has been the leading advocate for the rights of d/Deaf Americans (Moores, 2001). This is the first year in which a distinct Deaf epistemology may be identified. Deaf graduates of Gallaudet College worked and taught in those schools that employed d/Deaf workers, spread Gallaudet ASL throughout the country, were role models, and maintained the Deaf community in schools and through participation in deaf clubs and athletic activities. Movies were made of Deaf signers to preserve the language for future generations.

THE 21ST INTERNATIONAL CONGRESS ON EDUCATION OF THE DEAF (ICED) 2010 STATEMENT OF PRINCIPLE AND ACCORD FOR THE FUTURE

Statement of Principle

The legacy of the Milan conference has endured and the strength of the antisigning bias continues. Not until the 21st International Congress on Education of the Deaf (ICED) of 2010, *Partners in Progress*—130 years after the Milan Congress—were those resolutions finally rejected. The ICED 2010 Organizing Committee and the British Columbia Deaf community issued a statement of principles that rejected the principles of the 1880 Milan Congress, which denied the use of signs in the education of d/Deaf individuals. The statement of principles is as follows (Jamieson & Moores, 2011, pp. 26–27):

> In 1880 an international Congress was held in Milan to discuss education of the Deaf. At that time, the members passed several resolutions that affected the education and the lives of d/Deaf people around the world. These resolutions:
>
> - Removed the use of sign languages from educational programs for the Deaf around the world;
> - Contributed detrimentally to the lives of Deaf citizens around the world;
> - Led to the exclusion of Deaf citizens in educational policy and planning in most jurisdictions of the world;
> - Prevented Deaf citizens from participating in government planning, decision making, and funding in areas of employment, training, retraining, and other aspects of career planning;
> - Hindered the ability of deaf citizens to succeed in various careers and have prevented many of them from following their own aspirations; and
> - Prevented the opportunities for many Deaf citizens to fully demonstrate their cultural and artistic contributions to the diversity of each nation.
>
> *Therefore we:*
>
> - Reject all resolutions passed at the ICED Milan Congress in 1880 that denied the inclusion of sign languages in educational programs for Deaf students;
> - Acknowledge and sincerely regret the detrimental effects of the Milan conference; and
> - Call upon all nations of the world to remember history and ensure that educational programs accept and respect all languages and all forms of communication.

Accord for the Future

Immediately following the statement of principle, representatives of the ICED 2010 Vancouver Organizing Committee, the British Columbia Deaf community, the Canadian Association of the Deaf, and the World Federation of the Deaf issued the following Accord for the Future:

> Let it be stated that we, the undersigned,
>
> - Call upon all nations of the world to ratify and adhere to the principles of the United Nations, specifically those outlined in the Convention of Rights of Persons

with Disabilities, which states that education is to be delivered with an emphasis on acquisition of language and academic, practical, and social knowledge;

- Call upon all nations to endorse the regulations adopted by the World Federation of the Deaf at its 15th congress in Madrid in 2007, specifically those that promote and support equal and appropriate access to a multilingual/multicultural education;
- Call upon all nations to include the sign languages of their Deaf citizens as legitimate languages of those nations and to treat them as equal to those of the hearing majority;
- Call upon all nations to facilitate, enhance, and embrace their Deaf citizens' participation in all governmental decision-making processes affecting all aspects of their lives;
- Call upon all nations to involve their Deaf citizens to assist parents of Deaf infants, children, and youth in the appreciation of the Deaf culture and sign languages;
- Call upon all nations to support a child-centered approach in educational programs and a family-centered approach in all support services for both Deaf and hearing family members;
- Call upon all nations to refer all identified Deaf infants to regional and national organizations of the Deaf, schools and programs for the Deaf for support with early intervention;
- Call upon all nations to make every effort to ensure that their Deaf citizens obtain information about their human rights; and
- Call upon all nations of the world to recognize and allow all Deaf citizens to be proud, confident, creative, and enabling citizens in their respective countries.

THE TURNING POINT

It would be a mistake to assume that the Statement of Principle or Accord for the Future represented the viewpoint of all or even most educators of the d/Deaf, let alone attendees at ICED 2010. However, both documents show acknowledgment and acceptance of diversity, implicitly moving past a version of the standard epistemology to embrace some version of deaf epistemologies or multiple epistemologies.

The statements of ICED 2010 required a long germination period. As noted earlier, education of d/Deaf students went through a dark age from 1880 until the 1960s. The turning point in American education of d/Deaf students began to take shape in this decade, 80 years after the Milan conference and the establishment of the NAD, leading to the emergence of new deaf epistemologies. In 1960, there were no d/Deaf superintendents of day or residential schools for deaf students, and d/Deaf students still were not allowed in the Gallaudet graduate school, which was the only way to receive teacher certification. However, pressure for change was building, largely influenced by the civil rights movement. The graduate-level National Leadership Training Program (NLTP) for the d/Deaf was established with federal support in 1962 at San Fernando Valley College (now California State University, Northridge), and by its third year it was enrolling d/Deaf students. The same year, Gallaudet opened its graduate school to d/Deaf students, thus ensuring the creation of a large core of qualified and creative professionals. Federal legislation led to the establishment of the National Technical Institute for the Deaf (NTID) in the same decade, as well as establishment of vocational technical training programs for the d/Deaf within existing facilities for hearing students. The federally funded Model Secondary School for the Deaf was also established at Gallaudet during that period.

The prime mover for the most of these developments and others was a deaf man, Boyce Williams, whose impact in the last part of the 20th century was comparable to that of Clerc in the first part of the 19th century. Williams was employed by the federal government from 1945 to 1983 and worked his way up through the federal system to the position of chief of the Deafness and Communication Disorders Branch of the Rehabilitation Services Administration of the U.S. Office of Special Education and Rehabilitative Services. He funded research grants that led to the establishment of NTID and the vocational technical training centers as well as served as project officer for the NLTP grant (ensuring that potential d/Deaf leaders would be involved), in addition to grants for university PhD-level training in deafness. He was responsible for literally hundreds of workshops across the country and for the establishment and growth of vocational rehabilitation services and mental health programs for d/Deaf individuals. He was also responsible for the initial support for the National Theatre of the Deaf and the Registry of Interpreters for the Deaf and played a major role in the growth of the American Deafness and Rehabilitation Association. The last national census of the deaf population was conducted under his aegis. In sum, more than any other individual, he was responsible for the significant growth of opportunities and services for d/Deaf individuals and for the training of a large cadre of d/Deaf and hearing leaders.

In the 1960s and 1970s, deaf superintendents and other leaders in education and the professions began to take their rightful places. During that time, the Deaf community in America moved past the concept of maintaining Deafhood in the face of oppression to enlarging the concept of Deafhood. The contributions of d/Deaf leaders to the growth of Total Communication and the development of Signed English systems suggests a commitment at that time to working within the broader system of deaf education.

THE INDIVIDUALS WITH DISABILITIES EDUCATION ACT (IDEA) AND THE NO CHILD LEFT BEHIND ACT (NCLB)

Since the 1960s and 1970s, significant changes have occurred that have major implications for deaf epistemologies and deaf education. Two of the more pertinent ones are considered here. The primary impact has come from changes in educational placement and the second from the federal mandate for standard statewide curricula and standard grade-level assessment. Traditionally, d/Deaf students have been educated in residential schools or in separate day schools. Curricula were separate from those for hearing students. Changes began after the end of World War II with the population explosion and the unwillingness of state legislatures to build additional residential facilities. By 1970, more than half of all d/Deaf children were enrolled outside of residential schools.

The trend continued after the passage of the Education for All Handicapped Children Act of 1974, known in its present form as the Individuals With Disabilities

Education Act (IDEA), with its emphasis on placement in the least restrictive environment. The law effectively reduced the independence of education of the d/Deaf and moved it within the framework of a system serving significantly larger numbers of children, especially those with conditions such as learning disabilities and speech problems, whose needs are far different from those of d/Deaf children. At present, the number of d/Deaf children attending residential schools continues to decline, and schools in some states have closed or are close to closing. In many traditional residential schools, large majorities of students commute to schools from home on a daily basis, and in some cases residential schools have been converted completely to day schools with 100% of students commuting. The term *center school* is replacing *residential school* to reflect this reality.

The situation has been compounded by passage of the No Child Left Behind Act, which mandates rigorous standards for learning and statewide grade-level testing for all students, including those who are d/Deaf, with very few exceptions. Such mandates further limit the ability of programs to address the individual needs of children, which supposedly was guaranteed by IDEA. The most recent data (Gallaudet Research Institute, 2008) indicate that the largest single setting for d/Deaf students (60%) is in a regular school with hearing children, with 41% being served on a part-time basis by an itinerant teacher of the d/Deaf and 53% receiving speech therapy. Services typically involve a pullout model, under which the student receives instruction and/or therapy perhaps once a week for 30 to 60 minutes. The fact that more children receive itinerant speech therapy than itinerant educational services may indicate a hidden hearing epistemological bias.

Another factor is universal neonatal screening, which itself is a positive thing. However, in many states the follow-up may be through a state department of health, with no educational involvement and no participation of d/Deaf professionals. Although states are supposed to present all options to parents concerning communication modes and languages, this is not always the case.

HOW DO DEAF LEARNERS LEARN?

Several issues have been raised, in the form of questions or statements of fact. Put into statement form, they include the following:

1. Deaf learners are visual learners and process information differently from hearing learners, who are auditory learners.
2. The d/Deaf brain or mind is different from the hearing brain or mind.
3. A natural language such as ASL should be the main means of communication and instruction.

Any one of these statements requires book-length treatment, so only general issues are raised here. On first examination, the statement that d/Deaf students are visual learners should be true on its face. However, the 2007–2008 Annual Survey of Deaf and Hard of Hearing Children and Youth (Gallaudet Research Institute, 2008) found that more than 30,000 children reported a range of hearing loss. Only 8,519 (28%) had profound hearing losses (more than 90 dB, unaided). An additional 4,283 (14%) had severe losses (71–90 dB). Presumably, amplification would increase the speech reception of at least some of these children. Also, many children with less than severe hearing losses are placed in programs for d/Deaf students on the basis of educational decisions, not audiometric results.

While many students in programs for the d/Deaf are visual learners, the extent to which they may rely on either modality can vary. The question of d/Deaf and hearing brains or minds must be addressed on a much more complex level, inevitably leading to issues of cognition and intelligence (e.g., see Marschark & Hauser, 2009). Very briefly, d/Deaf learners receive, process, store, and access information in a completely or primarily visual mode. As such, the brains of d/Deaf and hearing people may be structured somewhat differently. Prelingual deafness might set some brain processes along different developmental tracks from those of hearing people. However, in a review of sign language and the brain, Campbell, MacSweeney, and Waters (2008) reported that evidence to date indicates that sign languages are structured and processed in a manner similar to that for spoken languages; both sign and spoken languages appear to depend on the same cortical substrate. Therefore, they may be considered functionally equivalent in terms of their cognitive and linguistic bases. Sign, which can use space to encode language, may employ more right-hemisphere processing, but the fundamentals seem to be the same.

The essential issue is not the possible differences between d/Deaf and hearing brains or minds. The brains of males and females may be structured differently to some degree, but the evidence suggests that they both function effectively in receiving and expressing information in a normal manner, although different pedagogical approaches may be called for. If d/Deaf learners have the same intellectual capacity as hearing learners, are there different learning styles to the extent that instruction in literacy, science, and mathematics should be organized and presented differently?

In a review of 20th-century research on intelligence and cognitive functioning of d/Deaf individuals, I have identified three stages (Moores, 2001). In stage 1, roughly the first third of the century, Pintner, Eisenson, and Stanton (1941) summarized the available data and concluded that d/Deaf individuals were inferior in intelligence to hearing individuals. In stage 2, Myklebust and Brutten (1953) concluded that d/Deaf individuals were not necessarily inferior intellectually, but that the deafness restricts the child functionally to a world of concrete objects and things. In stage 3, Vernon (1967) reviewed 31 research studies of the intelligence of d/Deaf individuals. He reported that in 13 studies, d/Deaf participants had mean scores superior to either test norms or the scores of control hearing participants, whichever were used. In seven studies, the scores did not differ significantly, and in the remaining 11 studies the scores of the d/Deaf participants were lower. Vernon concluded that d/Deaf children do as well as hearing children on intellectual tasks and are normal intellectually.

Marschark, Convertino, and La Rock (2006) proposed an additional stage that summarizes the data to the first years of the 21st century. They concluded that d/Deaf individuals are normal intellectually, but that they show some differences from hearing individuals in the ways they function, although the differences are not deficiencies—they are merely differences. This possibility must be explored in more detail. If there are differences, not deficiencies, in learning, then there should be differences in teaching. This calls into question the predominant mainstreaming and inclusion model for d/Deaf students in education. Unless regular education can be completely inclusive and respond to individual differences, it may not be appropriate for large numbers of d/Deaf students.

There appears to be consensus on this position. Deafness, per se, places no limitations on the potential of d/Deaf learners to acquire language, either spoken or signed, or on the potential to perform at grade level in mathematics, science, or social studies, yet the evidence is clear in the United States and across the world that this does not happen for the majority of d/Deaf students (Moores, 2001; Moores & Martin, 2006). Many reasons have been advanced for this lag in spoken language literacy and academic achievement. Chief among these is the argument that there is a critical period for language acquisition (Lenneberg 1967; see also Paul, Chapter 10), that late identification of deafness restricts the linguistic development of d/Deaf children and, by extension, their success in school. However, universal newborn screening for hearing loss is now common in many countries. In some cases follow-up is immediate, often with cochlear implants before one year of age (Hyde, 2009). Although there are reports of progress, early identification, intervention, and implantation have not proven to be panaceas (Priesler, 2007).

Other educators have addressed the language of instruction. Johnson, Liddell, and Erting (1989) stated that the low educational achievement of d/Deaf children—the failure of education of d/Deaf students—was due to a failure to use ASL as the means of instruction and that English-based sign systems should be banned. They argue that reliance on ASL would open the curriculum and allow d/Deaf children to achieve at grade level. In my opinion, ASL should be an integral part of instruction for most d/Deaf children. Whether it should be used alone or in some sort of coordination with an English-based sign system, as advocated by Stewart (2006), should be a matter of investigation. Although ASL-only programs have been in existence since around 1990 (Walworth, Moores, & O'Rourke, 1992), no experimental, quasi-experimental, or causal-comparative studies have been published in the ensuing years to investigate the effectiveness of ASL-only instruction relative to other approaches.

Similarly, there has been growing interest in the possible importance of phonology and phonological awareness in the development of literacy in d/Deaf students. Luckner, Sebald, Cooney, Young, and Goodwin Muir (2005/2006) found no studies between 1963 and 2003 that employed phonemic instruction or phonemic awareness as an intervention strategy. Since 2003, Trezek and colleagues have reported developments in research on the effectiveness of instruction in phonics and phonemic awareness (Trezek & Malmgren, 2005; Trezek & Wang, 2006; Trezek, Wang, Woods, Gampp, & Paul 2007). Their findings suggest that by combining phonics instruction with Visual Phonics and direct instruction, phonics awareness and phonics instruction can be modified to meet the beginning and remedial needs of young d/Deaf students. Wang, Trezek, Luckner, and Paul (2008) have proposed procedures to employ phonics-bases instruction to students who are d/Deaf; the results are promising. The key is to ascertain if such instruction will eventuate into true literacy, that is, comprehension, in later grades.

Unfortunately, the lack of research on ASL and phonological awareness is not an isolated case. The field suffers from a lack of data and is ruled by opinion. In a summary of reading comprehension research with d/Deaf students, Luckner and Handley (2008) concluded that there was an urgent need to increase the quantity and improve the quality of research undertaken in the field of deaf education. Their review, like previous reviews, highlighted areas where research was absent or limited.

CONCLUSION

Without considering the unique needs of d/Deaf students, it is possible that the focus on the regular education framework will result in constraints on teaching and assessment and have major implications for academic achievement. It is undeniable, and sadly ironic, that at a time of increasing societal acceptance of diversity, as evidenced by widespread acceptance of ASL, the education of d/Deaf students has lost much of its independence and distinctive character. The curriculum essentially is the regular education curriculum, assessment predominantly follows standardized state testing, and placement increasingly is in inclusive settings where a d/Deaf child may be the only one in a room or even a school.

There are no empirical data that support the efficacy of a regular curriculum over that of any other. There is no support for the position that a one-size-fits-all assessment model is beneficial. There is no research that suggests that placement of a child who is d/Deaf in an environment where all of his or her peers are hearing is of benefit academically or socially. Despite the fervent wishes of some people, d/Deaf students do not process information through the auditory channel, and most cannot speechread advanced academic material. However well-intentioned lawmakers and regular education leaders may be, the result can only be detrimental to at least some—and in my estimation, most—d/Deaf students. It reflects a version of the standard epistemology that conflicts with deaf epistemologies, however defined.

Although scholars may disagree on the meaning of deaf epistemology or epistemologies, they agree on the importance of ASL, visual learning, and the presence of d/Deaf professionals working with children and families from time of identification. The environment should be d/Deaf friendly. Families with hearing members should be aware that deafness is normal and is a social construct, not a pathology or sickness. Children should be exposed to and interaction with other d/Deaf students of similar and different ages and integrate into the Deaf community. Deaf children can be bicultural.

We are faced then with providing d/Deaf children with a free and appropriate public education, to quote IDEA. For generations, leaders in general education have talked about the benefits of a child-centered education built on the needs and characteristics of children. Drawing from the premises of deaf epistemologies, a d/Deaf child-centered educational system would have several characteristics that would differentiate it from public education. It would be visually oriented and visually stimulating. Groups would meet in circles rather than rows, even at older ages. Many or most of the teachers and aides would be d/Deaf. Much or all of the instruction would be in ASL.

The curriculum would be geared toward characteristics of d/Deaf children, and there would be a significant Deaf studies component. Assessment for understanding and mastery of subject matter would occur through both English and ASL.

Public schools, at present, are not set up to provide this type of education. Most d/Deaf children in these schools are the only d/Deaf student in a whole class or may have one class with other d/Deaf students; they are surrounded by hundreds of hearing students in their school. The regular classroom teachers are hearing, and the curriculum is designed for hearing children and has been developed to help children pass statewide exams. Communication is primarily in English and the important tests are given in English, perhaps with some accommodation but little or no modification.

Some of the bilingual–bicultural (bi–bi) programs in existence today meet many of these criteria. However, after more than 20 years of existence, they serve only about 11% of the d/Deaf population (Gallaudet Research Institute, 2008) and are concentrated in residential schools, which are facing declining enrollments.

There is need for further theorizing and research in a number of areas such as the effects of the following on teaching and learning activities involving d/Dhh students:

- Specific instructional strategies associated with the content areas such as mathematics, science, and social studies.
- The use of a general education curriculum with the focus on content standards and standardized assessments.
- The benefits and disadvantages of educational placements.
- The role of bi–bi programs.
- The education and training of teachers of d/Deaf children and adolescents.
- The involvement of parents in the education of their children.

If d/Deaf children are to thrive, both residential and public schools must embrace new models and paradigms; both must be flexible enough to experiment with new models. If not, the Deaf community will face serious challenges, the understanding of deaf epistemologies may change, and the concept of Deafhood may revert back to maintaining itself in the face of an oppressive world. We should all bend our efforts to prevent that.

REFERENCES

Boyd, R., & Van Cleve, J. (2007). Deaf autonomy and deaf dependence: The early years of the Pennsylvania Society for the Advancement of the Deaf. In J. Van Cleve (Ed.), *The deaf history reader* (pp. 153–173). Washington, DC: Gallaudet University Press.

Campbell, R., MacSweeney, M., & Waters, D. (2008). Sign language and the brain: A review. *Journal of Deaf Studies and Deaf Education, 13*(1), 1–20.

Clerc, L. (1851). Some hints to teaching the deaf. In *Proceedings of Second Convention of American Instructors of the Deaf and Dumb* (pp. 64–75). Hartford, CT: Case Tiffany.

Freire, P. (1970). *Pedagogy of the oppressed.* New York, NY: Continuum.

Gallagher, J. (1968). Organization and special education. *Exceptional Children, 34,* 485–491.

Gallaudet Research Institute. (2008). *Regional and national summary report of data from the 2007–2008 Annual Survey of Deaf and Hard of Hearing Children and Youth.* Washington, DC: Gallaudet University.

Gannon, J. (1981). *Deaf heritage: A narrative history of deaf America.* Silver Spring, MD: National Association of the Deaf.

Gannon, J. (1989). *The week the world heard Gallaudet.* Washington, DC: Gallaudet University Press.

Hairston, E., & Smith, L. (1983). *Black and deaf in America: Are we that different?* Silver Spring, MD: T. J. Publishers.

Holcomb, T. (2010). Deaf epistemology: The deaf way of knowing. *American Annals of the Deaf, 154*(2), 471–478.

Hyde, M. (2009). Inclusion in an international context. In D. Moores & M. Miller (Eds.), *D/deaf people around the world: Educational and social perspectives* (pp. 351–367). Washington, DC: Gallaudet University Press.

Individuals With Disabilities Education Improvement Act (IDEIA). (2004). Public Law 108–446, 118 Stat. 2647.

Jamieson, J., & Moores, D. (2011). Partners in education. In D. Moores (Ed.), *Partners in Education: The 21st International Congress on the Education of the Deaf* (pp. 20–28). Washington, DC: Gallaudet University Press.

Johnson, R., Liddell, S., & Erting, C. (1989). *Unlocking the curriculum: Principles for achieving access in deaf education* (Gallaudet Research Institute Working Paper No. 89-3). Washington, DC: Gallaudet University Press.

Kelly, A. (2008). Where is Deaf herstory? In H. D. L. Bauman (Ed.), *Open your eyes: Deaf studies talking* (pp. 35–41). Minneapolis, MN: University of Minnesota Press.

Kirk, S. (1983). Autobiographical remarks. In G. Harris & W. Kirk (Eds.), *The foundations of special education: Selected papers and speeches of Samuel A. Kirk.* Reston, VA: Council for Exceptional Children.

Ladd, P. (2003). *Understanding Deaf culture: In search of Deafhood.* Clevedon, UK: Multilingual Matters.

Ladd, P. (2008). Colonialism and resistance: A brief history of Deafhood. In H. D. L. Bauman (Ed.), *Open your eyes: Deaf studies talking* (pp. 44–52). Minneapolis, MN: University of Minnesota Press.

Lehrer, K. (2000). *Theory of knowledge* (2nd ed.). Boulder, CO: Westview.

Lenneberg, E. (1967). *Biological foundations of language.* New York, NY: Wiley.

Luckner, J., & Handley, C. (2008). A summary of the reading comprehension research undertaken with students who are deaf or hard of hearing. *American Annals of the Deaf, 153*(1), 6–36.

Luckner, J., Sebald, A., Cooney, J., Young III, J., & Goodwin Muir, S. (2005/2006). An examination of the evidence-based literacy research in deaf education. *American Annals of the Deaf, 150*(5), 443–456.

Marschark, M., Convertino, C., & La Rock, D. (2006). Optimizing academic performance of d/d/deaf students: Access, opportunities, and outcomes. In D. Moores & D. Martin (Eds.), *Deaf learners: Developments in curriculum and instruction* (pp. 179–200). Washington, DC: Gallaudet University Press.

Marschark, M., & Hauser, P. (Eds.). (2009). *Deaf cognition: Foundations and outcomes.* New York, NY: Oxford University Press.

Moores, D. (2001). *Educating the deaf: Psychology, principles, and practices* (5th ed.). Boston: Houghton Mifflin.

Moores, D. (2011). Waist deep in the big muddy: The Individuals With Disabilities Education Act (IDEA) and the No Child Left Behind Act. *American Annals of the Deaf, 155*(5), 523–525.

Moores, D., & Martin, D. (Eds.). (2006). *Deaf learners: Developments in curriculum and instruction.* Washington, DC: Gallaudet University Press.

Myklebust, H., & Brutten, M. (1953). A study of visual perception in deaf children. *Acta Oto-Laryngologica, 105*(Suppl.), 1–126.

No Child Left Behind Act. (2001). Public Law 107-110, 20 U.S.C. Special Character 6301 et seq. (2002).

Paul, P., & Moores, D. (2010). Perspectives on Deaf epistemologies. *American Annals of the Deaf, 154*(2), 417–420.

Pintner, R., Eisenson, J., & Stanton, M. (1941). *The psychology of the physically handicapped.* New York, NY: Crofts.

Popper, K. (1977). *The logic of scientific discovery.* London, UK: Routledge.

Preisler, G. (2007). The psychological development of deaf children with cochlear implants. In L. Komesaroff (Ed.), *Surgical consent: Bioethics and cochlear implants* (pp. 120–136). Washington, DC: Gallaudet University Press.

Reis, M. (2007). A tale of two schools: The Indiana Institution and the Evansville Day School, 1879–1912. In J. Van Cleve (Ed.), *The deaf history reader* (pp. 85–115). Washington, DC: Gallaudet University Press.

Stedt, J., & Moores, D. (1990). Manual codes on English and American Sign Language: Historical perspectives and current realities. In H. Bornstein (Ed.), *Manual communication: Implications for education* (pp. 1–20). Washington, DC: Gallaudet University Press.

Stewart, D. (2006). Instructional and practical communication: ASL and English-based signing in the classroom. In D. Moores & D. Martin (Eds.), *Deaf learners: Developments in curriculum and instruction* (pp. 207–220). Washington, DC: Gallaudet University Press.

Trezek, B., & Malmgren, K. (2005). The efficacy of utilizing a phonics treatment package with middle school deaf and hard of hearing children. *Journal of Deaf Studies and Deaf Education, 10*(3), 256–271.

Trezek, B., & Wang, Y. (2006). Implications of utilizing a phonics-based reading curriculum with children who are deaf or hard of hearing. *Journal of Deaf Studies and Deaf Education, 11*(2), 202–213.

Trezek, B., Wang, W., Woods, D., Gampp, T., & Paul, P. (2007). Using visual phonics to supplement beginning reading instruction for students who are deaf/hard of hearing. *Journal of Deaf Studies and Deaf Education, 12*(3), 373–384.

Vernon, M. (1967). Relationship of language to the thinking process. *Archives of Genetic Psychiatry, 16*(3), 325–333.

Walworth, M., Moores, D., & O'Rourke, T. (Eds.). (1992). *A free hand: Enfranchising the education of deaf learners.* Silver Spring, MD: T. J. Publishers.

Wang, Y., Trezek, B., Luckner, J., & Paul, P. (2008). The role of phonology and phonologically related skills in reading instruction for students who are deaf or hard of hearing. *American Annals of the Deaf, 153*(4), 396–407.

SUGGESTIONS FOR FURTHER READING

Kuhn, T. (1996). *The structure of scientific revolutions* (3rd ed.). Chicago, IL: University of Chicago Press.

Ladd, P. (2003). *Understanding deaf culture: In search of Deafhood.* Clevedon, UK: Multilingual Matters.

Marschark, M., & Spencer, P. (Eds.). (2010). *Oxford handbook of Deaf studies, language, and education.* New York, NY: Oxford University Press.

Moores, D., & Miller, M. (Eds.). (2010). *d/Deaf people around the world: Educational and social perspectives.* Washington, DC: Gallaudet University Press.

7

Paving the Way for Reform in Deaf Education

Thomas K. Holcomb

> In education, power is transmitted through social relations, representations, and practices, which determine whose language and cultural experiences count and whose do not, which students are at the center and, therefore, which must remain in the periphery.
>
> —Luis Moll, 2010, p. 454

The standard epistemology requires the use of scientific methods to gain knowledge and discover the truth but it is often at the expense of children who are different. For instance, in the case of educational practices, it is obvious that the formulation of educational theories and policies should be data driven. But who is designing the studies? What theories are "driving the data?" Enter the notion of deaf epistemologies.

Defined as a "way of knowing" that relies heavily on the Deaf community's personal testimonies, personal experiences, and personal accounts to document knowledge, deaf epistemologies have often been used as a basis for advocating for policy changes to address the chronic poor performance of deaf children (see Bragg, 2001; Jankowski 1997; Ladd, 2003; Lane, Hoffmeister, & Bahan, 1996; Van Cleve & Crouch, 1989, for reviews).

Deaf epistemologies incorporates what Moll (2010, p. 454) terms as the "language and cultural experiences that count." Without deaf epistemologies, the field of deaf education is at risk of continuing practices that ignore the identity, life and learning experiences, and the language and cultural needs of the very community it wants to educate (Lane et al., 1996; Simms, Rusher, Andrews, & Coryell, 2008). As such, the inclusion of a signed language in the education of deaf children is a hallmark of deaf epistemologies. In recent years, several deaf schools and institutions of higher education have adopted deaf-centric policies shaped by deaf epistemologies in an effort to improve academic performance of deaf students and to develop leaders who can impact policy. *Deaf-centric* is defined as educational practices that incorporate the language and culture of the Deaf community[1] (Lane et al., 1996).

In response to federal laws that mandate that all schools, including schools for deaf students, demonstrate accountability in the performance of their students, data regarding student outcomes is becoming increasingly available for public scrutiny. The preliminary data from three well-known deaf schools is showing emerging evidence of the effectiveness of pedagogical approaches that can be linked to standard epistemology. It is my contention that deaf epistemologies and the standard epistemology should not be viewed mutually exclusive.

EPISTEMOLOGY DEFINED

Epistemology has been defined in many different ways. All the definitions basically encompass three aspects of knowledge—belief, truth, and justification (see also Paul & Moores, Chapter 1). In a nutshell, epistemology addresses the question, *How do we know what we know?* In the case of the Deaf world and the field of deaf education, what constitutes true beliefs or justified beliefs? One goal of epistemology is to determine the criteria for knowledge so that we can know what can or cannot be known. For deaf epistemologies, this begs the question, *What are the criteria for knowledge that are crucial for educating deaf students?*

To better address the issue of deaf epistemologies, it is productive to consider the epistemologies of various minority, oppressed, or disenfranchised communities such as feminist, African American, Latino American, Native American, and queer/gay epistemologies. Epistemologies of minority, oppressed, or otherwise disenfranchised groups usually focus on opposing and rectifying oppression (Bakari, 1997; Freire, 1970; Moll, 2010; Spencer, 2008; Wright, 2003). Within these companion epistemologies, it has been posited that only members of such groups can acquire knowledge on the truth associated with their cultural beliefs and experiences. In this sense, the epistemology of the minority consists of theories of knowledge created by members, about members' modes of knowing, for the purpose of liberating members (Anderson, 1995; Bakari, 1997; Freire, 1970; Koertge, 1996; Ladd, 2008; Moll, 2010; Spencer, 2008).

Similarly, it has been the perspective of some Deaf leaders that the quality of deaf education can be improved only when justified beliefs and knowledge vis-à-vis deaf epistemologies are better understood and embraced (Andrews & Covell, 2006/2007; Geeslin, 2007; Jankowski, 1997; Ladd, 2008; Lang, 2003; Simms & Thumann, 2007; Stone, 2000). To this end, Bragg (2001) compiled a collection of essays written by Deaf individuals since 1852 and published them in a book titled *Deaf World: A Historical Reader and Primary Sourcebook*. This type of book demonstrates the importance of the Deaf voice, and is not unlike the epistemological work of various minority and disenfranchised groups. Such works begin as testimonials, develop into case studies and qualitative studies, and, as data accumulate, develop into larger scaled quantitative studies.

The work of Margaret Beale Spencer with African American youth in the education system and Luis Moll with the Latino American communities are good examples of this process. In both of these examples (Moll, 2010; Spencer, 2008), the roles of the communities' language and culture were considered critical to academic achievement of African American and Latino American youths. Thus, their respective epistemologies helped to shape educational research and practices in these communities.

In a vein similar to Spencer's and Moll's work, which "listen to the community's voice," Ladd (2003) suggests that deaf epistemologies provides an opportunity for people to understand clearly "Deaf ways of being in the world, of conceiving that world and their own place within it, both in actuality and in potentiality" (p. 19). One striking example is in the area of cognitive development and the wide range of cognitive abilities in deaf people, which are often inferior to those of their hearing peers. Even though this can easily be documented, there is no clear neurological explanation for the consistently poor academic achievement of deaf students (Hamers, 1998; Heiling, 1995; Maller, 2003; Moores, 2001). Many Deaf people, their allies, educators, and researchers feel that knowledge from the Deaf community has been neglected, dismissed, minimized, or misapplied in an effort to understand deaf children's potential and to increase their educational success (Bahan, 2008; Hoffmeister, 1990; Humphries, 2004; Lang, 2003; Nover, Andrews, Baker, Everhart, & Bradford, 2002; Pahz & Pahz, 1978; Simms & Thumann, 2007).

DEAF EPISTEMOLOGIES IN THE MAKING: "DEAF WAYS OF KNOWING"

Based on their own personal experiences and struggles through the educational system, Deaf people have long believed that they *know* what the problems were with the educational system, and yet they are silenced (Bauman, 2008; Reagan, 2010; Stone, 2000). Fleischer (2008) explains, "deaf people rarely spoke out for their rights to demand what they knew to be the best way in terms of critical pedagogy. We were silenced for a long time and let things pass by to appease the 'worldly knowledge' of hearing educators for their decision making" (p. 160). Prior to 1965, Deaf people were not allowed positions of authority within the deaf education setting. Although Deaf people worked in schools for the deaf, there were no opportunities for them to assume leadership roles, to take part in the political structure of the school, or to have any policy-making influence. Consequently, many Deaf educators want greater roles in shaping educational policies (Andrews, Martin, & Rusher, 2009; M. S. Holcomb, personal communication, May 30, 2008; Humphries, 2004; Lang, 2003; H. Larson, personal communication, June 12, 2008; Woll & Ladd, 2003).

This was not always the case. In the 1800s, Deaf leaders were actively involved in creating opportunities for their fellow deaf citizens to lead productive lives. This was exemplified in the educational arena by Laurent Clerc and Thomas Gallaudet, the first Deaf-hearing team who cofounded the American School for the Deaf in 1817. Consequently, during the 1800s, Deaf and professional teams founded and ran more than 24 schools—schools that employed many Deaf teachers and utilized American Sign Language (ASL) and English in the education of deaf children (Baynton, Gannon, & Bergey, 2007; Gannon, 1981; Marschark, Lang, & Albertini, 2002). When threatened by the oral-only advocates, such as the proclamation made at the 1880 Milan Conference, Deaf Americans organized a national political organization, the National Association of the Deaf (NAD). The NAD was established to assert that Deaf Americans knew best how to educate deaf children. However, by the early 1900s, the tactics of the oral extremists were powerful enough to completely exclude Deaf people from the decision-making process in the deaf education system (Moores, 2010). In response, papers were published in Deaf periodicals such as *The Silent Worker* and *The Deaf American* from the 1950s into the 1990s supporting the role of Deaf teachers in the classroom (Andrews & Franklin, 1996/97; Bjorlee, 1954; Boatner, 1952; Vernon, 1970).

After 80 years of educational catastrophe when deaf children struggled to obtain education through the oral means, the time was ripe for a revolution in which educational policies could be shaped with the active involvement of Deaf people rather than for deaf people (Marschark & Spencer, 2003; Pahz & Pahz, 1978; Wilcox, 2004). Humphries (2008, p. 37) described this as a coming-out process for Deaf people in which they were able to "develop a sustaining voice, one that sustains the individual and the group alike." Today, there are growing number of schools and programs shaped by Deaf epistemologies.

Higher education has also played a role in opening doors to Deaf adults so that they may earn the teaching and administration credentials to participate in the running of schools for the deaf. Ironically, Gallaudet College, the world's only higher education institution for Deaf students, was not the leader in this effort. Rather, the National Leadership Training Program (NLTP), established in 1962 at San Fernando Valley State College (now known as California State University, Northridge), took the lead.

With the inclusion of Deaf students in 1964, the NLTP ushered in a new era in which the Deaf voice was heard for the first time in a long time in higher education (Boyd, 1987; Scouten, 1984). In addition, it was the very first time that support services such as interpreters and notetakers were provided to allow Deaf students equal access to classroom instruction in a mainstream environment (Boyd, 1987; Stewart, 2007). Throughout the program, perspectives of both Deaf and hearing educators were solicited on how to improve the quality of deaf education. The collaborative efforts of Deaf and hearing educators being fomented and encouraged in the creation and design of innovative educational practices were powerful. Opposing perspectives were freely debated in the safety of the classroom under the guidance of experienced, progressive professors (G. Gustason, personal communication, June 5, 2008; M. S. Holcomb, personal communication, May 30, 2008; H. Larson, personal communication, June 12, 2008).

As a result, southern California was considered a *hotbed* of innovations in deaf education practices during the 1960s (G. Gustason, personal communication, June 5, 2008; M. S. Holcomb, personal communication, May 30, 2008; H. Larson, personal communication, June 12, 2008). Deaf people's *knowledge* was being put to use in the reform of the deaf education system. The big push for improved access to English, barrier-free communication environments, and effective pedagogical practices for use with deaf children was made possible once Deaf individuals and their hearing classmates began graduating from NLTP.

These innovations enjoyed widespread support among Deaf people and educators of the Deaf during the 1970s (Pahz & Pahz, 1978). As Pahz and Pahz wrote, recalling the excitement of those days, "It is hard to hide one's enthusiasm when a philosophy such as Total Communication, which so greatly enhances the deaf child's opportunities to learn, is known" (p. viii).

The pioneers of those days included several Deaf educators individuals who initiated new trends in deaf education. One was David Anthony, who developed Seeing Essential English (SEE). Others were Gerilee Gustason, who pushed the development of Signing Exact English (SEE2); Herb Larson, who was instrumental in transforming the mainstreaming experience to include the Deaf perspective; and Roy K. Holcomb, who formalized the concepts of Total Approach and Total Communication.

Although David Anthony was not a graduate of NLTP, he was surrounded by people who were. The initial concept of a manually coded English system began in Michigan before his arrival in southern California; however, he formalized the system with the input of Deaf and hearing educators in the area and eventually implemented the system at a deaf program in a public school setting to reverse the oral tradition of the deaf education system. Confounded by differing philosophies of how English should be presented manually, Gerilee Gustason, an NLTP graduate, along with other supporters, both Deaf and hearing, split from Anthony's group and developed a different system of representing English in signs. Regardless of differing philosophies, the basic premise of both systems was to make language visible to those who could not hear (Hoffmeister, 1990; Scouten, 1984; Stedt & Moores, 1990). Both Anthony and Gustason *knew* that more needed to be done to make language more accessible to deaf children and that it was practically impossible to master the nuances of English without being explicitly and visually exposed to the language (D. Anthony, personal communication, July 15, 2008; G. Gustason, personal communication, June 5, 2008).

Herb Larson also knew that the mainstream experience could not remain the status quo if deaf students were to benefit fully from the public school environment (H. Larson, personal communication, June 12, 2008). For this reason, he accepted a position within a public school system in southern California, thus becoming the first Deaf administrator of a mainstream education program. Based on his experiences as a Deaf person, Larson ushered in a new way of creating a more positive setting for deaf students to succeed in the mainstream setting by promoting full access to mainstream instruction. This included hiring sign language interpreters, allowing teachers to sign with Deaf students, and employing Deaf teachers, all of which were a radical shift.

In a similar vein, Roy K. Holcomb, another graduate of NLTP, knew that deaf children needed full access to communication, both at school and at home, to have an impact on the educational success of these children (Scouten, 1984). Based on this knowledge, he devised two complementary philosophies related to the totality of the communication experience of deaf children. Although Total Communication has since become synonymous with Simultaneous Communication, or speaking and signing at the same time (Pahz & Pahz, 1978; Tompkins, 2004), Holcomb's premise was more geared toward the fact that deaf children needed full access to communication (Roy K. Holcomb, personal notes, undated). He reasoned that one reason for the limitations in deaf children's educational success was the insufficient access to communication, and therefore it was necessary that deaf children be provided with full, or total, access to communication. To accomplish this, he argued that deaf children needed to see what hearing children hear and therefore that people must sign at all times in the presence of deaf children to provide them with the "Total Communication" experience that hearing children automatically enjoy (Scouten, 1984). Otherwise, deaf children would be doomed to limited academic success because of lost opportunities for incidental learning.

Holcomb also developed a second model, which he called Total Approach, wherein the communication method employed by classroom teachers should be flexible and eclectic enough to meet the specific needs of their students. More specifically, teachers should be able to utilize whatever strategies necessary to make it possible for Deaf students to understand the materials being presented. These include any and all forms of communication methods and language modalities, whether they be ASL, manually coded English, written English, spoken English, or fingerspelling. The point was to allow the Deaf student to understand and master the concepts being presented. This philosophy was intended to eliminate the rigidity and restrictiveness of specific communication philosophies so that the business of teaching could be the focus and function of the classroom.

Roy K. Holcomb's work gained immediate widespread acceptance in the academic community and among Deaf individuals. Jordan, Gustason, and Rosen (1976) surveyed the communication practices of the 970 identified programs serving deaf and hard of hearing students in the United States. With 82% of the 970 programs reporting, it was discovered that 43% of the respondents had recently made a change in their school's communication practice, with almost all of them making the shift from oralism/auralism to Total Communication. The survey also showed that 4,619 classrooms with deaf children were using Total Communication by 1976, some eight years after the philosophy was originated, as opposed to the oralism/auralism method, which was still being used in 2,370 classrooms.

The shift to Total Communication was formally endorsed by NAD and the National Fraternal Society of the Deaf in the 1970s (Pahz & Pahz, 1978). Additionally, Boyce R. Williams, the highest-ranking Deaf official in the U.S. Rehabilitation Services Administration, issued an official statement in 1971 about the Total Communication philosophy: "Total communication represents the great emancipation of deaf people from an inadequate, sterile educational system" (cited in Pahz & Pahz, 1978, p. 101).

Somehow, along the way, the Total Communication philosophy was transformed into the policy of requiring teachers and students to sign and speak simultaneously (Valli, 1990). This, in effect, eliminates the use of ASL or alternative communication methods that might be more suitable to help the Deaf child grasp the concept being taught. As a result, a restrictive environment for the Deaf child was once again created. This counters Roy K. Holcomb's two original premises: *Total Approach*, in which any and all approaches should be made available and used as appropriate, and *Total Communication*, which requires that Deaf children be given full access to communication taking place around them. In this sense, his knowledge has been discarded in favor of convenience for hearing teachers and parents and the traditional emphasis on oral skill development (Gertz, 2008; Simms & Thumann, 2007; Woll & Ladd, 2003). Once again, deaf epistemologies have been discounted in shaping educational policies for deaf children.

All these historical accounts make it appear that deaf epistemologies do not uphold the rigor that would be expected of the standard epistemology, that is, dependence on scientific evidence purporting to support the effectiveness of a practice or belief. However, it is important to note that in epistemologies of disenfranchised groups, testimony has been considered a valuable source and a reliable way of gaining knowledge (Klein, 2005). Deaf epistemologies is no different (Bechter, 2008).

To this end, Ladd (2003) discussed the importance of employing subaltern research methodology, which calls for the use of common folks as subjects, in understanding and validating the Deaf experience. Through this knowledge, pedagogical practices can be better implemented with increased potential for success. The importance of deaf epistemologies in shaping educational policies has been advocated by Lang (2003, p. 18), who stated, "By finding ways to circumvent the numerous barriers they have faced as learned individuals, deaf people lay claim to being more than pupils or victims of oppression, but contribute to the advancement of the field of deaf education as a science."

FAST-FORWARD 40 YEARS TO THE PRESENT

Deaf educators and their hearing allies in the 1960s focused on making English visible for deaf children, engineered mainstream environments to be more Deaf friendly, insisted that communication be totally accessible to deaf people, and encouraged flexible communication and language usage with deaf students. By 1980, in spite of widespread support for these efforts, deaf education practice had reverted to hearing-centric approaches in which the core of Deaf cultural values has been de-emphasized or devalued (Andrews & Covell, 2006; Nover & Andrews, 1998; Simms & Thumann, 2007; Stone, 2000).

Carol Padden, a leading Deaf scholar, examined and documented the core values of the Deaf community (Padden, 1980). She discussed how one unique, predominant value of the Deaf community departs significantly from the beliefs of the general, hearing public. While the hearing public places a premium on one's ability to speak, by contrast, the Deaf community has a disassociation from speech by which a person is not judged based on the ability to speak. In this sense, whether a deaf person can speak has no bearing on his or her status in the Deaf community, while it is often the primary focus of the larger, hearing-centric society (Bauman, 2008). Consequently, competing educational philosophies are largely influenced by these two divergent views on the value of speech in the education of deaf children, with speech development heavily emphasized by the hearing-centric administration in contrast to the focus on full, visual access to communication and language espoused by many Deaf individuals and their hearing allies (Lane, 2008; Marschark et al. 2002).

This conflict caused the rise of a new movement utilizing *Deaf knowledge* to address the continued poor performance of deaf students in academic arenas and to maximize their potential, particularly in reading and language (Bailes, 1999; Jankowski, 1997; Levesque, 1991; Nover & Andrews, 1998; Stone, 2000; Woll & Ladd, 2003). Such knowledge has been used in the past two decades, during which the bilingual/bicultural philosophy, the language planning model, and the Deafhood movement have been considered the best practices by many Deaf people and their hearing allies, including educators, administrators, linguists, and researchers (Ladd, 2003; Mahshie, 1995; Parasnis, 1998; Reagan, 2010; Simms & Thumann, 2007).

In actuality, the bilingual/bicultural philosophy should not be viewed as theory bound. It is much more. Francois Grosjean, a bilingual education scholar, asserted that for Deaf individuals, "bilingualism is a necessity not a choice" (2008, pp. 230–237). In other words, regardless of differing educational philosophies on how deaf children should be taught, Deaf people need the two languages, ASL and English, and need two cultures because the reality of their lives is that they live in at least two communities, those of Deaf people and hearing people. They lead a bilingual or even multicultural existence and travel between the Deaf community and the larger, predominately hearing society to meet their cultural, social, and educational needs. Breivik (2005) and Ladd (2008) have described this as hybridity between communities.

To this end, several progressive schools for the deaf have recognized the value of incorporating Deaf knowledge in their pedagogical endeavors and revised their educational philosophies accordingly. In these cases, ASL became the language of instruction and English became the written medium with the goals of providing Deaf children with increased access to content areas and helping them become fluent in both languages. Deaf epistemologies are reflected in the California School for the Deaf's Statement of Belief, which states, "The California School for the Deaf, Fremont has made a commitment to be a Deaf-centered environment in which the design of learning and the language of instruction are consistent with a Bilingual-Bicultural approach to educating Deaf children." Similarly, the mission statement of the Maryland School for the Deaf states that it "provides excellence in education in a bilingual environment to prepare all students to be contributing citizens."

In several parts of the country where there was resistance from existing schools and programs to incorporating Deaf knowledge, the leaders of the Deaf community proceeded to work with parents of deaf children and progressive educators to establish charter schools in their areas. For example, the Colorado Association of the Deaf and the Utah Association of the Deaf took lead roles in getting the charter school established in the Denver and Salt Lake City areas (M. Baer, personal communication, January 27, 2011; C. Moers, personal communication, February 10, 2011; M. Wilding-Diaz, personal communication, January 24, 2011; Rocky Mountain Deaf School, n.d.; Utah Association, n.d.). The Deaf leaders in the Twin Cities also worked closely with the parents and teachers of deaf students in the area to launch the Metro Deaf School in Minnesota (A. Hile, personal communication, January 18, 2011; D. Sherwood, personal communication, January 13, 2011; Metro Deaf School, n.d.). Interestingly, the Metro Deaf School is recognized as the second charter school of any kind to open in the United States. Similarly, the Jean Massieu School was among the first three charter schools to open in Utah. These schools as well as other charter schools serving deaf students based their mission on deaf epistemologies and adopted the bilingual model, in which the focus is on full access to instructional materials via the accessible, visual language (ASL) and a strong foundation in English through the written form (Berke, 2009).

Other charter schools include Jean Massieu Academy in Texas, Las Vegas Charter School of the Deaf in Nevada, and Sequoia School for the Deaf and Hard of Hearing in Arizona. The mission statement of the Las Vegas Charter School exemplifies the mantra of Deaf epistemologies associated with deaf education: "providing students with an educational program within a bilingual framework that enhances literacy (reading and writing), signacy (ASL) and oracy (speech)" (Las Vegas Charter School for the Deaf, n.d.). Deaf epistemologies is also reflected in Rocky Mountain Deaf School's vision statement: "As a high-performing, innovative educational program for students who are deaf, we are deeply committed to providing a rigorous, standards-based curriculum. We prepare each deaf student to be literate, academically successful, and technologically competent. We provide a linguistically rich learning environment through the acquisition of American Sign Language and English both inside and outside the classroom" (Rocky Mountain Deaf School, n.d.).

DEAF WAYS OF KNOWING—INFORMING DEAF WAYS OF TEACHING

On a different front in higher education, Deaf academics also have been working closely with hearing educators to transform the preparation of teachers who will work with deaf children (Andrews et al., 2009; Andrews & Covell, 2006; J. Andrews, personal communication, January 24, 2011; J. Coryell, personal communication, January 23, 2011). Instead of the traditional approach of viewing deaf children as subjects in need of intervention in the form of special education, leadership and teacher preparation programs at Boston University, California State University, Northridge, Gallaudet University, Lamar University in Texas, McDaniel College in Maryland, University of California San Diego, and other universities base their program philosophies on deaf epistemologies.

For example, Lamar University has been aggressive in seeking federal funding to develop graduate programs based on deaf epistemologies. Over the past few years, the U.S. Department of Education awarded Lamar University grants worth more than $5 million to prepare future teachers and leaders who have knowledge and skills related to Deaf culture, ASL, and bilingual strategies (J. Andrews, personal communication, January 24, 2011). Another example can be found in Boston University's philosophy statement: "The philosophy of the program incorporates a bilingual/bicultural approach (ASL/English) to educating Deaf children. The program views Deaf adults as competent individuals from a minority culture, not as a handicapped population" (Boston University, n.d.). Similarly, at McDaniel College, their commitment is reflected through their mission statement: "Philosophically, the program views deaf students from a bilingual perspective. For graduates, that translates into a genuine acceptance of and respect for the language and culture of deaf people, as well as a driving commitment to provide students with experiences that encourage literacy development and academic achievement." (McDaniel College, n.d.)

All these university programs are developed and delivered by those who have Deaf epistemologies coupled with academic preparation. They all have Deaf faculty working closely with hearing colleagues in preparing new generations of teachers, leaders, and researchers who are well versed in applying deaf epistemologies to the education of deaf children. In contrast, traditional programs often exclude Deaf people as professionals, teachers, students, and researchers by erecting potential barriers such as lack of appropriate support services and mentoring along with English-based examinations (e.g., the Graduate Record Examination), which have been determined to be biased against Deaf test takers (Andrews et al., 2009).

In pre-K–12 programs, there have been promising efforts to develop curriculum and professional training at the preservice and in-service levels (Nover et al., 2002), and at the early childhood level (Simms & Moers, 2009), at the preservice and in-service levels of master's degree programs (Humphries & Allen, 2008; Rusher, Martin, Gentry, Jackson, & Andrews, 2009; Simms & Thumann, 2007) and at the doctoral program level (Andrews et al., 2009). All of these programs emphasize deaf epistemologies, which is embedded and embraced in all coursework including research methodology courses.

Clearly, Deaf people are no longer silenced when it comes to the education of deaf children. Deaf people are "speaking out." Deaf people are playing an active role in liberating deaf children from oppressive and ineffective pedagogical practices of the past by ensuring that Deaf knowledge be acknowledged and integrated. With the push for pedagogical approaches shaped by deaf epistemologies comes the need for data-driven outcomes of these programs.

DEAF WAYS OF KNOWING—REFOCUSING THE LENS OF ASSESSMENT TO MEASURE DEAF WAYS OF KNOWING

As is true of most epistemologies of disenfranchised groups, deaf epistemologies is often viewed as insufficiently scientific. Interestingly, these claims have been made by opponents of African Americans and Latino American epistemologies in public schools where mainstream white American practices have dominated, despite changing demographics and increases in the numbers of minority children in the school systems (Moll, 2010; Spencer, 2008).

Rather than dismissing deaf epistemologies, a more productive approach is to launch scientific hypotheses to test Deaf-centered teaching practices. Viewed in this light, deaf epistemologies is a necessary part of the continuum from "ways of Deaf knowing" to ways of teaching.

Many professionals feel that the benchmarks that are indicators in the standard epistemology are necessary to document *true* knowledge, as opposed to the justified truth that is often found in deaf epistemologies, which relies heavily on the truths that are consistently evident in testimonies from Deaf individuals. However, this criticism regarding insufficient scientific data has rarely been directed toward the oral approaches that have been employed in deaf education settings for the past century.

In fact, poor results of deaf education system are well documented (Babbidge, 1968; Commission on Education of the Deaf, 1988; Marschark et al., 2002; Marschark &

Spencer, 2010; Rose, 2006). However, the practice of excluding Deaf culture and sign language and emphasizing oralism or monolingual English-only teaching continues to dominate deaf education and deaf education policy (Heiling, 1995; Scouten, 1984; Simms & Thumann, 2007). Lang (2003, p. 15) explained how Deaf people viewed those failures: "Deaf people themselves largely rejected the faddism and dreamy idealisms of the oralists and viewed oralism as an implausible ideology, surrounded by failure."

The value of deaf epistemologies is its intrinsic ability to inform researchers and policy makers. Armed with this knowledge, they can subject ideas gathered from deaf epistemologies to the rigors of scientific inquiry through applied classroom and empirical research. This has become urgent because of recent federal mandates such as the No Child Left Behind Act: All schools, including deaf schools, are now held accountable for the academic achievement of their students (Moores, 2010).

The challenge is to find a valid and reliable way to measure deaf students' academic growth and schools' overall performance. At present, assessment tools, in spite of their "universal design," are fraught with inherent bias against deaf students, making the test results unreliable and suspect (see Cawthon, 2009; Johnson, 2001; Johnson & Mitchell, 2008; Marschark et al., 2002; and Rose, 2006, for reviews). Most instruments assess knowledge and skills in one language—English—and neglect to assess actual knowledge and skills void of language barriers. They rarely assess the sign language abilities of Deaf children because there are few standardized sign language assessments suitable for assessing Deaf children's language. Grosjean (2008) views this as presenting a "fractional view" of the bilingual by focusing on only one language.

Regardless, the assessment based on standard epistemology has become the norm in measuring the effectiveness of individual programs, and deaf schools are not exempt in spite of the unique challenges associated with educating and testing deaf children (Cawthon, 2009). To date, the data specific to deaf children are relatively limited and difficult to obtain because of methods of collecting, compiling, and reporting the test scores of deaf students vary by individual state (Cawthon, 2008). For instance, in some states, such as Indiana, the scores of deaf students are not separated from those of the larger special education population, and in other states, such as Maryland, the scores of students attending a school for deaf students are not included in the statewide reports and therefore are not available on the Web. Understanding student performance is further complicated by the fact that many deaf students' test results are excluded in their school results. The percentage can be as high as 18% in California among mainstreamed students (Becker & Walters, 2007), whereas practically all students at the California School for the Deaf participate in the state-mandated testing program (H. Klopping, personal communication, October 17, 2008), making it difficult to compare the results.

Further clouding the issue is what Bosso (2008) described as deaf students failing their way into deaf schools, which makes school accountability complicated for these schools. More specifically, Bosso discussed the impact of the lack of early language access and the limited access to world knowledge among many deaf students. This results from the inability of parents to communicate effectively with their deaf children. After years of failure, many of these children are sent to a deaf school as a last resort. Consequently, this has created a difficult teaching situation for older deaf students with limited academic background. However, these schools are still held accountable for all of those students, including those deaf students who have recently transferred into a deaf school environment after years of failure in a mainstream program (Andrews & Covell, 2006; Raimondo, 2008).

Also complicating the matter of school accountability is the language used for high-stakes testing (Rose, 2006). Because most tests are developed in written English, many deaf people have difficulties passing these examinations because of language barriers rather than subpar knowledge or skills. Case (2008) explains why deaf students fare poorly on standardized tests: "For most deaf students, the fact is that standardized tests presume more familiarity with common English usage than these students generally attain in comparison with hearing peers of the same age" (p. 52).

The unique situation of the deaf population is often overlooked in all phases of the assessment process including the development of tests, the administration of the tests, and the provision of testing accommodations, resulting in subpar performance of deaf students (Bosso, 2008; Lollis, 2008; Thurlow, Johnstone, Thompson, & Case, 2008). For example, in California, a large portion of the second-grade test questions on the California Standards Test (CST) along with test items on California High School Exit Examination (CAHSEE) are sound-based items that ask about rhyming or appropriate syllabication (Moore, 2008). If a student takes a standardized test using ASL, this is considered a modification and thus invalidates the results. To illustrate, if a student takes the English-Language Arts test, part of CAHSEE, and has test questions signed, it is a modification and therefore that student did not pass the test. That student must then apply for a waiver rather than acknowledging that he performed well in his primary language (California Department of Education, n.d.). All of this has a potential negative impact on the test results for deaf children because they cannot fully access the test, especially when questions (for younger grades in particular) are sound-based and inherently biased in their presentation. This, subsequently, has an impact on the overall test scores at schools for the deaf (M. Berke, personal communication, January 20, 2011).

DEAF WAYS OF KNOWING—DOCUMENTING INDICATORS OF SUCCESS

Deaf students as a whole perform poorly on standardized English tests whether they are mainstreamed in a public school or attend a school for deaf students (Holt, Traxler, & Allen, 1997; Mitchell, 2008; Traxler, 2000). The database documenting language development among Deaf children in bilingual classrooms is meager but growing. The data on graduates of a school whose policies have been shaped by deaf epistemologies show that these students are performing at a higher level than their deaf peers elsewhere. For example, in California, students are required to pass both the English and mathematics components of CAHSEE to receive a high school diploma. Although on average only 46% of the graduates California School for the Deaf (an ASL/English bilingual program) passed the CAHSEE in the past four years (California School for the Deaf, 2010), there is a dramatic difference in the passing rate of students who began their academic careers at CSD prior to age seven, 80% of whom were able to pass the CAHSEE (H. Klopping, personal communication, December 1, 2010). In comparison, deaf students in the California mainstream programs are doing even worse, with only 10% of these students passing the CAHSEE (Becker & Walters, 2007).

Similar promising data are emerging from the Maryland School for the Deaf (MSD), another ASL/English bilingual program in which deaf epistemologies has been used to shape educational policies and practices. The majority of Deaf students are passing the Maryland State Assessment in the areas of English, mathematics, science, and social studies (Cawthon, 2008; Cronk-Walker, 2007/2008; J. Tucker, personal communication, July 15, 2008). Graduates of the Indiana School for the Deaf also have done relatively well compared to the national deaf population on the Stanford Achievement Test–Hearing Impaired between 1996 and 2003, with an average reading grade level of 8.25 (Geeslin et al., 2003). Furthermore, the differences between Indiana School for the Deaf students with deaf parents and those with hearing parents became less significant as the children got older. In cases in which students stayed seven years or more at the school, there was no significant difference in language and reading scores between students with deaf parents and those with hearing parents (Geeslin, 2007).

These results closely parallel the findings of the ASL/English bilingual project (Star Schools Project), led by sociolinguist Stephen Nover and his colleagues. Although not labeled deaf epistemologies, the focus of the five-year project, funded by the U.S. Department of Education, was to bridge the knowledge and beliefs espoused by Deaf educators and their hearing allies regarding deaf epistemologies using the scientific rigor expected of the standard epistemology. More specifically, the project attempted to move the knowledge and beliefs of the Deaf community regarding the development of literacy skills among deaf children from a theoretical framework to scientific, data-driven models and applications for effective teaching of deaf students.

In the Star Schools Project's 2002 final report submitted to the Department of Education and data reported in Andrews and Rusher (2010), it was noted that the 542 students who had teachers trained in bilingual methodologies performed at a significantly higher level than the national norms of deaf students on the English vocabulary and English language subtests of the ninth edition of the Stanford Achievement Test (SAT-9). More striking is the fact that the differences between students who had deaf parents and those with hearing parents vanished as students spent more time in the program (Nover et al., 2002). This project has since been absorbed by Gallaudet University and is operating under the Center for ASL/English Bilingual Education and Research (CAEBER) with the goal of building and strengthening empirical foundations for bilingual applications for classrooms where deaf children are educated.

In another research based on deaf epistemologies, a small-scale descriptive study was conducted in a public mainstream school with seven young deaf children (ages five to eight). Researchers reported that ASL/English bilingual teachers were effective in bringing these deaf children up to first grade level (Andrews, Ferguson, Roberts, &

Hodges, 1997). Another study conducted by DeLana, Gentry, and Andrews (2007) examined 25 deaf children in a mainstream setting. DeLana found that over a seven-year period, when taught by teachers trained in the use of bilingual strategies, Deaf children improved their test scores in English reading and language achievement using the SAT-9, with a statistical correlation between the years of ASL usage and the reading comprehension scores on the SAT-9 [r (22) = .508, $p < .05$] (DeLana et al., 2007).

In addition to these results discussed, studies have demonstrated the superiority of deaf children of deaf parents in achieving academic success (see Erting, 2003, for review). Other studies have produced empirical findings demonstrating the effectiveness of Deaf-centric practices that go beyond the deaf child/deaf parent superiority (e.g., DeLana et al., 2007; Mayer & Akamatsu, 2003; Strong & Prinz, 2000).

Although these findings are encouraging, the academic performance level of deaf students continues to be unsatisfactory across the board in light of their cognitive and linguistic potential. It is noteworthy that the work of Deaf scholars vis-à-vis deaf epistemologies continues to show the necessity of taking a holistic approach in measuring the effectiveness of a program and the success of its graduates. In addition to researching academic achievement, Deaf scholars are documenting the survival techniques of deaf people in the relatively hostile environments of hearing families and hearing-centric educational programs, focusing on their psychosocial, emotional, and linguistic needs rather than solely on academic achievement.

For example, data on deaf children's childhood experiences provide valuable information on how deaf students can be best supported in their educational endeavors (Oliva, 2004; Sheridan, 2001; Holcomb, 1998). More specifically, Oliva documented the experiences of mainstreamed deaf students. Sheridan focused her research on the social development and self-concept of deaf children, whereas I collected and examined data on deaf students' experiences in their attempts to become socially accepted by their peers at school, in both deaf schools and mainstreamed programs. In this sense, deaf epistemologies offer insights that help take a more comprehensive look at developmental strengths and challenges of deaf students by examining academic as well as social, emotional, linguistic, and cultural aspects of education.

CONCLUSION

I return to the question posed at the beginning of this chapter: What are the criteria for knowledge that are crucial for educating deaf students?

Deaf epistemologies are critical in identifying these criteria. Indeed, testimonies are an important component of the epistemologies of disenfranchised groups in general and in deaf education in particular. One only has to search the ERIC database on titles of doctoral dissertations to see the increasing numbers of studies that apply principles of deaf epistemologies or Deaf-centric perspectives in research design. Increasing numbers of Deaf professionals are staffing parent–infant programs, K–12 programs, postsecondary programs, and teacher-preparation programs.

Although deaf epistemologies rely heavily on personal testimonies, personal experiences, and observed outcomes that embody the justified beliefs of the Deaf community, they are critical components in gathering ideas, concepts, and ideologies that can then be tested with scientific precision. With the emerging community of Deaf researchers and their hearing peers seeking to quantify and qualify the effectiveness of Deaf-centric practices, deaf epistemologies need to be supported by additional across-the-board data-rich findings from empirical studies that meet the rigor of the standard epistemology. Such knowledge is now being made available through doctoral dissertations, research projects led by university professors, federal grant documents, school accountability reports, referred journal articles, and other publications.

While it has been argued that deaf epistemologies are based on old-school methods, this is not necessarily true. For instance, deaf children today have the benefit of the latest forms of technology, such as digital hearing aids and cochlear implants. These devices allow deaf children to utilize their hearing in ways that could never have been imagined before (Harkins & Bakke, 2003). Nevertheless, they have limitations, as there is nothing currently on the market that fully restores hearing for deaf children. Consequently, Deaf children continue to be impaired by barriers to their access to language and communication. These gaps will continue to prove devastating in terms of academic success if they are not remedied.

The field can look to deaf epistemologies for knowledge on how to use visual as well as auditory technologies, describe these communicative and linguistic gaps effectively, or even maximize the intrinsic communication and linguistic abilities of all deaf students. Deaf epistemologies provide knowledge on how deaf people can optimally use their visual strengths and to best compensate for their limited access to hearing. Deaf epistemologies also provide valuable insights for effectively and efficiently developing language and literacy competence, academic achievement, and successful integration into both Deaf and hearing societies. Deaf epistemologies provide knowledge on how family dynamics within families with a deaf child can be enhanced, expanded, and broadened. The vast knowledge generated by the collective experience of Deaf people, all of whom have varying degrees of hearing and speaking capabilities, has the potential to provide the information needed to achieve improved educational success for all deaf children.

With the individual and collective experiences and knowledge possessed by Deaf people regarding their lives in general and educational upbringings specifically, Benedict and Sass-Lehrer (2007), Harris, Holmes and Mertens (2009), and others have proposed that it is unethical not to actively include them and their perspectives in research endeavors and policy-making process. As Fred Schreiber, a tireless leader (and deaf epistemologist) of the National Association for the Deaf, aptly said, "The basic reason for becoming involved with deaf adults: we are your children grown. We can, in many instances, tell you the things your child would like to tell you, if he had the vocabulary and the experiences to put his feelings and needs into words" (Schreiber, 1969, cited in Schein, 1981, p. 57).

Harris et al. (2009) utilized Guba and Lincoln's (2005) paradigmatic model based on transformation, human rights, and social justice in designing a model that advocates for increasing Deaf people's voice in research design and data analysis. Such research can pick up where deaf epistemologies leaves off. One important part of Guba and Lincoln's model calls for transformative epistemology that requires a close collaboration between researchers and community members (not necessarily leaders but rather average people). Using this model, Deaf people are viewed as coresearchers, and their perspectives and knowledge are solicited in developing research questions, designing research, and analyzing data. In this way, Deaf knowledge vis-à-vis deaf epistemologies can serve as a basis for new knowledge gained through the standard epistemology.

In closing, it is obvious that many people in the field of deaf education, including educators, parents, and members of the Deaf community, seek knowledge that could translate into effective pedagogical practices with deaf children, knowledge that could elevate literacy levels among deaf children, knowledge that could consistently eliminate poor academic achievements of deaf children, and knowledge that could produce well-rounded Deaf adults. It is my contention that the knowledge represented by deaf epistemologies could launch us into years of productive research that empirically defines, tests, refines, and retests Deaf-centered beliefs, ideas, concepts, and ideologies. Although the standard epistemology uses scientific methods to gain such knowledge, deaf epistemologies must come first because they provide firsthand accounts on which "Deaf" knowledge is based. Clearly, both avenues are critical and should be considered valuable tools in developing policies and practices focused on improved quality of education and life for deaf children. For this reason, a relationship between the standard epistemology and deaf epistemologies should not be viewed as conflicting beliefs but as existing along a continuum that places deaf epistemologies in the forefront in the earnest pursuit of "truth."

My recommendations for further theorizing and research are as follows:

- In the pursuit of knowledge and truth related to "what works" in educating deaf children, the pedagogy of deaf students should be built on evidence-based practices informed by deaf epistemologies. Both quantitative and qualitative methods should be used for analysis.
- In the age of accountability, it is surprising that data for deaf students in the mainstream is not readily available. To analyze these data, a federal mandate is needed to make their scores known and hold both the schools for deaf students and mainstream programs accountable. The practice of concealing or collapsing mainstreamed deaf students' scores with other special education students needs to be discontinued.
- Data should be collected in different ways. Analysis should look at variables such as comparing students who have attended the program for their entire educational experience to those who have not, ASL skills of students and parents, effect of socioeconomic status of the family, how students of color perform compared to white students, and so on.
- With the majority of deaf students today graduating from a mainstream environment, deaf epistemologies can and should help shape future pedagogical practices in those programs regardless of the type of assistive technology, if any, the students have.

NOTE

1. The term *deaf* can be applied in many different ways. For the sake of clarity and specificity in the present chapter, *deaf* is used to refer to individuals whose hearing level warrants specialized services that are typically provided through deaf education. In following the convention within the field of Deaf studies, *Deaf* with capital D is used to specify deaf individuals who are also members of the Deaf community and use sign language as their primary mode of communication, regardless of their hearing level and ability to speak.

REFERENCES

Anderson, E. (1995). Feminist epistemology: An interpretation and a defense. *Hypatia, 10*(3), 50–84.

Andrews, J., & Covell, J. (2006). Preparing future teachers and doctoral-level leaders in deaf education: Meeting the challenge. *American Annals of the Deaf, 151*(4), 464–475.

Andrews, J., Ferguson, C., Roberts, S., & Hodges, P. (1997). What's up, Billy Jo? Deaf children and bilingual–bicultural instruction in east-central Texas. *American Annals of the Deaf, 142*(1), 16–25.

Andrews, J., & Franklin, C. (1996/1997). Why hire deaf teachers? *TEJAS: Texas Journal of Audiology and Speech Pathology, 12*(1), 120–131.

Andrews, J., Martin, G., & Rusher, M. (2009). *Shaping the river: Training doctoral level leaders in deaf education* (Office of Special Education Personnel Preparation Grant 2009–2012). Washington, DC: U.S. Department of Education.

Andrews, J., & Rusher, M. (2010). Codeswitching techniques: Evidence-based instructional practices for the ASL/English bilingual classroom. *American Annals of the Deaf, 155*(4), 407–424.

Babbidge, H. D. (1965). *Education of the deaf in the United States: A report to the secretary of health, education and welfare by his advisory committee of education of the deaf.* Washington, DC: U.S. Government Printing Office.

Bahan, B. (2008). Upon the formation of a visual variety of the human race. In H.-D. L. Bauman (Ed.), *Open your eyes: Deaf studies talking* (pp. 83–99). Minneapolis, MN: University of Minnesota Press.

Bailes, C. N. (1999). Deaf-centric teaching: A case study in ASL-English bilingualism. In. L. Bragg (Ed.), *Deaf world: A historical reader and primary sourcebook* (pp. 211–233). New York, NY: New York University Press.

Bakari, R. S. (1997). *Epistemology from an Afrocentric perspective: Enhancing black students' consciousness through an Afrocentric way of knowing.* Retrieved July 1, 2008, from DigitalCommons@University of Nebraska–Lincoln: http://digitalcommons.unl.edu/pocpwi2/20

Bauman, H.-D. L. (2008). Introduction: Listening to Deaf studies. In H.-D. L. Bauman (Ed.), *Open your eyes: Deaf studies talking* (pp. 1–34). Minneapolis, MN: University of Minnesota Press.

Baynton, D., Gannon, J., & Bergey, J. (2007). *Through Deaf eyes: A photographic history of an American Deaf community.* Washington, DC: Gallaudet University Press.

Bechter, F. (2008). The Deaf convert culture and its lessons for Deaf theory. In H.-D. L. Bauman (Ed.), *Open your eyes: Deaf studies talking* (pp. 60–82). Minneapolis, MN: University of Minnesota Press.

Becker, D. E., & Walters, C. (2007). *Independent evaluation of the California High School Exit Examination (CAHSEE): 2007 evaluation report.* Alexandria, VA: Human Resources Research Organization.

Benedict, B., & Sass-Lehrer, M. (2007). Deaf and hearing partnerships: Ethical and communication considerations. *American Annals of the Deaf, 152*(3), 275–282.

Berke, J. *Education—Charter schools for the deaf.* Retrieved January 11, 2011, from the About.com website: www.deafness.about.com/cs/schooling/a/charterschools.htm

Bjorlee, I. (1954, October). Deaf teachers of the deaf: Yesterday, today, tomorrow. *Silent Worker*, pp. 16–17.
Boatner, E. (1952, February). Deaf teachers of the deaf. *Silent Worker*, pp. 3–6.
Bosso, E. (2008). Testing, accountability, and equity for deaf students in Delaware. In R. C. Johnson & R. E. Mitchell (Eds.), *Testing deaf students in an age of accountability* (pp. 167–180). Washington, DC: Gallaudet University Press.
Boston University (n.d.). Retrieved on January 13, 2011, from http://www.bu.edu/sed/academics/graduate/cags/eddeaf/
Boyd, B. (1987). The National Leadership Training Program in the area of deafness: Its development and impact. *American Rehabilitation, 13*(3), 2–6.
Bragg, L. (2001). *Deaf world: A historical reader and primary sourcebook*. New York, NY: New York University Press.
Breivik, J. K. (2005). *Deaf identities in the making: Local lives, transnational connections*. Washington, DC: Gallaudet University Press.
California Department of Education. (n.d.). *Q and A for test variations*. Retrieved on January 30, 2011, from http://www.cde.ca.gov/ta/tg/hs/qandatestvar.asp#Q3
California School for the Deaf. (2010). *School accountability report card*. Retrieved on August 4, 2010, from http://www.axiomadvisors.net/livesarc/Presentation/SARCAdministration/Portals/Tabs/Portal.aspx?CDS=01316170131763&LanguageID=1&Preview=False&HidePDF=True
Case, B. (2008). Accommodations to improve instruction and assessment. In R. C. Johnson & R. E. Mitchell (Eds.), *Testing deaf students in an age of accountability* (pp. 51–62). Washington, DC: Gallaudet University Press.
Cawthon, S. W. (2008). No child left behind and schools for the deaf: Integration into the accountability framework. In R.C. Johnson & R. E. Mitchell (Eds.), *Testing deaf students in an age of accountability* (pp. 92–114). Washington, DC: Gallaudet University Press.
Cawthon, S. W. (2009). Professional development for teachers of students who are deaf or hard of hearing: Facing the assessment challenge. *American Annals of the Deaf, 154*(1), 50–61.
Commission on Education of the Deaf (COED). (1988). *Toward equality: Education of the deaf.* Washington, DC: U.S. Government Printing Office.
Cronk-Walker, N. (2007/2008, Winter). On deck for state assessments. *Maryland Bulletin*, pp. 4–5.
DeLana, M., Gentry, M. A., & Andrews, J. (2007). The efficacy of ASL/English bilingual education: Considering public schools. *American Annals of the Deaf, 152*(1), 73–87.
Erting, C. (2003). Language and literacy development in deaf children: Implications of a sociocultural perspective. In B. Bodner-Johnson & M. Sass-Lehrer (Eds.). *The young deaf or hard of hearing child: A family-centered approach to early education* (pp. 373–402). Baltimore, MD: Brookes.
Fleischer, L. (2008). Critical pedagogy and ASL videobooks. In H.-D. L.. Bauman (Ed.), *Open your eyes: Deaf studies talking* (pp. 158–168). Minneapolis, MD: University of Minnesota Press.
Freire, P. (1970). *Pedagogy of the oppressed*. New York, NY: Continuum.
Gannon, J. (1981). *Deaf heritage: A narrative history of deaf Americans*. Silver Spring, MD: National Association of the Deaf.
Geeslin, D., Charlebois, L., Fitzpatrick, L., Geeslin, H., Hazel-Jones, D., & Lawrence, C. (2003, August). *Can a deaf child have it all? Bilingual/bicultural philosophy*. Address to the conference of the American Speech-Language-Hearing Association, Chicago, IL.
Geeslin III, J. D. (2007). Deaf bilingual education: A comparison of the academic performance of deaf children of deaf parents and deaf children of hearing parents (Doctoral dissertation, Indiana University). *ProQuest Digital Dissertations*, 3287372.
Gertz, G. (2008). Dysconscious audism: A theoretical proposition. In H.-D. L. Bauman (Ed.), *Open your eyes: Deaf studies talking* (pp. 219–234). Minneapolis, MN: University of Minnesota Press.

Grosjean, F. (2008). *Studying bilinguals*. New York, NY: Oxford University Press.
Guba, E., & Lincoln, Y. (2005). Paradigmatic controversies, contradictions, and emerging confluences. In N. K. Denzin and Y. S. Lincoln (Eds.), *Handbook of qualitative research* (3rd ed.) (pp. 191–216). Thousand Oaks, CA: Sage.
Hamers, J. F. (1998). Cognitive and language development of bilingual children. In I. Parasnis (Ed.), *Cultural and language diversity and the Deaf experience* (pp. 51–78). Cambridge, UK: Cambridge University Press.
Harkins, J. E., & Bakke, M. (2003). Technologies for communication: Status and trends. In M. Marschark & P. E. Spencer (Eds.), *The Oxford handbook of Deaf studies, language, and education* (pp. 406–419). New York, NY: Oxford University Press.
Harris, R., Holmes, H., & Mertens, D. (2009). Research ethics in sign language communities. *Sign Language Studies, 9*(2), 104–131.
Heiling, K. (1995). *The development of deaf children: Academic achievement levels and social processes*. Hamburg, Germany: Signum.
Hoffmeister, R. J. (1990). ASL and its implications for education. In H. Bornstein (Ed.), *Manual communication: Implications for education* (pp. 81–107). Washington, DC: Gallaudet University Press.
Holcomb, T. (1998). Social assimilation of deaf high school students: The role of school environment. In I. Parasnis (Ed.), *Cultural and language diversity and the Deaf experience* (pp. 181–198). New York, NY: Cambridge University Press.
Holt, J. A., Traxler, C. B., & Allen, T. E. (1997). *Interpreting the scores: A user's guide to the 9th Edition Stanford Achievement Test for educators of deaf and hard-of-hearing students* (Technical Report 97-1). Washington, DC: Gallaudet University, Gallaudet Research Institute.
Humphries, T. (2004). The modern deaf self: Indigenous practices and educational imperatives. In B. J. Brueggemann (Ed.), *Literacy and deaf people: Cultural and contextual perspectives* (pp. 29–46). Washington, DC: Gallaudet University Press.
Humphries, T. (2008). Talking culture and culture talking. In H.-D. L. Bauman (Ed.), *Open your eyes: Deaf studies talking* (pp. 35–41). Minneapolis, MN: University of Minnesota Press.
Humphries, T., & Allen, B. (2008). Reorganizing teacher preparation in deaf education. *Sign Language Studies, 8*(2), 160–180.
Jankowski, K. A. (1997). *Deaf empowerment: Emergence, struggle, and rhetoric*. Washington, DC: Gallaudet University Press.
Johnson, R. C. (2001, Spring/Summer). High stakes testing and deaf students: Some research perspectives. *Research at Gallaudet*, pp. 1–6.
Johnson, R. C., & Mitchell, R. E. (2008). *Testing deaf students in an age of accountability*. Washington, DC: Gallaudet University Press.
Jordan, I. K., Gustason, G., & Rosen, R. (1976). Current communication trends at programs for the deaf. *American Annals of the Deaf, 121*(6), 527–532.
Klein, P. D. (2005). Epistemology. In E. Craig (Ed.), *Routledge encyclopedia of philosophy* (pp. 524-532). London, UK: Routledge.
Koertge, N. (1996). Feminist epistemology: Stalking an un-dead horse. In P. Gross & N. Levitt (Eds.), *The flight from science and reason* (pp. 413–419). Baltimore, MD: Johns Hopkins University Press.
Ladd, P. (2003). *Understanding Deaf culture: In search of Deafhood*. Clevedon, UK: Multilingual Matters.
Ladd, P. (2008). Colonialism and resistance: A brief history of Deafhood. In H.-D. L. Bauman (Ed.), *Open your eyes: Deaf studies talking* (pp. 42–59). Minneapolis, MN: University of Minnesota Press.
Lane, H. (2008). Do deaf people have a disability? In H.-D. L. Bauman (Ed.), *Open your eyes: Deaf studies talking* (pp. 277–292). Minneapolis, MN: University of Minnesota Press.
Lane, H., Hoffmeister, R., & Bahan, B. (1996). *A journey into the Deaf-World*. San Diego, CA: DawnSignPress.

Lang, H. (2003). Perspectives on the history of deaf education. In M. Marschark & P. E. Spencer (Eds.), *The Oxford handbook of deaf studies, language, and education* (pp. 9–20). New York, NY: Oxford University Press.

Levesque, J. (1991, August). Do we continue this tragedy? *DCARA News*, p. 2.

Lollis, J. (2008). High-stakes testing of deaf students in North Carolina. In R. C. Johnson & R. E. Mitchell (Eds.), *Testing deaf students in an age of accountability* (pp. 136–148). Washington, DC: Gallaudet University Press.

Mahshie, S. N. (1995). *Educating deaf children bilingually*. Washington, DC: Gallaudet University Press.

Maller, S. J. (2003). Intellectual assessment of deaf people: A critical review of core concepts and issues. In M. Marschark & P. E. Spencer (Eds.), *The Oxford handbook of deaf studies, language, and education* (pp. 451–463). New York, NY: Oxford University Press.

Marschark, M., Lang, H., & Albertini, J. (2002). *Educating deaf students: From research to practice*. New York, NY: Oxofrd University Press.

Marschark, M., & Spencer, P. E. (2003). Epilogue: What we know, what we don't know, and what we should know. *The Oxford handbook of deaf studies, language, and education* (pp. 491–494). New York, NY: Oxford University Press.

Marschark, M., & Spencer, P. E. (2010). *The Oxford handbook of deaf studies, language, and education*, Vol. 2. New York, NY: Oxford University Press.

Mayer, C., & Akamatsu, C. T. (2003). Bilingualism and literacy. In M. Marschark & P. E. Spencer (Eds.). *The Oxford handbook of deaf studies, language, and education* (pp. 136–150). New York, NY: Oxford University Press.

McDaniel College. (n.d.) Retrieved on January 13, 2011, from http://www.mcdaniel.edu/deaf_education.htm

Metro Deaf School. (n.d.). Retrieved on January 13, 2011, from http://www.mdsmn.org/about-us/history/

Mitchell, R. (2008). Academic achievement of deaf students. In R. Johnson & R. Mitchell (Eds.), *Testing deaf students in an age of accountability* (pp. 38–50). Washington, DC: Gallaudet University Press.

Moll, L. (2010). Mobilizing culture, language, and educational practices: Fulfilling the promise of Mendez and Brown. *Educational Researcher, 39*(6), 451–460.

Moore, P. (2008). The potential harm to deaf students of high stakes testing in California. In R. Johnson & R. Mitchell (Eds.), *Testing deaf students in an age of accountability* (pp. 217–238). Washington, DC: Gallaudet University Press.

Moores, D. F. (2001). *Educating the deaf: Psychology, principles, and practices* (5th ed.). Boston, MA: Houghton Mifflin.

Moores, D. F. (2010). Epistemologies, deafness, learning, and teaching. *American Annals of the Deaf, 154*(5), 447–455.

Nover, S. M., & Andrews, J. F. (1998). *Critical pedagogy in deaf education: Bilingual methodology and staff development* (USDLC Star Schools Project Report No. 1). Santa Fe, NM: New Mexico School for the Deaf.

Nover, S. M., Andrews, J. F., Baker, S., Everhart, V. S., & Bradford, M. (2002). *Star School USDLC Engaged Learning Project No. 5: ASL/English bilingual staff development project in deaf education: Evaluation and impact study, final report 1997–2002*. Santa Fe, NM: New Mexico School for the Deaf.

Oliva, G. (2004). *Alone in the mainstream*. Washington, DC: Gallaudet University Press.

Padden, C. (1980). The Deaf community and the culture of deaf people. In C. Baker & R. Battison (Eds.), *Sign language and the Deaf community* (pp. 89–104). Silver Spring, MD: National Association of the Deaf.

Pahz, J. A., & Pahz, C. S. (1978). *Total Communication: The meaning behind the movement to expand educational opportunities for deaf children*. Springfield, IL: Thomas.

Parasnis, I. (1998). On interpreting the Deaf experience within the context of cultural and language diversity. In I. Parasnis (Ed.), *Cultural and language diversity and the deaf experience* (pp. 3–19). Cambridge, MA: Cambridge University Press.
Raimondo, B. (2008). Accountability in the education of deaf students under the Individuals With Disabilities Education Act and No Child Left Behind. In R. C. Johnson & R. E. Mitchell (Eds.), *Testing deaf students in an age of accountability* (pp. 17–37). Washington, DC: Gallaudet University Press.
Reagan, T. (2010). *Language policy and planning for sign languages*. Washington, DC: Gallaudet University Press.
Rocky Mountain Deaf School. (n.d.). Retrieved on January 11, 2011, from http://www.rmdeafschool.net
Rose, S. (2006). *Monitoring progress of students who are deaf or hard of hearing*. Retrieved from the National Center on Student Progress Monitoring website: http://www.studentprogress.org
Rusher, M., Martin, T., Gentry, M., Jackson, K., & Andrews, J. (2009). *Continuing the deaf mosaic: Training highly qualified deaf educators to service EC-12 deaf children in Texas and Louisiana* (Personnel Preparation Training Grant). Washington, DC: US Department of Education.
Schein, J. (Ed.). (1981). *A rose for tomorrow: Biography of Frederick C. Schrieber*. Silver Spring, MD: National Association of the Deaf.
Scouten, E. L. (1984). *Turning points in the education of deaf people*. Danville, IL: Interstate Printers and Publishers.
Sheridan, M. (2001). *Inner lives of deaf children: Interviews and analysis*. Washington, DC: Gallaudet University Press.
Simms, L., & Thumann, H. (2007). In search of a new, linguistically and culturally sensitive paradigm in deaf education. *American Annals of the Deaf, 152*(3), 302–311.
Simms, L., Rusher, M., Andrews, J., & Coryell, J. (2008). Apartheid in deaf education: Examining workforce diversity. *American Annals of the Deaf, 153*(5), 517–522.
Simms, L., & Moers, L. (2009, April). ASL/English Bilingual Early Childhood Project. Conference held at Gallaudet University, Washington, DC.
Spencer, M. (2008). Lessons learned and opportunities ignored since *Brown v. Board of Education*: Youth development in a color-blind society. *Educational Researcher, 37*(5), 253–266.
Stedt, J. D., & Moores, D. F. (1990). Manual codes on English and American sign language: Historical perspectives and current realities. In H. Bornstein (Ed.), *Manual communication: Implications for education* (pp. 1–20). Washington, DC: Gallaudet University Press.
Stewart, J. Y. (2007, March 3). Wayne McIntire, 95, helped establish CSUN as a model in the field of deaf education. *Los Angeles Times*, p. B8.
Stone, R. (2000). A bold step: Changing the curriculum for culturally Deaf and hard of hearing students. In P. E. Spencer, C. J. Erting, & M. Marschark (Eds.), *The deaf child in the family and at school* (pp. 229–238). Mahwah, NJ: Erlbaum.
Strong, M., & Prinz, P. (2000). Is ASL skill related to English literacy? In C. Chamberlain, J. Morford, & K. Mayberry (Eds.), *Language acquisition by eye* (pp. 131–141). Mahwah, NJ: Erlbaum.
Thurlow, M., Johnstone, C., Thompson, S., & Case, B. (2008). Using universal design research and perspectives to increase the validity of scores on large-scale assessments. In R. Johnson & R. Mitchell (Eds.), *Testing deaf students in an age of accountability* (pp. 63–75). Washington, DC: Gallaudet University Press.
Tompkins, L. B. (2004). Cultural and linguistic voice in the deaf bilingual experience. In B. J. Brueggemann (Ed.), *Literacy and deaf people: Cultural and contextual perspectives* (pp. 139–156). Washington, DC: Gallaudet University Press.
Traxler, C. (2000). The Stanford Achievement Test, 9th edition: National norming and performance standards for deaf and hard of hearing students. *Journal of Deaf Studies and Deaf Education, 5*, 337–348.
Utah Association for the Deaf. (n.d.). Retrieved on January 21, 2011, from http://www.uad.org

Valli, C. (1990). A taboo exposed: Using ASL in the classroom. In M. Garretson (Ed.), *Eyes, hands, voices: Communication issues among deaf people*, pp. 129–131. Silver Spring, MD: National Association of the Deaf.

Van Cleve, J. V., & Crouch, B. (1989). *A place of their own: Creating the deaf community in America.* Washington, DC: Gallaudet University Press.

Vernon, M. (1970). The role of deaf teachers in the education of deaf children. *Deaf American, 22*, 17–20.

Wilcox, S. (2004). Struggling for a voice: An interactionist view of language and literacy in deaf education. In B. J. Brueggemann (Ed.), *Literacy and deaf people: Cultural and contextual perspectives* (pp. 157–191). Washington, DC: Gallaudet University Press.

Woll, B., & Ladd, P. (2003). Deaf communities. In M. Marschark & P. E. Spencer (Eds.), *The Oxford handbook of deaf studies, language, and education* (pp. 151–163). New York, NY: Oxford University Press.

Wright, H. K. (2003). An endarkened feminist epistemology? Identity, difference, and the politics of representation in educational research. *Qualitative Studies in Education, 16*(2), 197–214.

SUGGESTIONS FOR FURTHER READING

Brueggemann, B. J. (Ed.). (2004). *Literacy and deaf people: Cultural and contextual approaches.* Washington, DC: Gallaudet University Press.

Christensen, K. (Ed.). (2000). *Deaf plus: A multicultural perspective.* San Diego, CA: DawnSignPress.

Lindgren, K. A., DeLuca, D., & Napoli, D. J. (Eds.). (2008). *Signs and voices: Deaf culture, identity, language, and arts.* Washington, DC: Gallaudet University Press.

Padden, C., & Humphries, T. (2005). *Inside deaf culture.* Cambridge, MA: Harvard University Press.

8

Deaf Worldviews, Views of the Deaf World, and the Role of Deaf Children of Hearing Parents in Creating a Deaf Epistemology

Margery Miller

Epistemology is part of the field of philosophy, which examines what is considered to be knowledge: what we know about something or someone (see also Paul & Moores, Chapter 1). Epistemological studies attempt to determine what is "true" knowledge, which can be verified, what is unknown, and what can be verified as a so-called fact but in actuality has no basis in truth whatsoever. Some scholars try to combine these parts, which are viewed as being based in truth from someone's perspective (because rarely is there absolute truth), to produce a coherent, holistic, and defensible theory (Bradie, 1994; Raskin, 2002). This theory includes the pieces of knowledge but is actually greater than the sum of the truths, and it can be thought of as a stronger theory or view than one based on the component "weaker" truths. An interesting element of one view of epistemology is that "truth" is viewed as being relative, fluid, interactive, and context dependent.

In the past, truth was viewed as more fixed, stagnant, rigid, and absolute. Many people have come to see truth, perspectives, worldviews, views of the world, and facts as changing and interacting with the environment—or multiple environments. Thus, epistemology, the field of discovering what we know, must be fluid itself and analytically reactive to multiple environments (Kukla, 2000; Sexton, 1997).

CONSTRUCTIVISM

There are many different types of epistemological approaches, but the two that form the basis for this essay are *individual constructivism* and *group constructivism*. Individual constructivism views knowledge as coming from a person, who has come to "know" something. It is created through the eyes and existing constructs of a person, which influence interpretations (Sexton, 1997). With this model, nothing is assumed to be a universal truth and information is neither objective nor factual (Raskin, 2002). Your view or your reality may or may not have anything to do with an external reality, but it still exists and is your personal, constructivist view of the world—your own epistemology. This constructivist view has strong reflections of relativism: It is futile to search for universal truths and any model or epistemological construct is as worthy and accurate as any other. Thus, it would be impossible to search for what is true and what is falsely claimed as true, because all truth would be individually constructed and relative to the perspectives, interpretations, and views relative to that one person.

Lest we be led to believe that there is no pattern to constructing a personal notion of truth, we are only referring to individual truths and theories that have come about as the person becomes aware of important inconsistencies a notion or fact may have relative to other knowledge or facts that the individual has come to believe. If a notion is too different from previously held strong notions of truth, the new information will be rejected as false. If, however, a new construction can adjust enough to integrate prior notions of truth or theories viewed as facts and knowledge, then both the new piece of information and older notions can exist and form a larger epistemological truth. This is similar in many ways to the Piagetian principles within cognitive development where our concepts change and evolve as we accommodate and assimilate our conceptualizations to new incoming facts and experiences (Duncan, 1995; Smith, 1993).

Social constructivism, on the other hand, only recognizes the worth of an individual's view of a "truth" or way of knowing if many other people agree with it (Kukla, 2000; Searle, 1995). Thus if there is an agreement among people about knowledge constructions, then it becomes a truth or a reality merely because most of the individuals who make up a social group view it that way. Social constructivism is one possible explanation of why strongly held beliefs about the "truths" of educating d/Deaf or hard of hearing children[1] appear in radically different forms, each one pushing in a drastically different direction.

No new facts or supportive evidence will alter these ways of knowing or views of the language and life issues of people who are d/Deaf or hard of hearing, because there are sufficient numbers of people who hold the same beliefs, thus perpetuating the existence of parallel but incompatible deaf epistemologies. Examples abound, but the classic ones are the strongly held beliefs about the best educational methods for d/Deaf students, including oralism or manualism; Manual Codes on English (MCE), American Sign Language (ASL), or other "natural" sign languages from other countries; and inclusionary educational practices or uniquely designed separate educational practices.

Perhaps they are all true for some, perhaps not. Perhaps one is the "truth" and the other views are "false." Perhaps none of these views represent the real truth and are mere socially constructed epistemologies because they are beliefs held by enough people to make them viable. Research results in this area vary and often muddy the waters more than they illuminate the "truth."

EVOLUTIONARY EPISTEMOLOGY

Another important view is *evolutionary epistemology*. This idea includes important notions of individual and social constructivism, in that reality is not absolute and truth does not exist independently from the people viewing it, but evolutionary epistemology also states that the purpose of arriving at these relative truths (individually or in a group) is clear. We construct these truths to support us as we adapt to our environment as a totality. Construction is a continuous process of adaptation to one's environment, and it is processed at the biological, psychological, and/or social levels of our beings (Bradie, 1994). The psychological and the social ways we humans adapt as we try to make sense of our own perceived realities are propelled by our selective attention to pieces of knowledge. When held in combination with other truths, they assist us in surviving in our piece of the world. That is, we choose to attend to and place our own interpretation on observations, feelings, events, and perceived patterns.

MEMETICS

A variation on constructivism is called *memetics* (see also Raike, Chapter 12). Although in memetics individual or group constructivism is important, it also recognizes the permanence of knowledge. That is, knowledge does not need to be constructed by every human being independently; it can be passed from person to person without individuals coming to "know" these truths on their own as an adaptive life function. If enough people believe a transmitted piece of knowledge is a useful truth, it continues to exist and draw followers and believers, even if this fact or worldview is not actually supportive of survival at a biological, psychological, or social level.

The mere notion that a factual interpretation is widely held by others in a group or by a highly respected individual will influence some others to hold this belief as fact, even if it is in direct opposition to what would be most beneficial to the person's survival physically or emotionally. Therefore, this belief will be held to be true in spite of the fact that its premises, predictions, and "truths" can be proven wrong in many ways (Heylighen, 1992).

Studies on friendships tend to show that although we may differ on the surface from our friends, we tend to select friends who believe what we believe and interpret life and other people's behavior in ways similar to our ways (Aboud & Mendelson, 1996). Thus, we use the worldviews of our friends to validate our own, perpetuating our notion of truth and closing out other possibilities.

Although they are similar, there is a fine but important line between social constructivism and memetics. Constructivism views knowledge or truths as coming from the socially held and communicated beliefs of key groups, where memetics sees the groups or communities holding certain beliefs, as the creators of truth and knowledge (Heylighen, 1992). Memetics includes the notion that individuals can transmit a cognitive or behavioral pattern to other people in a way similar to the evolutionary transmission of genes (Dawkins, 1976; Moritz, 1990).

Dawkins described three of the critical components for a way of knowing to become a meme (a transmitted belief) that will be transferred to others (Dawkins, 1976; Moritz, 1990):

1. The "truth" being disseminated to others in the group must remain faithful to the original concept. If the transmitted belief is similar to the belief of the newer members of the social group, the "copy" will be more consistent with the original.
2. *Fecundity* is the concept that the speed of the spreading contributes to the strength of the meme.
3. The longevity (the length of time a notion or worldview has been in existence) contributes to its strength and frequency among the social group.

Even those who adhere to the existence of evolutionarily established truths admit that there is a mitigating factor where individuals do exert some kind of rational (also subjective) judgment on the accuracy or usefulness of various truths. It is the use of these personal intuitions, partly from experiences and partly from reviews of more objectively based "evidence," that mitigates the unbridled replication of memes among newer group members. Not only are our senses of knowing about ourselves and our culture subject to the views of others, but they also are shaped by our personal levels of independent thinking and our personal strengths for taking unique, more "truthful," and often unpopular stands.

DEAF EPISTEMOLOGIES AND SELF-IDENTITY

Deaf individuals, like other human beings, have multiple identities and are influenced by a variety of factors. Sometimes the identities are integrated, and sometimes they are fragmented. As noted by many scholars (Hauser, O'Hearn, McKee, Steider, & Thew, 2010; Holcomb, 2010; Miller, 2010; Moores, 2010; Wang, 2010; see also De Clerck, Chapter 2, and Parasnis, Chapter 4), Deaf people have numerous identity pressures and typically face more complex situations, in that most of the systems in which they find themselves are under the control of hearing/speaking people, organizations, and agencies (Corker, 1994).

Society imposes external pressures on deaf people to take on certain identities, to behave, think, and feel one particular way or another. These pressures influence deaf people, who strive to belong to select groups, such as their families. Corker (1994, p. 18) states, "All deaf people, whether they choose to affiliate with other deaf people, or not, work within hearing systems, use hearing interpreters, teachers, doctors, and solicitors, teach sign language to hearing people and (usually) have hearing parents. Despite the fact that all systems begin and end with the individual, the power and influence of the majority system cannot be denied."

It is important that the large majority of deaf (and hard of hearing) children are born to hearing parents and raised most often with hearing siblings. Erikson (1959, 1966), in particular, has stressed the critical importance of early and continued relations between the child and parents and other family members. Given the pressure from the majority hearing culture for "inclusion" of these children into hearing classrooms, with the belief that exposure to hearing role models will result in improved speech, English language skills, academic achievement, and social competence, one might expect that the presence of a d/Deaf or hard of hearing child in predominantly hearing families would lead to children who are comfortable in the hearing world. Of course, often this is not the case; instead, it may be the seed of discontent at an early age: In the eyes of other family members, they may be considered disabled or poor copies of the hearing prototype, of which other family members are masters.

Even the phrases "a deaf child in a hearing family" or "a deaf child in a hearing classroom" signifies an unconscious bias and denigration of the deaf family or class member. There cannot be a deaf child in a hearing family; it is a family with deaf and hearing members. There cannot be a deaf student in a hearing class; it is a class with deaf and hearing students. Anything less than this is prejudicial. A deaf child may have parents and siblings who can hear, but the "truth" is that it is no longer a hearing family once a deaf child is born into it. Lack of acknowledgment of this truth creates possible negative feelings and self-perceptions in deaf children of hearing parents, especially those who rarely interact with other people who are deaf.

MEMBERSHIP IN THE DEAF CULTURE

As might be expected, there are differences in what characteristics are requisite for membership in Deaf culture or the Deaf community. Deaf professional leaders such as Ladd (2003) and Padden and Humphries (1988, 2005), as well as hearing professionals such as Bauman (2008) and Lane (1992, 2008), have addressed the issue at length. Padden and Humphries (2005) illustrate the complexity as follows:

> Self-identification with the group and skill in ASL should be important diagnostic factors in deciding who is Deaf. But the bounded distinction between the terms Deaf and deaf represents only part of the dynamic of how Deaf people talk about themselves. Deaf people are both Deaf and deaf, and their discussions, even arguments, over issues of identity show that these two categories are often interrelated in complex ways. (p. 3)

Some Deaf people and some hearing people have worldviews that make distinctions between groups such as those born deaf or deafened at a very early age and those who are deafened later in life. For example, the medical model is usually viewed negatively when applied to those born deaf or who became deaf at a very early age (usually prelingually) but may be viewed as the right model for adults deafened once past early childhood or adolescence because they really have suffered a loss, as opposed to Deaf people, who are linguistically and culturally unique from the start (Corker, 1994).

Lane (1992) exemplifies this position:

> An embarrassment for the medical model of cultural deafness heretofore was that this "pathology" had no medical treatment. With cochlear implants, however, the medical specialty of otology has been expanding its traditional clientele beyond adventitiously deafened hearing people who seek treatment for whom an infirmity model is appropriate to include members of the Deaf community, for whom it is not. (p. 226)

This leads to the somewhat contradictory conclusion that a person who is born deaf is not disabled because he or she has never heard, but a person who loses his or her hearing *is* disabled because he or she once heard. Corker (1994, p. 28) commented that Lane's implication is that deafened people are not deaf and they are not hearing; therefore, they must be disabled as opposed to deafened and certainly are not part of the "real" Deaf community.

APPLICATIONS OF EPISTEMOLOGICAL FOUNDATIONS TO THE CULTURAL TRANSMISSION PROCESS OF BELIEFS IN THE DEAF COMMUNITY

It is important to point out that as a hearing person attempting to describe observed patterns and to understand the Deaf culture and identity epistemologies, I am keenly aware of several things. I cannot know what it means to be Deaf. The philosophical notion of subjectivism must be even more rigorously applied to me and my thoughts on the subject as someone outside of the culture. The only thing we can be sure of, and even that is uncertain according to some philosophers, is the knowing of ourselves, our conscious acts, and our personhood (Potter, 1994). Some even doubt that we can really know if there is a world outside of ourselves, so commenting on these observed or perceived observed "realities" may be a nonreal pursuit.

Often, researchers talk about the natural language of the Deaf community in the United States, American Sign Language (ASL), as coming largely from Deaf adults who make up this social and linguistic group, and it is passed on one of two ways. There is direct and immediate transmission from parents who are Deaf and members of this sociolinguistic group of ASL users to their Deaf (and often to their hearing) children, just as the culture(s) and language(s) used in China, the United States, France, Nigeria, and so on are passed from hearing parents to their hearing children within their families. Thus, when searching for the source of most of our "Deaf epistemologies," that is, their views of the world, most would look to the Deaf parent with Deaf children as being the most common source of transmission.

The residential schools for the Deaf are another source of language and culture transmission in the United States even when the parents of the Deaf child are not Deaf. With many Deaf role models working in the dormitories and classes, it seems likely that these institutions and the Deaf children of Deaf parents are rich sources of epistemologies for this social group and for transmission of widely held beliefs of Deaf culture. The beliefs change only to the degree that the Deaf adults with Deaf children, or who had Deaf parents themselves, change their truths, beliefs, and views of the world—which behavior patterns or choices characterize Deaf culture, which characterize the "hearing" world and how their members view Deaf people, and which characterize institutions that have both Deaf and hearing members.

Deaf children of Deaf parents are viewed as the prototypical and developmentally "ideal" deaf children (Miller, 2006), having close to "normal patterns of development in social, linguistic, and cognitive domains relative to hearing peers" (Marschark, 1993, p. 7). Some researchers would argue that with early identification of a deaf or hard of hearing child, early and appropriate intensive intervention, and an intact central nervous system and cognitively related genetic structures (that is, normal intelligence), deaf children of hearing parents develop as well as Deaf children of Deaf parents (Yoshinaga-Itano, Coulter, & Thomson, 2000; Yoshinaga-Itano, & Downey, 1996).

Regardless of the comparative course of development, on the surface, Deaf children of Deaf parents will become potential transmitters of Deaf culture and deaf epistemologies, as compared with deaf children of hearing parents who lack exposure to the Deaf adult community or their Deaf children. Scholars and leaders of Deaf culture often emphasize that Deaf children of Deaf adults are the important source of the existence and transmission of the language and culture of the signing Deaf adult community. These authors often describe the "beliefs," "preferences," and "values" of the Deaf adult community without data-based evidence to support these descriptions, although there are some exceptions.

Miller (2003) and others described a different view of the transmission process of Deaf culture or Deaf identity. For example, Miller, Moores, and Sicoli (2003) investigated college students' preferences for the hearing status of their future children with participants from a college known for its Deaf culture and bilingual environment. This was an attempt to verify or refute the commonly held belief that Deaf adults prefer to have deaf children rather than hearing children, in spite of the fact that most Deaf adults will in fact have hearing children. The results of this study indicated that 97% of the Deaf college age participants stated they had no preference in terms of the hearing/deaf status of their future offspring. The results did not seem to substantiate the long-held belief that among those in Deaf culture environments a strong preference for having deaf children would be found.

Marschark (1993, p.19) has called descriptions such as these "largely anecdotal," and although that is currently changing with an increase in research to define the cultural beliefs of this unique sociolinguistic group, for the most part it still is true. Much of the sociocultural descriptions rely on the views and described epistemologies of Deaf adults of Deaf parents or of Deaf adults who have come to embrace and internalize these perceived values of the culture, even if their parents were hearing and they themselves were late recipients of Deaf culture exposure and influences. Like any other culture, the Deaf adult community is a dynamic culture with coordinated changes in epistemologies. For example, as more deaf and hard of hearing students become educated in public school systems in the counties in which they reside and fewer students are educated in residential schools for the deaf, beliefs may shift.

As cochlear implants become more common, even for some Deaf children of Deaf parents and for some Deaf adults, the notion that hearing people (who view being deaf as a disability instead of as a sociocultural and linguistic difference) are trying to erase the Deaf culture and apply a pathological model to the medical interventions (cochlear implants) for these children has to change. Cochlear implants are a significant medical procedure to "remove" the inability to hear and to "add" hearing acuity. If Deaf parents with Deaf children are now embracing cochlear implants for their children and sending them into mainstreamed settings or combined educational settings, then how does the epistemology of Deaf people still maintain that hearing parents who implant their very young children are seeing their children as "defective" when Deaf parents within the culture sometimes do the same thing?

New epistemologies need to emerge with new memes describing the differences between hearing parents who do this and Deaf parents who do this. The new "truth" might state that Deaf parents can still expose their children to ASL and Deaf culture. Thus, an even stronger "truth" may be that it is acceptable for deaf parents to have this surgery performed on their children, but it is still "wrong" for hearing parents to do so because they may not be exposing their deaf children to ASL and Deaf culture.

The new nuances of Deaf adult epistemologies will have to be redefined as behavior patterns of many of its leaders (Deaf adults of Deaf parents) change and appear to fit into the dominant culture's ways of viewing medical intervention with Deaf children. Distinctions will become part of a new Deaf epistemology. Rationalizations will be developed so that hearing parents and hearing medical and rehabilitation practices can still be viewed as advancing a pathological model of being deaf, and Deaf adults (even those who choose implants for their children or themselves) will not be viewed in the same way.

However, it may not be the Deaf children of Deaf adults who have been transmitting some of the stronger views about the dominant culture (hearing people) or deaf epistemologies. As Miller (2003) suggests, it may be a combination of these culturally affiliated Deaf parents and Deaf children, along with the many deaf children raised by hearing parents and taught by mostly hearing teachers. It is these children who have what Miller (2003) refers to as the "culture of shared experiences," which may be the major transmitting force for deaf epistemologies.

These common experiences, although they may include many positive ones, are often based on the negative experiences of linguistic/communicative exclusion from family discussions at meal time, holiday gatherings, and so on. The common experiences often include feelings of inferiority as they are labeled as "special education" students and interact with neighbors who may be warm but do not form intense and complex relationships because of communication access issues. Views of the hearing world's treatment of deaf people comes through as accommodations and changes may or may not happen as needed.

Marginalization of many deaf and hard of hearing children in public schools may take place inadvertently and contribute to personal epistemologies about what it means to be deaf. Watching younger but hearing siblings have more responsibility than deaf children for watching other children in the family shows how even loving parents view differing capabilities of deaf and hearing people. Once a deaf child raised in this kind of loving but not necessarily optimal environment becomes an adult, one of two things may happen. (1) They stay in the hearing world with their hearing extended family and they do not become part of the Deaf adult community. They see their lives as productive, positive, and similar to their hearing peers. They do not long for membership in a community defined by being Deaf and they are certainly not carriers of Deaf epistemologies. (2) They sense that they are missing an important piece of themselves, much in the same way that adopted children may long to fill in the pieces of their own identities by learning about their biological parents. These teens and young adults who are deaf search for something that will make them Deaf: whole and joined with others who have a shared culture of common experiences.

Deaf teens and young adults who have been part of the Deaf community all along do not share many of the same experiences of deaf children who have largely functioned with hearing people. Deaf children of Deaf adults get a watered-down version of views against the dominant hearing culture. Although one can suggest that deaf children with hearing parents receive no version of this worldview, they live it every day, and when joined with others like themselves and with the larger Deaf adult community they realize that they do have a "culture of shared experiences," as Miller has described.

This is a more plausible explanation of one of the key components for deaf epistemologies: The transmission is experience itself. One often hears from people who try to reduce the importance of the Deaf culture on the development of Deaf and deaf children by saying that there is no way that the tenets of a culture can be transmitted without exposure to that culture. I am usually one of them. However, in the case of deaf children with hearing parents, they come to know some of these beliefs, because they are not beliefs but truths. They are truths—their truths—realized through a culture of common experiences.

Consideration of deaf epistemologies is in a nascent stage, and there is a need for a wide range of theorizing and research. Within the context of the current chapter, my recommendations are as follows:

- The individual and social epistemologies of Deaf children of Deaf parents and the individual and social epistemologies of deaf children of hearing parents should be studied for commonalities and differences.
- The individual and social epistemologies of Deaf individuals and deaf individuals should be studied for commonalities and differences.
- Educational inclusion, universal neonatal screening and early intervention, increases in cochlear implants, and revolutionary changes in technology present deaf individuals today with far different realities than in the past. Each of these separately and together should be investigated for epistemological implications.
- Similarities and differences related to age at onset, extent of hearing loss, educational experiences, racial/ethnic status, and so on should be studied.

NOTE

1. There is variation in the literature in the use of uppercase D and lowercase d in referring to individuals and groups, including terms such as *deaf, Deaf, d/Deaf,* and *D/deaf.* In some cases "and/or hard of hearing" is added. In this chapter, I use *deaf* to refer to individuals with an audiometric hearing loss and *Deaf* in a sociocultural sense to refer to those individuals who have a cultural attachment to a Deaf community.

REFERENCES

Aboud, F. E., & Mendelson, M. J. (1996). Determinants of friendship selection and quality: Developmental perspectives. In W. M. Bukowski, A. F. Newcomb, & W. W. Hartup (Eds.), *The company they keep: Friendship in childhood and adolescence* (pp. 87–112). New York, NY: Cambridge University Press.

Bauman, H.-D. L. (2008). *Open your eyes: Deaf studies talking*. Minneapolis, MN: University of Minnesota Press.
Berndt, T. J., & Murphy, L. M. (2002). Influences of friends and friendship: Myths, truths, and research recommendations. *Advances in Child Development, 30*, 275–310.
Bradie, M. (1994). Epistemology from an evolutionary point of view. In E. Sober (Ed.), *Conceptual issues in evolutionary biology* (2nd ed.) (pp. 453–475). Cambridge, MA: MIT Press.
Dawkins, R. (1976). *The selfish gene*. New York, NY: Oxford University Press.
Duncan, R. M. (1995). Piaget and Vygotsky revisited: Dialogue or assimilation? *Developmental Review, 15*, 458–472.
Erikson, E. (1959). *Identity and the life cycle*. New York, NY: International Universities Press.
Erikson, E. (1966). *Identity, youth, and crisis*. New York, NY: Norton.
Hauser, P., O'Hearn, A., McKee, M., Steider, A., & Thew, D. (2010). Deaf epistemology: Deafhood and deafness. *American Annals of the Deaf, 154*(5), 486–492.
Heylighen, F. (1992). Selfish memes and the evolution of cooperation. *Journal of Idea, 2*(4), 77–94.
Holcomb, T. (2010). Deaf epistemology: The deaf way of knowing. *American Annals of the Deaf, 154*(5), 471–478.
Kukla, A. (2000). *Social constructivism and the philosophy of science*. New York, NY: Routledge.
Ladd, P. (2003). *Understanding Deaf culture: In search of deafhood*. Clevedon, UK: Multilingual Matters.
Lane, H. (1992). *The mask of benevolence: Disabling the Deaf community*. San Diego, CA: DawnSignPress.
Lane, H. (2008). Do Deaf people have a disability? In H.-D. L. Bauman (Ed.), *Open your eyes: Deaf studies talking* (pp. 277–292). Minneapolis, MN: University of Minnesota Press.
Marschark, M. (1993). *Psychological development of deaf children*. New York, NY: Oxford University Press.
Miller, M. (2003). *A culture of shared experiences for Deaf children of hearing parents: Redefining the notion of culture and culture transmission*. Paper presented at the Fourth International Symposium on Bilingualism, Phoenix, AZ.
Miller, M. (2006). Individual assessment and educational planning: Deaf and hard of hearing students viewed through meaningful contexts. In D. Moores & D. Martin (Eds.), *Deaf learners: Developments in curriculum and instruction* (pp. 161–177). Washington, DC: Gallaudet University Press.
Miller, M. (2010). Epistemology and people who are deaf: Deaf worldviews, views of the Deaf world, or my parents are hearing. *American Annals of the Deaf, 154*(5), 479–485.
Miller, M., Moores, D., & Sicoli, D. (2003). Preferences of deaf college students for hearing status of their children. *Journal of the American Deafness and Rehabilitation Association, 32*, 1–8.
Moores, D. (2010). Epistemologies, deafness, learning, and teaching. *American Annals of the Deaf, 154*(5), 447–455.
Moritz, E. (1990). Memetic science I: General introduction. *Journal of Ideas, 1*, 1–23.
Padden, C., & Humphries, T. (1988). *Deaf in America: Voices from a culture*. Cambridge, MA: Harvard University Press.
Padden, C., & Humphries, T. (2005). *Inside Deaf culture*. Cambridge, MA: Harvard University Press.
Potter, V. G. (1994). *Understanding understanding: A philosophy of knowledge*. New York, NY: Fordham University Press.
Raskin, J. D. (2002). Constructivism in psychology: Personal construct psychology, radical constructivism, and social constructionism. In J. D. Raskin & S. K. Bridges (Eds.), *Studies in meaning: Exploring constructivist psychology* (pp. 1–25). New York, NY: Pace University Press.
Searle, J. (1995). *The construction of social reality*. New York, NY: Free Press.
Sexton, T. L. (1997). Constructivist thinking within the history of ideas: The challenge of a new paradigm. In T. L. Sexton & B. L. Griffin (Eds.), *Constructivist thinking in counseling practice, research, and training* (pp. 3–18). New York, NY: Teachers College Press.

Smith, L. (1993). *Necessary knowledge: Piagetian perspectives on constructivism.* Hove, UK: Lawrence Erlbaum.
Wang. Y. (2010). Without boundaries: An inquiry into deaf epistemologies through a metaparadigm. *American Annals of the Deaf, 154*(5), 428–434.
Yoshinaga-Itano, C., Coulter, D., & Thomson, V. (2000). The Colorado Newborn Hearing Screening Project: Effects of speech and language development for children with hearing loss. *Journal of Perinatology, 20,* S132–S137.
Yoshinaga-Itano, C., & Downey, D. (1996). The psychoeducational characteristics of school-aged students in Colorado with educationally significant hearing losses. *Volta Review, 98,* 65–96.

SUGGESTIONS FOR FURTHER READING

Kukla, A. (2000). *Social constructivism and the philosophy of science.* New York, NY: Routledge.
Ladd, P. (2003). *Understanding Deaf culture: In search of Deafhood.* Clevedon, UK: Multilingual Matters.
Searle, J. (1995). *The construction of social reality.* New York, NY: Free Press.
Sober, E. (Ed.). (1994). *Conceptual issues in evolutionary biology* (2nd ed.). Cambridge, MA: Harvard University Press.

9

Stories as Mirrors: Encounters With Deaf Heroes and Heroines

Donna M. McDonald

Despite being deaf[1] all my life, I know little about it other than my own experience of it. Like David Wright, "about deafness, I know everything and nothing" (1969, p. 5). I do not really know the extent to which my deafness has affected my life and the lives of others, in particular the lives of my family. When I left the School for the Deaf as an eight-year-old child to attend a regular school, I also left behind my childhood deaf world and thereafter was not exposed to the intimacies of deaf culture or the lessons of deaf history. Instead, I was positioned on a lifelong process of doing what it takes to fit into the hearing world. I made little effort until recent years to understand myself in relation to my deafness and my sense of deaf self.

When I began this task of self-reflection while writing my own memoir, *The Art of Being Deaf,* I thought about the books I had read as a child and all the books since then, whether for leisure or for education or for work. I reflected that literature surely had the capacity to influence my worldview; otherwise why read at all? (Or for that matter, why write?) I agreed with Ato Quayson (2007, p. 14) that "literature does not merely reflect any already socially interpreted reality, but adds another tier of interpretation" contingent upon both the historical and cultural contexts of the narrative as well as the reader's own history and culture. In this vein, I wondered whether stories of deafness in memoirs and fiction shape and expand our knowledge of what it means to be deaf or whether they simply respond to existing public perceptions—embracing stereotypes, myths, and Helen Keller–like legends—of deafness. It has also been claimed that most people are more likely to form their ideas about disability from books and films than from policies and personal interactions (Mitchell & Snyder, 2000). I worried about this because I had observed that the lives of people who are deaf tend to be portrayed, both fictively and memoiristically, as if their deafness is their dominant, defining feature. Thomas Couser (1997, p. 221) puzzles over this too when he writes, "Life writing can play a significant role in changing public attitudes about deafness," but then later asks (p. 225), "To what degree and how do the extant narratives of deafness rewrite the discourse of disability? Indeed, to what degree and how do they manage to represent the experience of deafness at all?"

Such uncertainty points to the mismatch between the rise of the disability memoir with the concomitant analysis of its role in shaping public attitudes and identity politics, on the one hand, and the specific study of representations of deafness and deaf people in fiction and memoir, on the other hand. The latter remains relatively unexplored in the field of literary disability, leaving idle a valuable resource for understanding the historical, cultural, social, and educational contexts that have shaped the lives of people who are deaf.

The heritage of diverse and extensive deaf fiction (much of which is hallmarked by the role of a deaf heroine), together with deaf memoirs, biographies, and life narratives (many of which are by women) acted as a prompt for my reflections upon my own deaf life and deaf self. In doing so, I answered my early musings about whether stories of deafness shape, or respond to, public perceptions. I found that they have the potential to do both: Careless writing can reinforce stereotypes (such as those evinced in Joanne Greenberg's 1970 novel, *In This Sign*) but thoughtful writing in any genre has the power to change attitudes. Certainly, my own attitudes about deafness changed. By reading other people's stories of deafness and deaf people's lives, I found that I became less judgemental of my own deaf self and more open to the possibilities of relaxing my guard and allowing other people into my private deaf self.

GESTURES: DEAFNESS IN FICTION

> So we arrive, at last at the pulse and purpose of literature: to reject the blur of the "universal"; to distinguish one life from another; to illumine diversity; to light up the least grain of being, to show who it is concretely individual, particularized from any other. . . . Literature is the recognition of the particular. (Ozick, 1983, p. 248)

But not, apparently, if the characters are deaf. Deaf characters in fiction tend to be used as generic symbols of alienation or serve as a source of special knowledge, saddled with stereotyped constructs of pity and crude assumptions about deafness, for example, *deaf and dumb, deaf mute* (Krentz, 2007; Miller 1992). Christopher Krentz, in *Writing Deafness* (2007), illuminates the cultural contexts for the competing renderings of deaf lives by hearing authors in 19th-century American literature (and also argues their significance in identity formation for both hearing and deaf people). Two anthologies, Trent Batson and Eugene Bergman's 1985 anthology, *Angels and Outcasts: An Anthology of Deaf Characters in Literature,* and Brian Grant's 1987 anthology, *The Quiet Ear: Deafness in Literature,* contribute substantially to our understanding of how deafness has historically been portrayed in fiction and memoir. However, this is not to be confused with improving our understanding of the experiences of deafness itself, as both anthologies are necessarily shaped by the limitations of the editors' worldviews of deaf identity politics and loss, respectively.

Brian Grant was partially deafened as a result of injury during his service in World War II, and so his anthology is shaped by his own sense of loss, leading him to introduce many of his excerpts with emotively laden words about the "suffering" of deaf people. For example, he observes that Harriet Martineau "was plagued by deafness from childhood" and "gave advice to her fellow sufferers" in her *Letter to the Deaf* (1987, p. 27). In contrast, Batson and Bergman, former Gallaudet University academics, are aggressive in their editorial approach, stripping their motivation of all sentiment. They claim their anthology makes it "possible to know much about the attitudes in the western world toward deaf people, and how these attitudes have changed" (p. ix). They also take the opportunity throughout their commentary to advance the cause of American Sign Language (ASL). Their polemical petticoats are evident in their attack on the deaf writer, Albert Ballin, when they judge his authorial voice in *The Deaf Mute Howls* to be limited by "the chains of deaf Uncle-Tomism" (1985, p. 269) because he "is too apologetic, too ambivalent" (1985, p. 269) in his efforts to describe his hardships. Their harsh judgment against Ballin assumes that there can only be one true and right "deaf voice" (a curious assessment given that Batson is hearing).

In view of Tillie Olsen's thesis about the silencing of women writers (1978), together with the repeated observation that deaf people tend not to write because of their purported language limitations (Couser, 1997; Kisor, 1990), the number of excerpts written by deaf women autobiographers in Brian Grant's anthology is surprising. They include the Victorian feminist Harriet Martineau's *Autobiography* (p. 27), deaf–blind writer Helen Keller's *The Story of My Life* (pp. 35–37), poet Dorothy Miles's *Gestures* (p. 51), writer Jessica Rees's *Sing a Song of Silence* (pp. 55–57), journalist Frances Warfield's *Keep Listening* (pp. 38–40), and actor Elizabeth Quinn's *Listen to Me* (p. 52). All these women lost their hearing as a result of childhood illnesses such as meningitis or scarlet fever. This imbues their writing with the melancholy of loss and the bravado of achievement.

Grant's anthology is not all gloom: it is also rich with historical, contemporary, literary and poetic depictions of deaf experiences. However, the theme of loss is the shadow in most of the fictional representations of deafness and deaf people by the hearing writers in his anthology. Many of the stories are bleak, tragic, dour, or comedic in a slapstick sort of a way, playing to culturally perceived stereotypes of deafness. For example, the excerpt from C. P. Snow's *Last Things* includes the observation, "Often she wore the expression, at the same time puzzled, obstinate, and protesting that one saw in the chronically deaf" (Grant, 1987, p. 143). Some of the images of the isolated deaf outcast are confronting. Alfred de Musset's short story "Pierre and Camille," which Brian Grant describes as a "classic of the fictional treatment of deafness" (Grant, 1987, p. 98), is set in France in 1760. "Unfortunately, at this time when so many prejudices were destroyed and replaced, there existed a most pitiless one against the poor creatures known as deaf-mutes. . . . They inspired more horror than pity" (Grant, 1987, p. 96). Similarly, the excerpt from Carson McCullers's novel, *The Heart Is a Lonely Hunter,* tells a dark tale of Singer and his friend Antonapoulos, who are both deaf. The latter is "mentally deranged" (Grant, 1987, p. 146) and committed to an asylum in a distant town. Singer misses his friend and is lonely. When he learns that Antonapoulos has died, he shoots himself in his chest from grief. McCullers's heightened portrayal of deafness and intellectual disability as an allegory of loneliness was deliberate and knowing. She refused to research these disabilities, preferring to rely on her own crude assumptions, which she intuitively knew would be readily accepted by her contemporary readers (Krumland, 2008, p. 35). Few of the fictional excerpts in the anthology ring with jubilation or exuberance. Charles Dickens's approach to writing about deafness provides the exceptions. For example, in *Great Expectations*, Pip meets the elderly and deaf but cheerful father of Wemmick, Mr. Jaggers's clerk. Wemmick is also jocular and practical in his interactions with his deaf father.

Robert F. Panara debates the perception that deaf people have been neglected in fiction and drama or that their image has been distorted. Panara, who lost his hearing through illness as a 10-year-old boy, published extensively on the subject of the deaf writer in America. His 1960 publication *The Silent Muse: An Anthology of Prose and Poetry by the Deaf* included 100 poetic and 28 prose works by American deaf writers between 1835 and 1960. (John Lee Clark's 2009 edition of *Deaf American Poetry: An Anthology* is the most recent addition to this genre.) It was the first such compilation of writing by deaf writers (Lang, 2007, p. 106). In his essays examining the use of deaf characters in fiction, drama, and science fiction, Panara defends several writers, including the 18th-century novelist Daniel Defoe, who created the first literary deaf character in his 1715 novel, *The History of the Life and Surprising Adventures of Duncan Campbell*. However, in this example, Panara concedes that the exploits of Duncan Campbell "are too sensational and exaggerated even to seem probable. For example, Duncan Campbell becomes so adept at speech and lipreading that he completely disguises his deafness whenever he so desires" (Panara, 1972, p. 3). Panara's other examples of "realistic" deaf characters include rogues, imposters, fakes, and charlatans. He concedes that these characterizations are melodramatic, thus apparently contradicting his claim about the realistic individuation of deaf characters.

Three contemporary novels, *An Equal Music* by Vikram Seth (1999), *Deafening* by Frances Itani (2003), and *Talk Talk* by T. C. Boyle (2006), differ markedly in their representations of deaf people and deafness, despite being published within a few years of each other. Their competing perspectives of deafness are shaped by their thematic concerns—music, history, and identity—and so they position the reader to respectively *witness*, be *immersed* in, and *navigate* experiences of deafness. (Curiously, in all three novels, the deaf heroines have romantic relationships with hearing men. In the real world, most deaf women tend to partner with deaf men. Krentz [2007, p. 105] has also observed that "most deaf characters in nineteenth century American canonical literature are children or women; in writing deaf people, hearing authors seemed to need to infantilize or feminize them. . . . We do not encounter strong deaf males in these pages.")

Vikram Seth's novel, *An Equal Music* (1999), tells the story of a renewed love affair (after a lapse of 10 years) between musicians, Michael and Julia, set in present-day England. Julia is a pianist and now married with a young son, and Michael is a violinist with the Maggiore, a string quartet. Following their reunion, Michael persuades Julia to play with the quartet on a European tour. Michael eventually discovers that Julia has recently lost her hearing and is still adapting to her loss. In most fictional stories featuring deafness and deaf people, the reader sees the life of the deaf character through the perceptions and experiences of the hearing narrator, and so it is in Seth's novel: The reader discovers the implications of Julia's deafness by witnessing Michael's grief-laden reactions and other people's responses to her different hearingness. Their grief is all the more sharp for taking place within the drama of music. However, Seth's portrait of love between the two musicians, Michael and Julia, shows that their love is flawed not by Julia's deafness but by Michael's self-absorbed temperament and Julia's marriage.

Seth subtly discloses Julia's hearing loss; Julia's secret is yielded bit by bit. Michael's eventual comprehension of Julia's deafness quickly translates into a practical awareness of its implications: "the light is going . . . if it is true, it will soon be too dark for her to see what I am saying" (p. 142). Michael then tries to imagine what Julia can and cannot hear: "Geese flee, honking. What of this could she hear? How much am I imagining of what she can and cannot? The cawing of a crow, the chacking of a magpie in a plane tree near the Bayswater Road, the buses roaring and sneezing—what can she hear?" (p. 143). By playing in this way with the variety of sounds we encounter all around us, Seth avoids the melodrama of assuming that Julia lives in the soundless world so often conjured up in the minds of hearing people when they contemplate deafness.

Seth's novel does not direct the reader's focus to the heroine's grief at the loss of her hearing but rather to other people's responses to her deafness. However, Seth does accord Julia a rare opportunity to give her insider account of deafness. For example, following Michael's discovery of her hearing loss, Julia writes a letter to him, in which she describes the sensations as first of being "muffled in cottonwool" (p. 151) and later as "suddenly things bang out at me" (p. 151). This twinned image conjures up both a silence of sorts and also confinement and fragility: Confinement because in not hearing the full range of sound, Julia would feel herself to be limited, and fragility because that limitation would give rise to a sense of danger, of knowing that sounds that she is not aware of but which are so necessary for her safety are "out there." In the next few sentences in Julia's letter, Seth conveys his understanding that deafness is a nuanced world of subdued sound and silences that become sound-sensations in themselves: "It was a strange transition from the world of sound to the world of deafness—not soundlessness, really, because I do hear all sorts of noises, only usually they are the wrong ones" (p. 152).

Michael sets about the task of researching deafness by buying a book on the subject. He also tries to imagine the sensation of deafness while listening to music: "I have put on a record of Schubert's string quintet and it is to the sounds of that music that I make my first acquaintance with the elaborate chaos that lies behind the tiny drumskins of my outer ears" (p. 156). However, when he contemplates the role of music in his love for Julia, Michael also raises the spectre of the role of sound in all its communicative power—and by implication, the desolation of silence—in forging and sustaining the bonds of love between two people.

Frances Itani's novel, *Deafening* (2003), takes place in the quiet of small town life in Canada and against the noise of the gunfire of the Great War in Europe. It can be read either as a story of love between a young deaf woman, Grania, and her hearing husband, Jim, or as a fictionalized account of a moment in history, the Great War, in which one of the characters just happens to be deaf. It can also be read as a fictionalized tutorial about deafness (based on Itani's memories of her deaf grandmother), portraying the early 1900s as a time when deafness was regarded as a most terrible affliction and when educational debates about signing versus oralism were intense and bitter.

In contrast to Seth's (1999) novel in which the reader *witnesses* some experiences of deafness from a third-person perspective (Michael), in Itani's novel, the reader is *immersed* in experiences of deafness through the narrative device of the interior monologue of the deaf heroine, Grania. This is supported by an omnipotent narrator's observations of other people's responses to Grania's deafness.

Itani's evocation of a deaf life is obsessively melancholy, but her observations of the things that make life different for a deaf person are authoritative. She tells the story of Grania's hearing loss through illness, the varied reactions of parental grief and sibling pragmatism to Grania's deafness; the dilemmas of speech, lipreading, and signing—"Tress and Grania have already begun to make up their own language, with their hands" (p. xiii); schooling; social reactions—"People will think she's stupid" (p. xiv); the marital stress experienced by Grania's parents; the power of the spoken word—"If you can say your name, you can tell the world who you are" (p. xiii); and the importance of inclusion. She even illustrates the emotion of lip movements when they are read by a deaf person, for example, "Bernard's lips smile when he says the end of her name" (p. xiii). Itani authenticates her story by prefacing several chapters with excerpts on deafness and hearing loss from a range of sources such as "Lecture, The Toronto Fair" (pp. 3, 68), Alexander Graham Bell (p. 77), *The Canadian* (a newsletter by the Ontario School for the Deaf, p. 103), and *Illustrated Phonics* (p. 219).

Unlike Seth's *An Equal Music* (1999), in which Julia's deafness is portrayed as just one element of her personality and her life, Itani's *Deafening* (2003) portrays Grania's deafness as an all-consuming shaper of her personality to the exclusion of other influences. Her deafness is cast as a shadow that falls across her whole life—socially, vocationally, and even in her prospects for marriage. Itani also portrays Grania's interior world as one that is dominated by her contemplation of her deafness throughout her entire life. Grania's self-absorption about her deafness is so persistent that it inevitably jars. It also has the effect of infantilizing Grania by not according her the maturity to look outside of herself and into the concerns of others. In fact, Itani reinforces Grania's childlike status throughout the entire novel by showing Grania conjuring up characters from her childhood storybooks in times of stress, with the character of Dulcie making frequent appearances.

In his discussion about parental biographies, Couser warns of this "reification of the image of the deaf *as* children, unable to speak for themselves, having to be represented by others" (1997, p. 241). Similarly, Christopher Krentz reminds us that the Latin word *infans* means "incapable of speech" and remarks that "speechless deaf characters . . . can appear as if infants, never growing to adulthood through speech, remaining permanently infantilized in silence" (2007, p. 105). Consequently, the character of Grania is so one-dimensional that she is really just a cipher for deafness.

Changing tack, T. C. Boyle's adventure novel, *Talk Talk* (2006), uses the crime of identity theft to *navigate* through issues of identity formation, not only for the deaf heroine, Dana Halter, but also for all the major characters in his novel. When Dana, who lost her hearing as a child, discovers that she is the victim of credit-card identity theft, she pursues the thief, Peck Wilson, across North America with her boyfriend, Bridger. In contrast to the other two novels, where the narrative tension arises from the impact of deafness upon the main characters' lives, Boyle's novel features a deaf heroine whose deafness is independent of the unfolding drama. Thus, Boyle meets the narrative challenge identified by Lennard Davis (2002, p. 45): "When characters have disabilities, the novel is usually exclusively about those qualities. [Yet] the disabled character is never of importance to himself or herself."

In *Talk Talk*, Boyle (2006) does not make Dana do the symbolic work of loss, loneliness, alienation, or oppression so often given to deaf characters in fiction. Instead, he treats the character of Dana with respect, giving her the multidimensional complexity that inheres in all of us. Boyle is not deaf, but he describes Dana and her day-to-day deaf experiences with authenticity, weaving his knowledge of deafness into his novel to support his ruminations on identity. Boyle quickly draws the reader into the deaf person's experience of sound in Chapter 1 by emphasizing Dana's quality of watchfulness before establishing, in an incisive paragraph, *Talk Talk*'s plot of Dana's wrongful arrest amid a confusion of identities. The story of *Talk Talk* subsequently spools out with Dana's detention in a courthouse jail, her court appearance and release, her dismissal from the school at which she teaches, her pursuit of the identity thief across North America, her boyfriend Bridger's meeting with Dana's mother, and their final confrontation with the identity thief.

Throughout this adventure, we learn about Dana's deaf-life, including her attempt to write a book about the Wild Child of Averyron, found at the age of 11 or 12 living ferally in Napoleonic France. We also learn about the impact of deafness on relationships, the politics of sign language versus oral speech, hearing technology such as cochlear implants, and the implications of these for Dana's sense of self. Boyle's treatment of all this material is more nuanced than this list might suggest. In particular, he captures the paradox of the occasional fragility of Dana's integration of her deaf-self into her generally exuberant personality. Dana's boyfriend, Bridger, reveals more about her in his reminiscences about the first time he met her in a dance club and in his continuing curiosity, sometimes clumsily expressed, about her deafness. For example, when Dana recounts the joy of a deaf couple upon learning that their baby was deaf— "'Thank God,' they said, 'she's one of us'"—Bridger asks, "And what do you mean by that?" (p. 40). Their conversation becomes strained with Bridger's confusion and Dana's hurt.

> "But that isn't you," he said, fumbling around the issue. "I mean, you're not like that."
> "I don't understand."
> "You're not—I mean, you weren't born like that. Right?"
> She'd looked as if she was going to cry, but now she forced a smile.
> "Born like what?"
> "Deaf." (p. 40)

Bridger's assertion, "you're not like that," carries the doubt of prejudice coupled with the connotation of a hearing person's superior sense of self when confronted with deafness. The question of whether Dana was born deaf or acquired it through illness is irrelevant to her. She *is* deaf, and her hearing loss was not just a single physiological, auditory incident. It continued to shape her sense of self in the wake of people's responses to her deaf characteristics, "her atonal voice, the non-sequiturs, the fluidity of her face when she spoke, as if every muscle under the skin were a separate organ of communication" (p. 38).

In contrast to Itani's portrayal of the relationship between Grania and Jim, which seems to be entirely sustained (and so stretches credulity) by their shared interest in Grania's deafness, Boyle normalizes the relationship between Dana and Bridger by showing them enjoying common interests such as music, dancing, and eating out at restaurants and by having them talk and argue on a range of topics other than deafness. At the same time, he repeatedly shows Dana asserting her allegiance to her deaf-self; for example, she argues with Bridger against having cochlear implants. By navigating the reader through Dana's own navigation of her deaf-self in her hearing world, Boyle adds a textural layer to his exploration of identity in general. In the end, Dana's strongly forged sense of self wins out in her pursuit of the thief, who has constructed his identity around other people's credit cards.

Different readers will have different responses to these three novels (and the previous historical examples of fictional representations of deafness and deaf lives). My own responses vary each time I reread them. My most consistent response to *An Equal Music* (1999) is to marvel at Seth's respectful representation of Julia's hearing loss. My emotions toward *Deafening* (Itani, 2003) are more complex: I feel resentful, angry, embarrassed, and sullen because I do not want *this* to be the story of deafness that is told today. At the same time, Itani's novel provides me with a historical perspective that I would not otherwise have, helping me to grasp the distance travelled in deaf education and opportunities since the turn of the 20th century (and the distance that has yet to be travelled). *Talk Talk* (2006) inspires me to take on the feisty, independent-minded qualities of the deaf heroine, Dana. However, my most telling response to all three novels as a reader who is deaf is the frisson of recognition: I see my deaf experiences reflected to a lesser or greater degree in each of these stories.

This quiver of recognition points to a clue for educators. Deafness and hearing loss are mysteries to hearing people. Just as deaf people do not know what hearing people can hear, hearing people do not know what deaf people cannot hear. They also cannot really know how this influences the way deaf people conduct their lives. The inclusion on the reading curricula of all students, hearing and deaf, of at least some novels that foreground the experiences of deaf people would be a valuable step toward guiding readers to an empathetic understanding of the complexities of deaf lives. While a disability literary discourse might be too advanced for school classrooms, it would be a creative way of engaging student teachers and educators in examinations of disability and culture. Indeed, embedding discussions of disability across all subject areas—not just literary studies—might go some way toward relocating disability from the margins to the center of our cultural life.

VOICES: DEAFNESS IN BIOGRAPHY, MEMOIR, AND AUTO/BIOGRAPHICAL FICTION

In examining memoirs, I am mindful of Christopher Jon Heuer's exhortation about the autobiographical task of the deaf writer: "The experience of deafness is so unique for each individual and is molded to such an extent by all the other forces operating on a person's life that, if one were to remove these other forces and components, the experience of deafness alone would be that of a vacuum" (2007b, p. 199). With this observation, Heuer brings an astringent clarity to his discussion of the tasks of writing and reading narratives of deafness, whether they are autobiographies or biographies or fictions. The image of disability in literature is so symbolically powerful that it can override everything else, even to the extent of trapping the autobiographical writers themselves into configuring their life stories within the enclosed box of their disability. "Being deaf" is particularly prone to being fixed to the page by the stiff pin of a one-dimensional identity.

As I have noted, early literary representations of deafness were dominated by hearing writers who brought their own fears, assumptions, and coping strategies, ranging from comedy to sorrow, to their interpretations of deaf people's lives. This helps to explain the potency of the early- to mid-20th-century memoirs by Helen Keller (*The Story of My Life*, 1996/1903), David Wright (*Deafness: An Autobiography*, 1969), and Frances Warfield (*Cotton in My Ears*, 1948, and *Keep Listening*, 1957). They were not only among the first personal insider stories of deafness (and blindness, in Keller's case), but they also held out success stories of integration into the hearing world—regarded by most hearing people as the ultimate quest of deaf people—through triumph over adversity and conversion through cure. Keller, an American writer and scholar, became such a world-renowned celebrity that she battled against the image of herself as a human hybrid of freak and angel. Wright, a South African poet, wrote somewhat dourly of his quest to dominate his deafness rather than allow it to dominate him. Frances Warfield, an American journalist and writer, wrote an early fictionalized memoir, *Cotton in My Ears* (1948) before writing a second reportage-style memoir, *Keep Listening* (1957), which takes place between 1933 and 1956.

Yet in the final decade of the 20th century, Henry Kisor (1990, p. 3) was still able to observe in his memoir account of his successful life and career as an American journalist, *What's That Pig Outdoors?*, that "there isn't a large body of literature about the deaf by the deaf." Bauman (1989, p. 47) surmised, "Deaf history may be characterized as a struggle for Deaf individuals to 'speak' for themselves rather than to be spoken about in medical and educational discourses." Couser (1997, p. 226) wrote that "this should not be surprising, for a number of factors militate against deaf autobiography . . . making them unlikely and rare entities." In addition, because most of these memoirists experienced their deafness (or family member's deafness) as a hearing loss, rather than as a sensory experience integral to the sense of self, it is possible to argue that their stories are not primarily about the experience of deafness but are more about their apparently heroic responses to their loss, grief, and subsequent journey toward acceptance. The fact that they (or a family member) lost their hearing somewhat clouds the issue, leading the average reader to therefore surmise that these "loss" experiences are representative of all deaf people. They are not, but sightings of the prelingually deaf memoirist are rare. Couser (1997, p. 283) warns that "the number of [published deaf] narratives is still so small that each new text is in danger of being taken as more representative than it could be."

In his essay "Signs of Life," a discussion of contemporary deafness narratives and their place within the genre of disability discourses, Couser (1997, p. 6) observes that "some groups of individuals . . . find powerful cultural obstacles to life writing." He notes that people with a disability or illness often have to contend with "pervasive cultural discourses" (p. 31) from which they must reclaim their life stories, even while he himself approaches deaf narratives as a question of defining the deaf identity, thus undermining his stated concern about those "pervasive cultural discourses." Couser's approach differs from Heuer (2007b), who tackles the task of deaf narratives more as a question of the writer's craft, of understanding the intention of what the writer wants to say. Indeed, Heuer's irreverent attitude to his own hearing loss in his anthology of essays, *BUG: Deaf Identity and Internal Revolution,* is startling: He provokes the reader into gasps of laughter and discomfort at the same time. While Heuer's anthology is arguably not a memoir, his essays nevertheless tell the reader much about one young man's responses to his deafness. He rails against the repercussions of his hearing loss with mordant humour, dismissing any difficulties the reader might have with his chaotic, conflict-embracing approach with the throwaway line, "Deal with it." Kleinman (1995, p. 5) describes the writer's task more elegantly:

> Living and writing at the margin of the wider society . . . can be a statement about what is and what is not at stake. Perhaps it is only at the margin that we can find the space of critical engagement to scrutinize how certain of the cultural processes that work behind our backs come to injure us all, constraining our possibilities, limiting our humanity. And perhaps it is at the margin, not the centre, where we can find authorization to work out alternatives that can remake experience, ours and others.

Although Couser (1997) points out the difficulty of autobiography in providing deaf people complete control over their self-presentation, he is complicit in this difficulty by imposing his hearing judgments on the deafness narratives in his analysis. A powerful example of this occurs when he writes, "The *desire* [my emphasis] of some deaf individuals to pass as hard of hearing, if not as hearing, suggests the continuing power of the stigma attached to deafness" (p. 224). Without disputing the power of stigma, I take exceptional issue with Couser's attribution of "pass[ing] as hearing" as the deaf person's *deliberate desire to hide* his or her deafness when most deaf people are not that self-absorbed about their deafness, and just simply lapse into the subconscious habits of survival against the stares and furrows of the hearing world. (Krentz, 2007, provides a more thoughtful, historically determined analysis of the concept of passing. Brenda Jo Brueggemann's October 1997 essay, "On (Almost) Passing," explores the same question). Couser also misses the irony of his admission that "deaf children are apparently damned if they do and damned if they don't try to talk" (p. 245), when he himself has a pathological script available to fit whatever choice the deaf memoirists make—denial, avoidance, faking, romanticizing, minimizing, but never the possibility of successfully integrating the deaf-self and hearing-orientation elements of their personalities. The one deaf writer he lets off the hook is Bernard Bragg (*Lessons in Laughter*, 1989), of whom he notes "the relative lack of introspection and reflection on what it is like to be deaf" (p. 273). (Couser's comment seems to suggest that Bragg was, perhaps, not an especially thoughtful person. However, given that both of Bragg's parents were deaf, his first language was American Sign Language, and he attended residential schools for the deaf and Gallaudet, Bragg was evidently enculturated in his deaf identity. To expect him to be introspective about his deafness would be akin to expecting hearing people to be introspective about their hearingness.)

Such a critical streak is not unusual, as Corker (1996, p. 108) records in one of her client narratives: "When I try to explain what my experience is, it is always disputed, it is never good enough for the [hearing] person who is on the receiving end of the explanation." Perhaps you have to be deaf to feel this particular sting, but there must be a space in which individual deaf people can write autobiographically and "gain recognition, acceptance, and affirmation of deafness, without assumptions about 'deaf identity' as the main driving force in their lives" (Corker, 1996, p. 61).

At the same time, deaf people cannot afford to be overly sensitive about this. If assumptions are to be shattered, they must be shattered by deaf people themselves; hearing people cannot take on the task, missionary-like, on their behalf. Deaf people must persist in their efforts to tell, write, show, illustrate, film, construct, and distribute their stories in whatever medium they can apply for whatever audience they can find.

In this context, I turn now to the reflective accounts of deafness in Frances Warfield's *Keep Listening* (1957); an extended essay-style memoir by Bainy Cyrus, "All Eyes," from *Deaf Women's Lives: Three Self-Portraits* (2006); and Hannah Merker's book of meditative essays, *Listening* (2000). I chose these because they offer competing insights into the impact of deafness and hearing loss on the authors' lives.

A keen advocate for the needs of deaf and hard of hearing people, Frances Warfield wrote extensively on this subject. Her fictionalized memoir, *Cotton in My Ears* (1948), and reportage-style memoir, *Keep Listening (1957)*, bear the hallmarks of her journalistic skills as she deftly converts the incidents of her life into stories replete with the tension of the diagnosis of hearing loss, drama of adapting to her hearing impairment, disappointment, and self-deprecatory humor as she stumbles from mishap to mayhem. Each has a happy ending, with a marriage proposal in the first fictionalized memoir and the restoration of her hearing through surgery in the second memoir.

The quality that sets Warfield apart from other writers of deafness (memoir or fiction) is her detachment from her subject, that is, herself. She writes with a historian's perspective and a journalist's lack of sentiment. Reading Frances Warfield's memoir of her deaf life was like reading letters from a much-loved aunt about the impact of her hearing loss on her life, and her relationship with her "hard-of-hearingness." Her story reached out to me down through the history of years to such an extent that I realized that I would have liked such a mentor in my own life. The force of this realization winded me. I felt the warmth of an imagined friendship with Warfield and the chill of its absence.

Warfield's memoir could be regarded as "a conversion narrative, with its sudden and profound change in the status of the narrator" (Couser, 1997, p. 233), but it is equally a narrative in which the heroine triumphs by deliberately *erasing* her "adversity." She makes the source of her adversity disappear, which might be comforting to the hard-of-hearing reader seeking such a solution, but by ending her memoir with the resurrection of her hearing, Warfield runs the risk of implying that the wholeness of her life is also resurrected. Fortunately, Warfield's memoir is more textured than either of these labels suggest because she tackles so many issues, giving them a historical sweep as well as an immediately personal perspective.

Her sense for history distinguishes her memoir from other deaf memoirs, which tend to be more inwardly directed, if not self-absorbed. She conveys a strong understanding of the historicity of the cultural and technological responses to her hearing loss, signaling not only her research into what has gone before but also her hopes for the future. This helps her to emerge from her memoir as a sympathetically decent character. She is flawed, funny, and brave in the face of her fears: "My strenuous busyness was convincing; even my good friends were taken in. But for all my gyrating, I was not moving; simply turning faster and faster inside my somewhat-loosened shell. Still hiding. Still afraid" (Warfield, 1957, p. 59).

The absence of self-pity in Warfield's writing is appealing as is her enthusiasm in sharing what she has learned about deafness, hearing technology, and cultural attitudes toward hearing loss. In fact, Warfield's advocacy is so insistent that it hints at the possibility that surgery may have delivered the sense of hearing to her but she is still, at heart, "a hard of hearing person," in the same way that deaf people who benefit from hearing technology or cochlear implants still regard themselves as "deaf."

Hannah Merker's book of essays, *Listening* (2000), is not strictly a memoir, as "that is another book" (Merker, 2000, p. 201). Rather, it unfolds itself as Merker's quest to understand the mystery of silence. Instead of revealing the ups and downs of her life, Merker has crafted her essays as meditative explorations of listening, drawn from her memories of sound. She is spartan in exposing information about her personal life both before and after her hearing loss as a result of a skiing accident when she was 39 years old, which she also recounts with stripped-bare simplicity. Despite the trauma, which would surely have been profound, Merker's self-consciously literary and exploratory book is shaped by her theme that "the world becomes larger as the mind reawakens to the soaring symphony of everyday life" (Merker, 2000, p. 2).

Merker signals her anthropomorphic approach to sound on the first page: "The silence around me is invisible" (Merker, 2000, p. 1). By describing it as an entity that cannot be seen, she makes silence a character in her story and uses the artist's skill of perceiving negative space to describe what she hears now, in the place of what she heard before. It is a poetic and unusual approach; inevitably, Merker does not succeed in disguising her longing for the return of her former world of sound despite her attempts to reconcile with her loss. By describing what emerges for her when she listens with *all* her senses, including her senses of memory and imagination, Merker inverts the usual story of hearing loss to make it a story of listening gain.

Bainy Cyrus's "All Eyes" is one of three essays by deaf women in an anthology titled *Deaf Women's Lives: Three Self-Portraits* (Cyrus, Katz, Cheyney, & Parsons, 2006). All three women attended oral deaf schools but their life stories depart from that unifying feature. Their stories have undoubtedly been chosen because of their diversity, which includes the experiences of a young Jewish deaf girl in wartime England (Eileen Katz) and the world travels of a proselytizing advocate for Total Communication (Frances Parsons). Cyrus provides an unadorned statement of the facts as she apparently remembers and experiences them, making her essay appear deceptively simple because of its linear, autobiographical approach and informative tone of voice.

A statement about the potency of influences in the first few years of any child's life, Cyrus's essay also emphasizes the role of her predominantly oral-deaf education during the 1960s and 1970s in determining the quality of her life. Her discussion of the oralism versus signing debate is restrained and compassionate, providing guidance to anyone trying to find his or her own response to it. In telling her life story, Cyrus is empathetic in talking about the impact of her deafness on her family and friendships, placing any hardships that she experienced within the social and historical contexts of her times. Her description of the changing nature of her friendships with her deaf friends draws particular attention. As they grew away from their shared childhoods of an exclusively deaf world toward adult lives that straddled different worlds, they renegotiated their friendships with each other. Toward the end of her essay, she implies that the apparent absence of doubt in her story may have been hard-won: "The more I learned [about deafness], the more I appreciated my own life as a deaf person. I was finally at ease with my disability" (Cyrus, 2006, p. 90). In an essay free of self-pity and triumphalism, Bainy Cyrus's clear-as-a-bell honesty increases her authority; she has the reader leaning into the page to learn more.

Frances Warfield, Bainy Cyrus, and Hannah Merker all write assertively and confidently about their experiences, providing the reader with varied insights into contemporary deaf lives. Cyrus exposes the shifts and strains in her relationships as a result of her deafness; Warfield whips up the mayhem of a busy urban life with its jangle of noise and confusion; and Merker backs away from such complexity as she set herself a different narrative quest, distilling her story to the rhythms of sounds.

In contrast, and despite his authorial reputation, David Lodge's 2008 autobiographical novel *Deaf Sentence* fails to "disrupt patterns of perceptions" (Fisher Fishkin, 1990, p. 133) because the novel's narrator, Desmond Bates, a professor nearing retirement, adopts an unrelievedly stale, grumpy-old-man approach in his reflections on his age-related deafness. As foreshadowed by the novel's title, David Lodge's narrator plays a one-note song of self-pity as he tells the story of his deteriorating hearing, yielding only once or twice to sardonic doubts about the authenticity of his reflections: "I was almost persuaded by my own story, moved by the pathos of my imagined plight" (Lodge, 2008a, p. 151).

Self-pity may be a predictable response to hearing loss, but it is an unattractive trait that leaves little room for new self-knowledge when sustained for the duration of the novel. While it would be unreasonable to expect any person, fictional or real, who has enjoyed hearing all his life to adapt quickly to his hearing loss and simultaneously develop a deaf consciousness, it is reasonable to assume that a writer of Lodge's stature and experience would have taken the time to bone up on his deaf literary predecessors with a view to enriching his own narrative. The sole deaf exemplar from whom the narrator, Professor Bates, draws some sort of companionable consolation is Beethoven—a too-oft-quoted example by hearing people seeking to establish a knowing empathy in conversations with deaf people, as if Beethoven is the only other deaf person in history.

It could perhaps be argued that David Lodge *is* disrupting "patterns of perception" in his novel. After all, how well does the general public understand the consequences of age-related hearing loss, let alone deafness? Certainly, I have already been taken to task for the severity of my judgment by colleagues who have reminded me the issues arising from elderly hearing loss are of a different order from the issues arising from congenital deafness such as mine. I agree. However, given that David Lodge has openly declared that he is losing his hearing and said in a *Sunday Times* interview (2008b) that he wrote this novel to explore the implications of that loss, the shallowness of the deaf narrator's reflections remains surprising. It is certainly a missed opportunity for a deeper and more rounded personal account of hearing loss, albeit fictionalized, instead of serving up the old "plight" story of deafness under the guise of comic satire (and, coincidentally, confirming Christopher Krentz's observation about the absence of strong deaf male characters in fiction [Krentz, 2007, p. 105]). Lodge's tin ear is particularly disappointing as his novel seems so unmindful of his writing predecessors—hearing and deaf, novelists and memoirists.

Mindful as I am of Couser's warning not to overstate the representative qualities of just a few published deaf narratives (Couser, 1997, p. 283), I hesitate to corral these memoirs and autobiographical novels into a single finding. However, we can glean some unifying themes.

The reader learns much about the historical, cultural, social, and educational attitudes toward, and perceptions of, deafness and deaf people in all the memoirs discussed in this chapter. Despite the long-standing perception of deaf people as "isolated," the deaf subject in memoir is placed firmly within the context of his or her times: The reader comes to know the deaf subject within the swirl of life taking place either around or with the deaf subject. Each memoir acts as a call to arms: In each, the memoirist advocates for a better understanding of the difficulties and possibilities of deaf lives. Each memoir also draws the reader's attention, either by allusion or by direct discussion, to the importance of education, work, and relationships (family and friendships) to the quality of deaf people's lives. Taken together, the works discussed in this chapter provide a historical sweep, illustrating the improved quality of deaf people's lives, notwithstanding their difficulties, and their ability to speak up for themselves—that is, to "own" and write their life stories.

THE RELUCTANT MEMOIRIST

While researching and writing my own memoir of deafness, *The Art of Being Deaf*, I took up Couser's puzzle about whether life writing can effect change by examining how stories of deafness and deaf people are told in fiction and memoir. I respected A. N. Wilson's (1988) warning that

> The sense of our own identity is fluid and tolerant, whereas our sense of the identity of others is always more fixed and quite often edges towards caricature. We know within ourselves that we can be twenty different persons in a single day and that the attempt to explain our personality is doomed to become a falsehood after only a few words. . . . And yet . . . works of literature, novels and biographies

> depend for their aesthetic success precisely on this insensitive ability to simplify, to describe, to draw lines around another person and say, 'This is she' or 'This is he' (p. 175).

Nevertheless, reading those fictional stories and memoirs helped me. They guided my task of self-examination in which I set about answering questions such as, Who am I in relation to my deafness? What does my being deaf mean in relation to other people? What additional tasks in developing my sense of self have I had to take on board (or avoided) because I am different from other people? (Corker, 1996).

It is true that the tropes of grief, trauma, and triumphalism dominate deaf narratives so much so that the casual reader could mistake these themes for being the only stories of deaf people's lives. In addition, deaf narratives can be blunt instruments in conveying the complexities of identity, in particular, the elusive deaf identity. The underlying premise of much deaf fiction and memoir is usually that deafness is something to be overcome lest you be defeated by it. The exceptions prove the rule. However, this does not mean that those deaf narratives do not tell us other things.

The considerable diversity of deaf narratives is especially compelling. My search for representations of deafness and deaf characters in fiction, biography, memoir, and autobiographical fiction revealed that deaf lives appear in a range of genres, a variety of occupations, at all levels of society from the impoverished to the more well-to-do, and around the globe. A close reading of these texts also reveals that the authorial concern about the quality of deaf people's lives is a recurrent, if sometimes subtle, characteristic of deaf narratives. What I initially took to be an unhealthy and somewhat maddening preoccupation with the characteristics of loneliness, alienation, and grief for deaf people I eventually understood to be the possibility of providing the "general reader" with insights into the lives of deaf people. Historical and contemporary fictional representations of deafness and memoirs of deaf people's lives can tell us much, not just about deafness and hearing loss, but also about the social, cultural, and educational values of the day. In other words, even when narratives of deafness might be contentious, inaccurate, exaggerated, or just plain silly, they also provide us with a rich resource of insights into d/Deaf epistemologies. Deaf narratives provide the general reader and specialists in a range of enterprises—such as education, health, social work, philosophy, and law—with fresh ways of understanding deafness and deaf people's lives. This is particularly significant given that the lives of deaf people seem to be mostly invisible to the general population.

I enjoyed the companionability of those deaf fictions and memoirs. I enjoyed seeing the multiple possibilities of my deaf-self/hearing-persona experiences reflected in, or challenged by, what I read. I found that stories from the Deaf community do not speak for me, as the framing of deafness as a separate linguistic and cultural entity has not shaped my life, and nor was I drawn to the militancy of identity politics that uses terms such as *oppression* and *oppressors* to deride the efforts of parents and educators to teach deaf children to speak (Lane 1984; Padden & Humphries 1998). Nevertheless, I found that this reading and then writing my own story of deafness changed not only my relationship with it but also changed my relationship with myself and others.

CONCLUSION

Just as knowledge is not absolute, so is identity mutable, fluctuating over time and in response to context and circumstance. We can learn much about the diversity of deaf experiences and the nuances of deaf identity by reading memoirs of deaf people and novels with deaf characters. Whether they are written by hearing or deaf writers, by providing different perspectives on deafness, they have something useful to say, demonstrate, and illustrate about deafness and the lives of deaf people.

For further research and theorizing to broaden our understanding of d/Deaf epistemologies, the following questions should be explored:

- What can we learn about differences and similarities in cultural responses to deafness and deaf people's lives by examining the literature of different cultures?
- To what extent does a foundation knowledge of deaf literary studies contribute to an improved sense of self or clarity of identity for the deaf student?
- How do deaf literary studies contribute to an improved understanding of the educational and psychosocial needs of deaf students?

NOTE

1. I use the word *deaf* here in the sense of how I have understood that word ever since I first became aware of my own deafness as a child—drawing on both its audiological sense and its social role—to include people whose hearingness is substantially less than what is understood to be normal or ideal; whose ability to participate in hearing-centered conversations is profoundly affected; who communicate by sign, speech, or a combination of both; and whose sense of identity is likely to be shaped by the experiences arising from their inability to hear a range of sounds. In addition, because I was born deaf—"moderate-severe, sloping to profound; unknown etiology," according to a recent audiological assessment—I understand my own deafness not as a loss but as an experience: It is an essential element in my sense of I-am-who-I-am even though I do not identify myself as a member of the deaf community.

REFERENCES

Batson, T. W., & Bergman, E. (1985). *Angels and outcasts: An anthology of deaf characters in literature.* Washington, DC: Gallaudet College Press.

Bauman, H. Dirksen-L. (1989). Voicing Deaf identity: Through the 'I's' and ears of an other. In S. Smith & J. Watson (Ed.), *Getting a life: Everyday uses of autobiography* (pp. 47–62). Minneapolis, MN: University of Minnesota Press.

Boyle, T. C. (2006). *Talk talk.* New York, NY: Viking.

Bragg, B. (1989). *Lessons in laughter.* Washington, DC: Gallaudet University Press.

Brueggemann, B. J. (1997). On (almost) passing. *College English, 59*(6), 647–660.

Brueggemann, B. J. (2009). *Deaf subjects: Between identities and places.* New York, NY: New York University Press.

Clark, J. L. (2009). *Deaf American poetry: An anthology.* Washington, DC: Gallaudet University Press.

Corker, M. (1996). *Deaf transitions: Images and origins of deaf families, deaf communities, and deaf identities.* Philadelphia, PA: Jessica Kingsley Publishers.

Couser, G. T. (1997). *Recovering bodies: Illness, disability, and life writing.* Madison, WI: University of Wisconsin Press.

Cyrus, B. (2006). All eyes. In B. Cyrus, E. Katz, C. Cheyney, & F. Parsons (Eds.), *Deaf women's lives: Three self-portraits* (pp. 1–90). Washington, DC: Gallaudet University Press.

Cyrus, B., Katz, E., Cheyney, C., & Parsons, F. (2006). *Deaf women's lives: Three self-portraits.* Washington, DC: Gallaudet University Press.

Davis, L. J. (2002). *Bending over backwards: Disability, dismodernism, and other difficult positions.* New York, NY: New York University Press.

Fisher Fishkin, S. (1990). The borderlands of culture: Writing by W. E. B. Du Bois, James Agee, Tillie Olsen, and Gloria Anzaldua. In N. Sims (Ed.), *Literary journalism in the 20th century* (pp. 133–183). New York, NY: Oxford University Press.

Grant, B. (1987). *The quiet ear: Deafness in literature.* London, UK: Deutsch.

Heuer, C. J. (2007a). *BUG: Deaf identity and internal revolution.* Washington, DC: Gallaudet University Press.

Heuer, C. J. (2007b). Deafness as conflict and conflict component. *Sign Language Studies, 7*(2), 195–199.

Itani, F. (2003). *Deafening.* New York, NY: Grove Press.

Keller, H. (1996). *The story of my life.* Mineola, NY: Dover (Original work published 1903).

Kisor, H. (1990). *What's that pig outdoors? A memoir of deafness.* New York, NY: Hill & Wang.

Kleinman, A. (1995). *Writing at the margin: Discourse between anthropology and medicine.* Los Angeles, CA: University of California Press.

Krentz, C. (2007). *Writing deafness: The hearing line in 19th-century American literature.* Chapel Hill, NC: University of North Carolina Press.

Krumland, H. (2008). A big deaf-mute moron: Eugenic traces in Carson McCullers's *The heart is a lonely hunter. Journal of Literary Disability, 2*(1) 32–43.

Lang, H. G. (2007). *Teaching from the heart and soul: The Robert F. Panara story.* Washington, DC: Gallaudet University Press.

Lodge, D. (2008a). *Deaf sentence.* London, UK: Harvill Secker.

Lodge, D. (2008b, April). *Living under a deaf sentence.* Retrieved April 30, 2008, from the Sunday Times (London) website: http://entertainment.timesonline.co.uk/tol/arts_and_entertainment/books/article3778988.ece

Merker, H. (2000). *Listening: Ways of hearing in a silent world.* Dallas, TX: Southern Methodist University Press.

Miller, J. (1992). The rustle of a star: An annotated bibliography of deaf characters in fiction. *Library Trends, 41*(1), 42–60.

Mitchell, D. T., & Snyder, S. L. (2000). *Narrative prosthesis: Disability and dependencies of discourse.* Ann Arbor, MI: University of Michigan Press.

Olsen, T. (1978). *Silences.* New York, NY: Delta/Seymour Lawrence.

Ozick, C. (1983). *Art and ardor.* New York, NY: Knopf.

Padden, C., & Humphries, T. (1998). *Deaf in America: Voices from a culture.* Cambridge,MA: Harvard University Press.

Panara, R. (1972). Deaf characters in fiction and drama. *Deaf American, 24*(9), 3–8. Retrieved from https://ritdml.rit.edu/bitstream/handle/1850/1336/RFPanaraPaper05-1972.pdf?sequence=1

Quayson, Ato. (2007). *Aesthetic nervousness: Disability and the crisis of representation.* New York, NY: Columbia University Press.

Seth, V. (1999). *An equal music.* London, UK: Phoenix House.

Warfield, F. (1948). *Cotton in my ears.* New York, NY: Viking.

Warfield, F. (1957). *Keep listening.* London, UK: Victor Gollancz.

Wilson, A. N. (1988). *Incline our hearts.* London, UK: Penguin.

Wright, D. (1969). *Deafness: An autobiography.* New York, NY: Stein & Day.

SUGGESTIONS FOR FURTHER READING

Gitter, E. (1992). Deaf-mutes and heroines in the Victorian era. *Victorian Literature and Culture, 20,* 161–177.

McDonald, D. (2007). I hear with my eyes. In J. Schulz (Ed.), *A revealed life: Australian writers and their journeys in memoir* (pp. 32–45). Sydney: ABC Books and Griffith Review.

McDonald, D., & Ferrier, E. (Eds.). (2010). Deaf [Special issue]. *Media and Culture Journal, 13,* 3. Retrieved from http://journal.media-culture.org.au/index.php/mcjournal/issue/view/deaf

Pajka-West, S. (2010). Representations of Deafness and Deaf people in young adult fiction. *Media and Culture Journal, 13,* 3. Retrieved from http://journal.media-culture.org.au/index.php/mcjournal/article/viewArticle/261

Zazove, P. (2009). *Four days in Michigan.* Dallas, TX: Durban House Press.

PART IV

EDUCATIONAL AND PHILOSOPHICAL PERSPECTIVES

10

The Qualitative-Similarity Hypothesis

Peter V. Paul

In this chapter, I present the underpinnings of the qualitative-similarity hypothesis (QSH) and a synthesis of a sample of research investigations on children and adolescents who are d/Deaf or hard of hearing (dDhh) (Paul 2008, 2009, 2010; Paul & Lee, 2010; Paul & Wang, 2012; Trezek, Wang, & Paul, 2010, 2011). dDhh children are those who have slight to profound hearing losses based on the pure-tone average in the better of their two unaided ears (e.g., Moores, 2001; Paul & Whitelaw, 2011). Children are identified as Deaf if they have Deaf parents who use American Sign Language (ASL) or if they use ASL themselves. These children, and others whose home language is not English, can also be classified as English language learners (ELLs), which is the common phrase used to refer to children who are learning English as a second language, especially in educational settings (e.g., Paul & Wang, 2012).

CONCEPTUAL FRAMEWORK OF THE QSH

An understanding of the underpinnings of the QSH requires integrating aspects from other broad entities such as the nature of discipline structure (e.g., literacy, mathematics) and the development of individuals' knowledge with respect to learning the contents of a discipline. In general, the QSH is grounded predominantly in behavioral and/or cognitive theories of learning such as information processing or parallel distributed processing (see discussions in Paul, 2008, 2009; Paul & Lee, 2010). Insights from social/contextual and affective models can be or have been incorporated to a certain extent (Paul & Wang, 2012).

Much of the research on the QSH has been conducted within the purview of a version of the standard epistemology, particularly with the application of an objective methodology and the concept of discovered knowledge involving the separation of the knower and the knowledge obtained (see Paul & Moores, Chapter 1). It is possible to utilize findings from other epistemologies, for example, deaf epistemologies (see Holcomb, Chapter 7), to assess the validity of the QSH. However, there needs to be agreement on the nature and outcomes of such research (e.g., defining and measuring reading comprehension) as well as on the implications of the underpinnings (e.g., fundamentals, discipline structure) of the QSH, discussed later in this chapter. In fact, a number of proponents of multiple epistemologies, based on social/contextual models, reject the separation of the knower and knowledge and the use of an objective methodology (for a readable account, see Noddings, 2007; Ritzer, 2001; see also, Paul & Moores, Chapter 1).

Regardless of the model, a certain level of cognitive ability is most likely a requisite for learning content areas such as literacy, science, or mathematics. However, it is not clear whether there is or should be strong relationships between the structure of cognition in individuals' minds (i.e., biological, neurological, information processing, etc.) and that of discipline (or knowledge) structures (e.g., Phillips, 1983; Phillips & Soltis, 2004). Nevertheless, a few cognitive constructs should be mentioned, for example, working memory, metacognition, self-regulation, and *rational* thinking, which are strongly connected to the acquisition of knowledge and the effective use of problem-solving skills in educational settings (Cartwright, 2009; Pickering, 2006; Shanahan, 2009). These cognitive constructs may be influenced by the debate on the structure of a discipline.

The Structure of a Discipline

What does it mean to say that a discipline has a structure? The layers of complexity become evident because the answer or answers to this question, in some scholars' eyes, is contingent on one's epistemology, which dictates the approaches, procedures, and methods for investigating this issue—and even influences the wording of the question itself (Noddings, 2007; Pring, 2004; Ritzer, 2001; see also, Paul & Moores, Chapter 1). On a simplistic level, it can be argued that a particular discipline has an internal, logical conceptual framework that impacts one's understanding at various levels because of the demands on cognition (e.g., Donovan & Bransford, 2005; Cartwright, 2009; Shanahan, 2009). Thus, some concepts and skills are easier to learn or acquire before others because of their inherent difficulty. For example, the concept of addition needs to be understood before a child can learn the concept of multiplication—which is conceptualized as repeated addition (Battista, 2001; English & Halford, 1995; Mayer, 1992).

From another perspective, it might be that discipline structures (often called knowledge structures) are contingent on an external psychological or developmental framework on *how individuals learn*—considering specifically the rate and manner of acquisition and optimal periods for development (e.g., Donovan & Bransford, 2005; Phillips & Soltis, 2004). That is, in the process of learning mathematics or science or in learning to read or write, there are skills that are easier or more difficult because of the complicated—often unpredictable—intertwinement of factors associated with the broad domains of cognitive (e.g., the structure of individuals' minds), sociocultural (e.g., interactions, home environment, social artifacts or institutions), and affective behaviors (e.g., motivation, interest, demeanor).

It is probably counterproductive to argue that the structure of a discipline is determined solely by either internal (i.e., inside the head) or external (e.g., teaching–learning) variables. More likely, it involves both broad groups of variables as well as computations of variables within the groups. Whether a discipline is coherently structured, is loosely structured, or has no real structure at all is an open question (see Spiro, Vispoel, Schmitz, Samarapungavan, & Boerger, 1987; see also, the discussion in Cartwright, 2009).

The question of discipline (or knowledge) structure is not merely an academic issue. The outcomes of the debates are critical because there are implications for educational practices, specifically the proffering of instructional methods and curricular contents (for a discussion, see Paul & Wang, 2012, Chapter 4). For example, clarifying the construct of discipline structure might be important to validate the existence and order of content standards associated with the range of school subjects in P–12 education. In addition, it might be possible to discern whether there should be a general education curriculum or instruction for all students rather than the differentiated special curricula and instruction varying according to either cognitive (e.g., learning styles, individual profiles, etc.) or cultural (e.g., ethnicity, disabilities, gender, etc.) factors.

The view adopted here is that there is a conceptual structure or framework associated with disciplines, which varies from being highly structured to loosely structured. To complete the discussion of the underpinnings of the QSH, two additional constructs are highlighted: critical period and fundamentals.

The Critical Period of Development: Language and Literacy

English as a First Language The debate on the structures (in this case, theoretical structures) of English language and English literacy has an illustrious and contentious history (e.g., McGuinness, 2004; Pence & Justice, 2008). Considering the crucial constructs of language (e.g., listening comprehension or general language ability), the relevant focus here is on its development and subsequent effects on the acquisition of literacy skills (e.g., Cain & Oakhill, 2007; Crystal, 1995; McGuinness, 2004, 2005; Rymer, 1992). With respect to language, one line of research has centered on the construct of a critical period (i.e., age period) for acquisition (Lenneberg, 1967; Rymer, 1992). Despite diverging views, especially those on optimal age ranges, there seems to be support for an optimal period for language growth. Specifically, language growth is considered to be faster and more complete in the early years (e.g., birth to age five), but slower and possibly fragmented after puberty.

The work of Lenneberg (1967) has influenced the discussion of and research on the language development of children with language/learning disabilities as well as that engendered by Stanovich's rendition of the *Matthew effects*, discussed later in this chapter. Specifically, Lenneberg (1967) hypothesized that the language development of children with developmental delays (i.e., cognitive or intellectual delays) differed quantitatively from that of typical children but was qualitatively similar with respect to mental age. This hypothesis seems to be tenable for many children with language/learning disabilities as well as cognitive/intellectual disabilities (e.g., Cain & Oakhill, 2007; Kamhi & Catts, 2012; Vellutino, 2003; see also the review in Chapters 6–9 of Paul & Wang, 2012).

English as a Second Language The research on the critical period construct has also been applicable to the learning of a second language, either sequentially (after the first language) or in a bilingual situation (learning two languages simultaneously) (e.g., see Felix [in Paul, 2001]; McLaughlin, 1984, 1985, 1987; see also Paul, 1985, 2009; Paul & Wang, 2012). The representative and long-standing exemplar is the work of Felix (in Paul, 2001), who attempted to explain the differences in achievement between individuals who acquired two languages fairly early in life (i.e., before puberty) and those who acquired a second language later in life. Felix argued that much of the differences between the two groups is due to the development and utilization of two different cognitive systems. Individuals who acquire two languages early (prior to puberty, but even prior to age five) are using cognitive structures that are most suitable for learning, whereas individuals who are attempting to acquire a language later may be employing two different cognitive systems—a language-specific one (i.e., the modular hypothesis, Fodor, 1983) and a cognitive problem-solving one. These two different systems compete with rather than facilitate each other, slowing down and fragmenting the acquisition of the second language.

From another perspective, Cummins (1979, 1984, 2007) has argued that the two languages can facilitate each other, but there must be a level of proficiency developed in *both* languages. Specifically, Cummins asserted that there need to be threshold levels of linguistic competence in both languages. The positive effects of the first language on the second language (and even on cognitive and academic achievement) do not materialize until individuals have attained a threshold level of competence in the second language. Cummins acknowledged that it is best to learn two languages at an early age (this is assumed to mean prior to puberty) to reap the benefits of the threshold effects.

In sum, the earlier the development of language proficiency, the most facilitative the effects on the acquisition of skills and knowledge in other content areas such as literacy, science, and mathematics. With respect to the QSH, the focus is on the development of foundational and conventional English language and literacy skills, which are critical for the comprehension of academic or discipline knowledge in English (e.g., Shanahan, 2009; for ELLs, see Birch, 2007). The construct of an optimal period for English literacy development has been examined by other scholars, most notably Stanovich (e.g., 1986, 1991, 1992) with his constructs of the *Matthew effects* and the *developmental lag hypothesis*.

Matthew Effects and Developmental Lag Stanovich (1986, 1991, 1992, 2000; Stanovich, Nathan, & Zolman, 1988) has proffered the Matthew effects, which also led to the developmental lag hypothesis and which has influenced a line of research on children with language/learning disabilities as well as children with other specific disabilities such as dyslexia. Both of these constructs contribute to the underpinnings of the QSH (e.g., see early discussion in Paul, 1985; see also Paul, 2010; Paul & Lee, 2010; Paul & Wang, 2012).

The Matthew effects is formulated simply as "the rich get richer and the poor stay the same or get poorer." With respect to reading development, this means that when children learn to read during an optimal period—typically, by grade 2 or 3—they can read to learn (i.e., get *richer*) and do so voraciously and widely. For these children, reading is pleasurable, and they grow linguistically and cognitively.

On the other hand, if children do not learn to read during this optimal period, then they cannot read to learn effectively and this negatively affects their subsequent language and cognitive development. The problems can accumulate to the point where they will read little and begin to lag behind the progress of their typical peers (i.e., get *poorer*). The longer this continues, the greater the lag. The developmental growth of these poor readers/writers may become stagnated and exhibit significant language and cognitive delays. There are little or no reciprocal or facilitative relationships between reading and cognition, between reading and language development, or even among language, cognition, and reading. The lag becomes greater mainly because the language and cognitive demands of literacy materials beyond the third-grade level pose an almost insurmountable barrier.

Based on the concept of the Matthew effects, Stanovich and his colleagues proposed the developmental lag hypothesis, which contains two versions: strong and weak (Stanovich, 1991, 1992, 2000; Stanovich et al., 1988). The strong version asserts that struggling readers (and possibly writers) do catch up to their peers who are developmentally typical. To make up for lost ground, however, this catching-up period needs to be relatively short with intensive and extensive, focused instruction, particularly in the problematic areas. These problematic areas might be those associated with decoding (e.g., word identification) or comprehension (e.g., making inferencing, prior knowledge, metacognition). Much of the emphasis of the developmental lag has been on problems related to the area of phonology or phonological processes (e.g., phonological and phonemic awareness), which impede the acquisition of emergent and mature reading comprehension processes (e.g., Stanovich, 1991, 1992, 2000; Stanovich et al., 1988).

Stanovich and colleagues noted that a substantial number of children have difficulty catching up, despite the richness of the instructional approaches. Beyond the early elementary grades, it seems almost impossible for children to recover the lost ground. As a result, Stanovich proposed a weak version of the developmental lag hypothesis, which states that some children, for whatever reasons, might not catch up or reach the level of their typical counterparts—albeit in theory they should. It should be noted that the weak version is not asserting that these children develop *differently* per se or that these children cannot make *any* progress in literacy.

The weak version has engendered another view, labeled the *deficit hypothesis* (e.g., see discussions in Francis, Shaywitz, Stuebing, Shaywitz, & Fletcher, 1996; O'Brien, Mansfield, & Legge, 2005; O'Shaughnessy & Swanson, 1998; Reimer, 2006; Snowling, Defty, & Goulandris, 1996). This version seems to be most applicable to the research on a number of children with severe dyslexia and those with severe cognitive or intellectual delays (e.g., McGuinness, 2005). Despite the best instructional or psychological intervention efforts, the barriers associated with learning to read effectively cannot be overcome or remedied—at least psychologically. It seems that the best-case scenario is that the reading skill of these children can be stabilized (e.g., maintained at a certain level with some growth). There are multiple reasons for this situation, and phonological processes play only one major role (see also the discussion in Paul & Wang, 2012).

Summary In sum, there seems to be an optimal, perhaps critical, period for developing a language, and this seems to influence the acquisition of subsequent conventional literacy skills—which also adheres to an optimal or critical time frame. The similarity—or, perhaps, commonality—of developmental problems in language and literacy suggests the viability of another construct pertinent to the QSH—that of *fundamentals.*

Fundamentals: Language and Literacy

One of the basic premises of the QSH is that there are developmental fundamentals that apply to all children attempting to learn the through-the-air or face-to-face aspects of the English language and its written counterpart (i.e., reading and writing). Given that neither the English language nor English literacy is a unitary construct, there is no all-encompassing fundamental to account for the entirety of development. Although there might be a group of fundamental attributes, the contributions of one or more attributes varies with intensity and age (e.g., early versus later development) and is subjected to multiple interactions involving language, cognitive, and the affective (e.g., motivation, etc.) domains (e.g., Cain & Oakhill, 2007; McGuinness, 2004, 2005; Stanovich, 1991, 1922, 2000; Stanovich et al., 1988).

In making the case for fundamentals, there are two major questions to consider:

1. What does it mean to know (be proficient in) a language, specifically a phonemic-based language such as English?
2. Is there a relationship between proficiency in the through-the-air form of English and its written counterpart?

A clear understanding of the responses to these questions should set the stage for interpreting the findings of research on both first-language and second-language development of English language and literacy. From another perspective, despite the evidence for the QSH, there is a substantial need for additional investigations utilizing more sophisticated research designs.

English Language: A Brief Rendition It is no simple feat to describe what it means to possess a bona fide language such as English. There are numerous theories within the purview of cognitivism, social, or environmental/behaviorism, including a range of computations or combinations (e.g., Paul, 2009; Pence & Justice, 2008). The discussion of this complex phenomenon here is simplified.

If an individual has proficiency in English, then s/he has developed a working intuitive understanding of the integrative use of major language components such as phonology, morphology, syntax, semantics, and pragmatics (Crystal, 1995, 2006; Pence & Justice, 2008). All language components are necessary for the full development of English, even though some theorists might place greater value on a particular component. What it means to reach a threshold level in each language component or with the integration of all components is, of course, not clearly understood.

Most children develop an adequate language level by the time they start formal schooling—at about age five or six—with the more difficult aspects of phonology accomplished by age eight or so (e.g., Crystal, 2006; Pence & Justice, 2008). After children have learned the basics of a language, then they can use language to learn. In other words, children can use their language (actually literate language) to not only acquire information in the various content areas such as social studies and science but also to grow in their understanding and use of more complex language structures, including vocabulary knowledge involving colloquial and academic nuances or meanings.

It has been argued—although it is controversial—that phonology represents the building blocks of a language (e.g., Crystal, 2006; Pence & Justice, 2008). Essentially, to learn or acquire a language—any language—one must access its phonology (spoken elements or signed elements), which seems to facilitate the acquisition of other language components. For a spoken language such as English, phonology entails segmentals (phonemes such as consonants and vowels) and suprasegmentals (prosodic features such as intonation, pauses, etc.). Phonology is highlighted here because of its necessary, but not sufficient, role (particularly phonological processes) in the development of emergent and foundational reading skills and its facilitation of higher-level conventional reading comprehension skills.

The structure of English involves the components of phonology, morphology, and syntax, whereas the meaning and use aspects involve semantics and pragmatics. With respect to the QSH (and Stanovich's developmental lag), much of the research has been focused on the acquisition of the structure of English as well as the relation of that structure to the development of reading/literacy skills. This is true not only for children with disabilities and dDhh children but also for ELLs.

English Literacy: A Brief Rendition Delineating the notion of fundamentals for the development of English literacy, particularly English reading, is no less complex. In fact, it might be even more complicated because English reading requires more than just English language development. With respect to the findings of the National Reading Panel (2000), National Early Literacy Panel (2008), and extant literacy research syntheses (e.g., Cain & Oakhill, 2007; Israel & Duffy, 2009; McGuinness, 2004, 2005; Ruddell & Unrau, 2004), the fundamentals include an understanding or competence in English (i.e., proficiency and processing) plus print access skills (e.g., decoding) and comprehension skills (e.g., vocabulary, prior knowledge, and metacognition). That is the simplified version for English literacy.

To make initial progress in early reading English—especially to learn to read—young children need to develop *metalinguistic awareness,* defined as awareness of print (pragmatics), sounds (phonemes), letters (graphemes), relationships between letters and sounds (phonics or sound–letter correspondences), word parts (morphemes), word order (syntax), and connected text structures (discourse) (Cain & Oakhill, 2007; Israel & Duffy, 2009; McGuinness, 2004, 2005; National Early Literacy Panel, 2008; National Reading Panel, 2000; Ruddell & Unrau, 2004). Competence in *any* language is helpful for the development of higher-level areas such as prior knowledge, metacognition, and breadth and depth of vocabulary knowledge. Nevertheless, for *readers of English* to develop and use these higher-level skills productively for reading to learn, they must have automatic lower-level skills often associated with word identification, including alphabet knowledge (knowledge of letters and sounds and the relationships between them) and morphological understanding (word parts). With rapid automatic word identification or decoding skills, readers of English print can expend the greater part of their efforts and resources on applying higher-level skills to make sense of and grow in their understanding of information from the text.

There are, of course, other cognitive areas of importance—such as attention and working memory (Cain & Oakhill, 2007; Pickering, 2006; Snow, Burns, & Griffin, 1998; Snow, Griffin, & Burns, 2005; Snowling & Hulme, 2005). An adequate working memory is related to proficiency in any language. With respect to the reading of English, the concern is on the development of working memory necessary for comprehension of symbols (print, etc.) based on the alphabetic principle. In other words, the processing of English syntax and longer discourse structures requires that readers hold specific textual aspects long enough in working memory to construct the meanings of phrases and sentences. In reading English, working memory is best facilitated by the use of phonology (e.g., phonological code, decoding into sounds, etc.; National Early Literacy Panel, 2008; for dDhh children, see reviews in Hanson, 1989; LaSasso, Crain, & Leybaert, 2010; Trezek, Wang, & Paul, 2010, 2011; Wang, Trezek, Luckner, & Paul, 2008).

In sum, the following areas seem to be fundamental and pertinent for the QSH:

- Knowledge of the language of print (i.e., components of English).
- Metalinguistic awareness of language- and print-related factors (e.g., of letters, sounds, letter–sound relationships [phonology, orthography], functions of print [pragmatics], words [semantics], sentences [syntax]).
- Phonological-based working memory or phonological memory (and processes).
- Comprehension capabilities (i.e., the development of textual, intertextual, and cultural prior knowledge, metacognitive, and self-regulatory skills).

RESEARCH ON OTHER POPULATIONS: CHILDREN WITH DISABILITIES AND ELLS

The debate on developmental or difference hypotheses and their educational implications has been ongoing for a number of years for children with language/learning disabilities and those who are learning English as a second language—that is, ELLs (e.g., Kamhi & Catts, 2012; McLaughlin, 1984, 1985, 1987; Paul, 2009; Paul & Wang, 2012; Stanovich, 1991, 1992). Most (but not all) of the data seem to support the basic premises of the QSH (or the developmental lag hypothesis). Demonstrating similarities within the QSH or a related similar framework does not obscure individual differences or issues that exist within each heterogeneous population for children with disabilities or for those who are ELLs (see Paul, 2008; Paul & Wang, 2012). The general findings should be considered as guidelines; otherwise, this becomes an oversimplification of the challenges associated with the various subgroups with each population.

Children With Disabilities

Dissension exists on whether there are distinct heterogeneous subgroups within the specific populations of children with disabilities (e.g., language/learning; cognitive/intellectual) that should be investigated separately or whether the attributes of these subgroups can be incorporated in a broad qualitative similarity framework for that group as compared to typical children with no identified reading or language disabilities (e.g., Kamhi & Catts, 2012; Stanovich, 1991, 1992; Vellutino, 1979; see also Paul & Wang, 2012). Despite the heterogeneity, it is possible to delineate certain patterns of development and problems.

Research seems to substantiate the assertions of not only the work of Lenneberg (1967) but also several of the findings from the early synthesis work of Vellutino (1979). Vellutino argued that the reading disabilities of these children were due to verbal ability in the primary language (in this case, English), not necessarily to visual or auditory processing difficulties. The difficulties were related to the problems in the various components of language, including phonology, morphology, syntax, and semantics. The bulk of the investigations has been conducted on these specific language components with most of the recent attention being devoted to phonology—specifically, phonological and phonemic awareness.

There is support for the fundamentals of English reading, presented previously. For example, fluency in word identification (i.e., decoding based on phonological processes, etc.) seems to be a prerequisite for higher-level reading comprehension skills (National Early Literacy Panel, 2008; National Reading Panel, 2000). As another example, many children might have inadequate vocabulary knowledge (semantics) and a range of comprehension processing problems, including prior knowledge, metacognition, and metalinguistic awareness of language and print reading factors.

It seems that more attention needs to be given to the language comprehension processes of English literacy; however, this means the language of English if one is to read in English (for dDhh children, see Mayer, 2007; Trezek et al., 2011). However, not all children with disabilities fit this conceptualization (e.g., Cain & Oakhill, 2007; Paul & Wang, 2012). These children seem to have additional difficulties (e.g., phonological processes, inferencing, etc.) that either contribute negatively to the development of English language or literacy skills or actually impede their development, despite years of instruction. As with any other complex entity, the contributions of the fundamentals for English and English literacy vary according to other social–cognitive and sociocultural developmental factors such as age, influences of the home and school environments, and so on.

English Language Learners (ELLs)

It should be no surprise that, similar to first language/literacy development, there is a complex array of factors that impact the acquisition of English by ELLs. The general findings here reflect the findings of the National Literacy Panel on Language-Minority Children and Youth (August & Shanahan, 2006), which seem to be the most recent and comprehensive synthesis of research on the literacy skills of ELLs (Paul & Wang, 2012).

These general remarks need to be interpreted with caution; otherwise, there is a risk of oversimplification. At the least, it can be argued that there are multiple factors that influence the acquisition of adequate English language and literacy skills such as age at which literacy skills are acquired, oral proficiency in both the first language and the language of English, print literacy skills in the first and second language, cognitive skills (e.g., working memory, phonological memory, metacognition), and sociocultural aspects such as home (e.g., parental involvement, socioeconomic status, etc.) and school environments (e.g., school resources, quality of teachers, etc.).

With respect to the discussion on dDhh children and adolescents, especially those who know ASL as a first language, one important construct is the notion of transfer (e.g., see the work of Cummins, 1979, 1984; see also Paul, 2001, 2009). The issues of transfer (from the first to the second language) and development (of the second language) are dependent on language and literacy fundamentals, mentioned previously, especially if one goal is the subsequent development of English reading and written language.

Support for the QSH can be gleaned from syntheses on ELLs in their acquisition of the components of English (e.g., see Cziko, 1992; McLaughlin, 1984, 1985, 1987; Paul, 1985, 2001, 2009) and English literacy (e.g., August & Shanahan, 2006; Bernhardt, 1991). For example, many ELLs acquire aspects of morphology and syntax in a manner that is developmentally similar (e.g., stages, errors, strategies) to that of younger native first-language learners. In addition, similar to children learning to read English as a first language, ELLs need to develop rapid automatic word identification skills (via decoding and orthography) to obtain adequate levels of reading comprehension. As with first language learners, English phonological processes (e.g., phonological coding, memory, etc.) are necessary but not sufficient for developing reading. ELLs need more intensive and extensive instructional focus on general language comprehension areas and processes such as word knowledge, prior knowledge, metacognitive skills, and so on.

Paul and Wang (2012) summarized these findings:

> It appears that the script or print literacy development of ELLs is qualitatively similar to that of English monolingual learners. That is, whether learning English as a first- or second- language, children need to acquire good decoding and orthographic skills before they can progress with accurate and fast word recognition skills, which are the prerequisites for subsequent adequate levels of reading comprehension. The findings are consistent with those on the literacy development of children with language/learning disabilities . . . , sensory disabilities . . . , and developmental disabilities. . . . In essence, the Qualitative-Similarity Hypothesis (QSH . . .) might be applicable to all children who are learning English, regardless of their sensory/cognitive abilities or cultural/linguistic backgrounds. (p. 299)

RESEARCH ON CHILDREN WHO ARE d/DEAF OR HARD OF HEARING (dDhh)

Much of the research on dDhh children has focused on their development of signed and written English as a first language, particularly in the areas of morphology and syntax. There are both empirical (evidence-based) and reason-based (e.g., reviews, meta-analyses) investigations on the role of phonology or phonological processes in English reading development (e.g., Allen, Clark, del Giudice, Koo, Lieberman, Mayberry, & Miller, 2009; Mayberry, del Giudice, & Lieberman, 2011; Wang et al., 2008; Paul, Wang, Trezek, & Luckner, 2009). Some of the research on phonology has also involved the role of working memory (e.g., Hanson, 1989; Paul, 2009; Trezek et al., 2011; Wang et al., 2008).

Hard of Hearing (hh) Students

From the work of Pintner and Lev (1939) to more recent syntheses (e.g., Moores, 2001; Paul, 2001, 2009; Spencer & Marschark, 2006), it has been documented that the degree of hearing impairment correlates negatively with academic achievement—even a slight hearing loss (e.g., up to 26 dB) can affect the development of spoken and written English language abilities. Although the development of hh students is quantitatively delayed or slower, they do proceed through learning stages of English speech and language that are similar to those of younger peers who have typical hearing.

To exemplify the notion of quantitative delays and qualitative similarities, consider the findings of early researchers (e.g., Davis & Blasdell, 1975; Davis, Shepard, Stelmachowicz, & Gorga, 1981; Pressnell, 1973; Wilcox & Tobin, 1974). Pressnell, Wilcox, and Tobin documented delays and similarities for the performance of students with moderate (about 56 dB) or greater hearing losses on acquiring or understanding aspects of the verb system of English (e.g., tense agreement, voice, etc.). Pressnell analyzed spontaneous language samples as well as the children's performance on the Northwestern Syntax Screening Test (Lee, 1969).

Davis and Blasdell (1975) examined the performances of young children, aged six to nine years with losses between 35 and 75 dB (again, average pure tone average [PTA] in the better unaided ear). These researchers focused on the children's ability to comprehend relative clauses that were embedded medially (as in "The woman *who chased the cat* fell down the slope"). The hh students made more errors than their hearing counterparts, and the gap increased with age. Nevertheless, the errors of the hh children were similar to those made by their younger peers.

In fact, since the work of Blair, Peterson, and Viehweg (1985) to the present (see reviews in LaSasso et al. 2010; Moores, 2001; Paul, 2009; Spencer & Marschark, 2006; Trezek et al., 2010, 2011), the findings have remained fairly consistent. However, as noted by Blair et al. (1985), the quantitative delays can be reduced with early intervention and amplification. The reduction of delays or the beneficial effects of early intervention and amplification still need to be investigated further and may not have strong research support (see Marschark & Spencer, 2010). Nevertheless, the notion of qualitative similarity for hh students has not been substantively challenged.

Children and Adolescents With Severe to Profound Losses

The developmental order of English morphemes has received considerable attention (Cooper, 1967; Crandall, 1978; Raffin, 1976; Raffin, Davis, & Gilman, 1978). For example, Cooper (1967) found that deaf children had more difficulty with derivational morphology (e.g., *deaf* to *deafness* or *ice* to *reice*) than with inflectional morphology (e.g., *slow* to *slowly* or *see* to *sees*), and these findings are similar to those reported in the studies on hearing children (e.g., see McGuinness, 2004, 2005). In another early study, Crandall (1978) reported that the production of inflectional morphemes did not increase significantly with age, which might also account for the difficulty in the use and development of inflectional morphemes by dDhh children in the series of investigations on Signed English (Bornstein & Saulnier, 1981). Relative to developmental order, Crandall (1978) documented that the first six morphemes used were similar to those documented for children with typical hearing (Brown, 1973).

Several investigators have focused on the acquisition and use of morphemes via exposure to a particular sign system. Raffin and associates (e.g., Gilman, Davis, & Raffin, 1980; Raffin, 1976; Raffin et al., 1978) examined the use of the sign morphological markers of Seeing Essential English. These markers represented a few of the most common English morphemes such as *–s* (plurality and third-person singular), *–ly* (adverb), and *–ed* (past tense). Again, the results indicated that the order of acquisition of the markers by dDhh students was qualitatively similar to that of the younger hearing children. dDhh students proceeded through the developmental stages at a slower rate, and the production of errors and the use of strategies were similar to those of the younger hearing children.

Quigley and his associates provided much of the evidence on the acquisition of syntax for different environments: negation, conjunction, verb processes, pronominalization, question formation, relativization, complementation, disjunction, and alternation (Quigley, Wilbur, Power, Montanelli, & Steinkamp, 1976; Russell, Quigley, & Power, 1976; see also the reviews in Paul, 2001, 2009) (see Table 1).This line of research detailed the performances of a national stratified and random sample of deaf

Table 1. **Examples of Syntactic Structures**

Structures	Examples
Negation	The girl will not read the book. The man did not kiss the woman.
Conjunction	I like football and soccer. She kicked and screamed at the dog.
Disjunction and alternation	I read the book, but not the magazine She is either sick or crazy.
Question formation	
Yes/no	Did you see that movie?
Wh-	Where is my pipe? Why are you happy?
Tag-	Mary loves John, doesn't she? (negative tag) This isn't right, is it? (positive tag)
Verb processes	
Passive voice	The dog was mauled by the cat.
Truncated passive	The window was hit.
Pronominalization	
Reflexive	Mother bought herself a diamond.
Relativization	The boy who kissed the girl ran away. The cat scratched the dog who stole its food.
Complementation	
That clause	That Mary was insane was obvious to her brother.
Infinitive	I would like for you to kiss my mother-in-law.

students (i.e., 90 dB or greater pure-tone average [PTA]) between the ages of 10 and 19 years old on tests of comprehension of syntactic structures presented in sentences and compared their performance with that of younger hearing students. It was found that the eight-year-old hearing students performed significantly better than the 18-year-old deaf students on most of the tasks.

Despite the quantitative delays, Quigley and associates reported that the acquisition of the structures by deaf students was similar to that of the hearing students. This was observed for the structures in general as well as within each structure itself. With respect to the former, the acquisition of negation (use of the negative, e.g., *not*) was easier than the development of relativization (use of relative clauses, e.g., *The boy who kissed the girl ran away*). For the latter, consider the condition of question formation. dDhh children found yes/no questions (*Do you want candy?*) to be easier than wh–questions (*Where do you live?*), and these, in turn, were easier than tag questions (e.g., *You like me, don't you?* or *You aren't eating that cookie, are you?*).

The notion of a quantitative delay–qualitative similarity was also observed by Payne and Quigley (1987) in the comprehension of verb–particles by both hearing and deaf (90 dB or greater PTA). The age design of the Payne and Quigley study was similar to that employed by the earlier research by Quigley on syntax. Payne and Quigley developed and tested an instrument containing 64 verb–particle items at three levels of semantic difficulty in five syntactic patterns. The three semantic levels were as follows:

- literal—*walks out*
- semi-idiomatic—*washes up*
- idiomatic—*gives up*

The five syntactic conditions were the following:

- SVA—subject, verb, adverb
- SVAO—subject, verb, adverb, object
- SVOA—subject, verb, object, adverb
- SVPO—subject, verb, preposition, object
- SVAPO—subject, verb, adverb, preposition, object

Hearing students performed significantly better than dDhh students on all semantic levels in all syntactic conditions. In general, there was a hierarchy of understanding moving from literal to idiomatic within each of the syntactic condition from the easiest (SVO) to the most difficult (SVAPO). Finally, Payne and Quigley (1987) reiterated the two general findings that seem to have stood the test of time with respect to research on dDhh children, particularly those with severe to profound hearing losses: (1) there is little improvement in the performance across ages and (2) performance is highly related to reading comprehension ability (Moores, 2001; Paul, 2009; Trezek et al., 2011).

There is even some evidence for the QSH for d/Deaf students who know Spanish as a first language and are ELLs (e.g., King, 1981). King (1981) examined the performance of (1) d/Deaf children with profound hearing losses and hearing students who were learning English as a first language and (2) Spanish d/Deaf children with profound hearing losses and hearing students who were ELLs. The screening and four diagnostic tests of the Test of Syntactic Abilities (Quigley, Steinkamp, Power, & Jones, 1978) were used. King reported that the order of difficulty on the syntactic tasks was similar for both groups of students. In addition, King provided an analysis of errors that seemed to reveal that the error types were also similar for both groups.

Summary

Clearly, there is a need for additional research on dDhh children who are ELLs and whose first language is ASL or some other language. For example, given the obvious differences in modality between ASL (sign only) and English (spoken and written), the transfer from the performance form of a sign language (ASL) to the written form of a spoken language (English) is neither automatic nor clear-cut. Second language learners do use their knowledge of the first language in acquiring information (e.g., grammar) about the second language. Nevertheless, acquiring adequate, independent literacy skills in a second language such as English requires at least an understanding of the alphabetic principle, which in turn is dependent upon access to phonology and morphology of English (e.g., Paul, 2009; Paul & Wang, 2012).

There is also a need for additional studies involving dDhh's English language comprehension processes, especially in relation to the development of reading. Several scholars have argued that reading difficulties might be due more to language comprehension processes rather than to print literacy processes (e.g., Marschark, Sapere, Convertino, Mayer, Wauters, & Sarchet, 2009; Mayberry et al., 2011). However, this might be a narrow view of the English literacy process (e.g., Cain & Oakhill, 2007; Israel & Duffy, 2009; McGuinness, 2004, 2005; National Early Literacy Panel, 2008; Storch & Whitehurst, 2002; Whitehurst & Lonigan, 2002). The focus for English reading should be on English language comprehension skills as well as on decoding or other print English literacy skills (e.g., Mayer, 2007; Paul, 2009; Paul & Wang, 2012; Trezek et al., 2010, 2011). The increased focus on English language comprehension is the impetus for the ongoing debate on the role of phonology.

THE PHONOLOGY DEBATE

As mentioned previously, phonology is the building blocks for the English language and facilitates the development of the other English structures (morphology, syntax) as well as vocabulary (semantics). Phonology and morphology work in tandem to facilitate the development of rapid automatic word identification or decoding skills. The existence of a strong relationship between rapid word identification skills and reading comprehension has been documented for dDhh adolescents at the secondary and postsecondary levels (e.g., see reviews in Paul, 2009; Trezek et al., 2011; Wang et al., 2008). The less-skilled readers are slower and produce more errors than do more-skilled readers. The nature of this relationship for *deaf* (i.e., profound hearing impairment) or Deaf readers is open to debate (Allen et al., 2009; Mayberry et al., 2011; Paul et al., 2009; Wang et al., 2008).

Although a few researchers have documented limited phonological processing (Allen et al., 2009) or that phonological processing seems to be a relatively low to moderate predictor for reading comprehension (Mayberry et al., 2011), there is ample evidence that d/Deaf readers, particularly the more-skilled readers, use phonological information during the reading comprehension process (Hanson, 1989; Paul, 2009; Trezek et al., 2010, 2011; Wang et al., 2008).

One line of research has focused on working memory, which is similar to the phonological memory process highlighted for the emergent literacy skills of children who have typical hearing (National Early Literacy Panel, 2008). The bulk of research findings reveals that dDhh children and adolescents who use predominantly a phonological code in working memory tend to be better readers than those who use predominantly a nonphonological code (Hanson, 1989; Paul, 2009; Perfetti & Sandak, 2000; Trezek et al., 2010, 2011; Wang et al., 2008). There are a few empirical and reason-based investigations that reported no strong relationship between phonological coding and reading skills (e.g., Allen et al., 2009; Mayberry et al., 2011). The reasons for the equivocal findings are not clear; however, it has been speculated that contributing factors include artifacts of the tests, the interpretations of the findings, or, more important, the role of phonology during the emergent literacy stages as opposed to the later conventional stage (Paul, 2009; Paul & Wang, 2012; Wang et al., 2008).

In sum, much of the controversy related to phonology or phonological processes is related to research on children with profound hearing losses, who may be predominantly dependent on signing—either English signing or ASL. From one perspective, similar to other populations mentioned in this chapter, phonology is necessary but not sufficient for English reading development (e.g., Paul & Wang, 2012; Wang et al., 2008). The role of phonology in young dDhh children, learning English literacy, from preschool to grade 3 has not been studied extensively.

CONCLUSION: FROM THE PAST TO THE FUTURE

The QSH is a broad hypothesis grounded mostly in behavioral and cognitive models using the scientific method, particularly one related to a version of the standard epistemology (see Paul & Moores, Chapter 1). There is some support from research motivated by social or sociocultural models (e.g., Williams, 2004, 2011). Most of the challenges to the QSH stem from research informed by sociocultural models, based on the tenets of multiple epistemologies—particularly the view that knowledge is shaped predominantly by social entities such as ethnicity, gender, race, or culture. Within the field of deafness, much of the dissension seems to be with d/Deaf children and adolescents who use sign predominantly. A few challenges are the result of misinterpretations of either second language literacy research (e.g., Mayer & Wells, 1996; Paul 2009; Paul & Wang, 2012) or extant theories of reading involving the role of phonology (e.g., see Paul et al., 2009; Trezek et al., 2011; Wang et al., 2008).

The QSH is a viable construct with important implications for the development of English language and literacy in dDhh children learning English as a first language or who are ELLs. Further research on the QSH should lead to refinements, and there is a need for more sophisticated research designs. Investigators should focus on the following items:

- Application of the QSH to other content areas such as mathematics and science.
- Relative contributions of English language comprehension processes to the development of emergent and conventional English literacy skills.
- Utility of constructs such as discipline knowledge, critical or optimal periods, and fundamentals for various subgroups of dDhh children and adolescents (i.e., varying across degree of hearing impairment, age, gender, language/communication modality, etc.).
- Role of phonology or phonological processes in the development of emergent and conventional literacy skills for dDhh children from preschool age (age three to five years) to the end of grades 3 or 4 (i.e., eight or nine years old).
- Influence of social and cultural factors on the basic assumptions of the QSH.

REFERENCES

Allen, T., Clark, M. D., del Giudice, A., Koo, D., Lieberman, A., Mayberry, R., & Miller, P. (2009). Phonology and reading: A response to Wang, Trezek, Luckner, and Paul. *American Annals of the Deaf, 154*(4), 338–345.

August, D., & Shanahan, T. (Eds.). (2006). *Developing literacy in second-language learners: Report of the National Literacy Panel on Language-Minority Children and Youth.* Mahwah, NJ: Lawrence Erlbaum.

Battista, M. (2001). Research and reform in mathematics education. In T. Loveless (Ed.), *The great curriculum debate: How should we teach reading and math?* (pp. 42–84). Washington, DC: Brookings Institution Press.

Bernhardt, E. (1991). *Reading development in a second language.* Norwood, NJ: Ablex.

Birch, B. (2007). *English L2 reading: Getting to the bottom* (2nd ed.). Mahwah, NJ: Lawrence Erlbaum.

Blair, J., Peterson, M., & Viehweg, S. (1985). The effects of mild hearing loss on academic performance of young school-age children. *Volta Review, 87,* 87–93.

Bornstein, H., & Saulnier, K. (1981). Signed English: A brief follow-up to the first evaluation. *American Annals of the Deaf, 126,* 69–72.

Brown, R. (1973). *A first language: The early stages.* Cambridge, MA: Harvard University Press.

Cain, K., & Oakhill, J. (Eds.). (2007). *Children's comprehension problems in oral and written language.* New York, NY: Guilford Press.

Cartwright, K. (2009). The role of cognitive flexibility in reading comprehension: Past, present, and future. In S. Israel & G. Duffy (Eds.), *Handbook of research on reading comprehension* (pp. 115–139). New York, NY: Routledge.

Cooper, R. (1967). The ability of deaf and hearing children to apply morphological rules. *Journal of Speech and Hearing Research, 10,* 77–86.

Crandall, K. (1978). Inflectional morphemes in the manual English of young hearing impaired children and their mothers. *Journal of Speech and Hearing Research, 21,* 372–386.

Crystal, D. (1995). *The Cambridge encyclopedia of the English language.* New York, NY: Cambridge University Press.

Crystal, D. (2006). *How language works.* London, UK: Penguin.

Cummins, J. (1979). Linguistic interdependence and the educational development of bilingual children. *Review of Educational Research, 49*(2), 222–251.

Cummins, J. (1984). *Bilingual and special education: Issues in assessment and pedagogy.* San Diego, CA: College Hill Press.

Cummins, J. (2007). Pedagogies for the poor: Realigning reading instruction for low-income students with scientifically based reading research. *Educational Researcher, 36*(9), 564–572.

Cziko, G. (1992). The evaluation of bilingual education: From necessity and probability to possibility. *Educational Researcher, 21*(2), 10–15.

Davis, J., & Blasdell, R. (1975). Perceptual strategies employed by normal-hearing and hearing-impaired children in the comprehension of sentences containing relative clauses. *Journal of Speech and Hearing Research, 18*, 281–295.

Davis, J., Shepard, N., Stelmachowicz, P., & Gorga, M. (1981). Characteristics of hearing-impaired children in the public schools, part II: Psychoeducational data. *Journal of Speech and Hearing Disorders, 46*, 130–137.

Donovan, M., & Bransford, J. (Eds.). (2005). *How students learn: History, mathematics, and science in the classroom.* Washington, DC: National Academies Press.

English, L., & Halford, G. (1995). *Mathematics education: Models and processes.* Mahwah, NJ: Lawrence Erlbaum.

Fenstermacher, G., & Soltis, J. (2004). *Approaches to teaching.* New York, NY: Teachers College, Columbia University.

Fodor, J. (1983). *The modularity of mind: An essay on faculty psychology.* Cambridge, MA: MIT Press.

Francis, D., Shaywitz, S., Stuebing, K., Shaywitz, B., & Fletcher, J. (1996). Developmental lag versus deficit models of reading disability: A longitudinal, individual growth-curve analysis. *Journal of Educational Psychology, 88*(1), 3–17.

Gilman, L., Davis, J., & Raffin, M. (1980). Use of common morphemes by hearing impaired children exposed to a system of manual English. *Journal of Auditory Research, 20*, 57–69.

Hanson, V. (1989). Phonology and reading: Evidence from profoundly deaf readers. In D. Shankweiler & I. Liberman (Eds.), *Phonology and reading disability: Solving the reading puzzle* (pp. 69–89). Ann Arbor, MI: University of Michigan Press.

Israel, S., & Duffy, G. (Eds.). (2009). *Handbook of research on reading comprehension.* New York, NY: Routledge.

Kamhi, A., & Catts, H. (2012). *Language and reading disabilities* (3rd ed.). Boston, MA: Pearson Education.

King, C. (1981). *An investigation of similarities and differences in the syntactic abilities of deaf and hearing children learning English as a first or second language* (Unpublished doctoral dissertation). University of Illinois, Champaign–Urbana.

LaSasso, C., Crain, K., & Leybaert, J. (Eds.). (2010). *Cued speech and cued language for deaf and hard of hearing children.* San Diego, CA: Plural Publishing.

Lee, L. (1969). *Northwestern syntax screening test.* Evanston, IL: Northwestern University Press.

Lenneberg, E. (1967). *Biological foundations of language.* New York, NY: Wiley.

Marschark, M., Sapere, P., Convertino, C. M., Mayer, C., Wauters, L., & Sarchet, T. (2009). Are deaf students' reading challenges really about reading? *American Annals of the Deaf, 154*(4), 357–376.

Marschark, M., & Spencer, P. (2010). The promises (?) of deaf education: From research to practice and back again. In M. Marschark & P. Spencer (Eds.), *The Oxford handbook of deaf studies, language, and education* (Vol. 2, pp. 1–14). New York, NY: Oxford University Press.

Mayberry, R., del Guidice, A., & Lederberg, A. (2011). Reading achievement in relation to phonological coding and awareness in deaf readers: A meta-analysis. *Journal of Deaf Studies and Deaf Education, 16*(2), 164–188.

Mayer, C. (2007). What really matters in the early literacy development of deaf children. *Journal of Deaf Studies and Deaf Education, 12*(4), 411–431.

Mayer, C., & Wells, G. (1996). Can the linguistic interdependence theory support a bilingual–bicultural model of literacy education for deaf students? *Journal of Deaf Studies and Deaf Education, 1*(2), 93–107.

Mayer, R. (1992). Mathematical problem solving: Thinking as based on domain specific knowledge. In R. Mayer (Ed.), *Thinking, problem solving, cognition* (pp. 455–489). New York, NY: Cambridge University Press.

McGuinness, D. (2004). *Early reading instruction: What science really tells us about how to teach reading.* Cambridge, MA: MIT Press.

McGuinness, D. (2005). *Language development and learning to read: The scientific study of how language development affects reading skill.* Cambridge, MA: MIT Press.

McLaughlin, B. (1984). *Second-language acquisition in childhood: Vol. 1. Preschool children* (2nd ed.). Hillsdale, NJ: Lawrence Erlbaum.

McLaughlin, B. (1985). *Second-language acquisition in childhood: Vol. 2. School-age children* (2nd ed.). Hillsdale, NJ: Lawrence Erlbaum.

McLaughlin, B. (1987). *Theories of second-language learning.* Baltimore, MD: Edward Arnold.

Moores, D. (2001). *Educating the deaf: Psychology, principles, and practices* (5th ed.). Boston, MA: Houghton-Mifflin.

National Early Literacy Panel. (2008). *Developing early literacy: Report of the National Early Literacy Panel.* Washington, DC: National Institute for Literacy. Retrieved from http://www.nifl.gov/earlychildhood/NELP/NELPreport.html

National Reading Panel. (2000). *Report of the National Reading Panel: Teaching children to read—An evidence-based assessment of the scientific research literature on reading and its implications for reading instruction.* Jessup, MD: National Institute for Literacy.

Noddings, N. (2007). *Philosophy of education* (2nd ed.). Boulder, CO: Westview Press.

O'Brien, B., Mansfield, J., & Legge, G. (2005). The effect of print size on reading speed in dyslexia. *Journal of Research in Reading, 28*(3), 332–349.

O'Shaughnessy, T., & Swanson, H. (1998). Do immediate memory deficits in students with learning disabilities in reading reflect a developmental lag or deficit? A selective meta-analysis of the literature. *Learning Disability Quarterly, 21*(2), 123–148.

Paul, P. (1985). Reading and other language-variant populations. In C. King & S. Quigley, *Reading and deafness* (pp. 251–289). San Diego, CA: College-Hill.

Paul, P. (2001). *Language and deafness* (3rd ed.). San Diego, CA: Singular/Thomson Learning.

Paul, P. (2008). Introduction: Reading and children with disabilities. *Balanced Reading Instruction, 15*(2), 1–12.

Paul, P. (2009). *Language and deafness* (4th ed.). Sudbury, MA: Jones & Bartlett.

Paul, P. (2010). Qualitative-similarity hypothesis. In R. Nata (Ed.), *Progress in education* (Vol. 20, pp. 1–31). New York, NY: Nova Science.

Paul, P., & Lee, C. (2010). Qualitative-similarity hypothesis. *American Annals of the Deaf, 154*(5), 456–462.

Paul, P., & Wang, Y. (2012). *Literate thought: Understanding comprehension and literacy.* Sudbury, MA: Jason & Barlett Learning.

Paul, P., Wang, Y., Trezek, B., & Luckner, J. (2009). Phonology is necessary, but not sufficient: A rejoinder. *American Annals of the Deaf, 154*(4), 346–356.

Paul, P., & Whitelaw, G. (2011). *Hearing and deafness: An introduction for health and educational professionals.* Sudbury, MA: Jason & Bartlett Learning.

Payne, J.-A., & Quigley, S. (1987). Hearing-impaired children's comprehension of verb–particle combinations. *Volta Review, 89*, 133–143.

Pence, K., & Justice, L. (2008). *Language development from theory to practice.* Upper Saddle River, NJ: Pearson/Merrill Prentice Hall.

Perfetti, C., & Sandak, R. (2000). Reading optimally builds on spoken language: Implications for deaf readers. *Journal of Deaf Studies and Deaf Education, 5*, 32–50.

Phillips, D. (1983). On describing a student's cognitive structure. *Educational Psychologist, 18*(2), 59–74.

Phillips, D., & Soltis, J. (2004). *Perspectives on learning.* New York, NY: Teachers College Press.

Pickering, S. (Ed.). (2006). *Working memory and education.* Boston, MA: Elsevier.

Pintner, R., & Lev, J. (1939). The intelligence of the hard-of-hearing school child. *Journal of Genetic Psychology, 55,* 31–48.

Pressnell, L. (1973). Hearing-impaired children's comprehension and production of syntax in oral language. *Journal of Speech and Hearing Research, 16,* 12–21.

Pring, R. (2004). *Philosophy of educational research* (2nd ed.). New York, NY: Continuum.

Quigley, S., Steinkamp, M., Power, D., & Jones, B. (1978). *Test of syntactic abilities: Guide to administration and interpretation.* Beaverton, OR: DORMAC.

Quigley, S., Wilbur, R., Power, D., Montanelli, D., & Steinkamp, M. (1976). *Syntactic structures in the language of deaf children* (Final Report). Urbana, IL: University of Illinois, Institute for Child Behavior and Development. (ERIC Document Reproduction Service No. ED 119 447).

Raffin, M. (1976). *The acquisition of inflectional morphemes by deaf children using seeing essential English* (Unpublished doctoral dissertation). University of Iowa, Iowa City.

Raffin, M., Davis, J., & Gilman, L. (1978). Comprehension of inflectional morphemes by deaf children exposed to a visual English sign system. *Journal of Speech and Hearing Research, 21,* 387–400.

Reimer, J. (2006). Developmental changes in the allocation of semantic feedback during visual word recognition. *Journal of Research in Reading, 29*(2), 194–212.

Ritzer, G. (2001). *Explorations in social theory: From metatheorizing to rationalization.* Thousand Oaks, CA: Sage.

Ruddell, R., & Unrau, N. (Eds.). (2004). *Theoretical models and processes of reading* (5th ed.). Newark, DE: International Reading Association.

Russell, W., Quigley, S., & Power, D. (1976). *Linguistics and deaf children.* Washington, DC: Alexander Graham Bell Association for the Deaf.

Rymer, R. (1992, April 13). Annals of science: A silent childhood—I. *New Yorker,* pp. 41–81.

Shanahan, C. (2009). Disciplinary comprehension. In S. Israel & G. Duffy (Eds.), *Handbook of research on reading comprehension* (pp. 240–260). New York, NY: Routledge.

Snow, C. E., Burns, M. S., & Griffin, P. (1998). *Preventing reading difficulties in young children.* Washington, DC: National Academy Press.

Snow, C. E., Griffin, P., & Burns, M. S. (2005). *Knowledge to support the teaching of reading: Preparing teachers for a changing world.* San Francisco, CA: Wiley.

Snowling, M., Defty, N., & Goulandris, N. (1996). A longitudinal study of reading development in dyslexic children. *Journal of Educational Psychology, 88*(4), 653–669.

Snowling, M., & Hulme, C. (Eds.). (2005). *The science of reading: A handbook.* Malden, MA: Blackwell.

Spencer, P., & Marschark, M. (Eds.). (2006). *Advances in the spoken language development of deaf and hard of hearing children.* New York, NY: Oxford University Press.

Spiro, R., Vispoel, W., Schmitz, J., Samarapungavan, A., & Boerger, A. (1987). Knowledge acquisition for application: Cognitive flexibility and transfer in complex content domains. In B. Britton & S. Glynn (Eds.), *Executive control processes in reading* (pp. 177–199). Hillsdale, NJ: Lawrence Erlbaum.

Stanovich, K. (1986). Matthew effects in reading: Some consequences of individual differences in the acquisition of literacy. *Reading Research Quarterly, 21,* 360– 407.

Stanovich, K. (1991). Word recognition: Changing perspectives. In R. Barr, M. Kamil, P. Mosenthal, & P. D. Pearson (Eds.), *Handbook of reading research* (2nd ed., pp. 418–452). White Plains, NY: Longman.

Stanovich, K. (1992). Speculations on the causes and consequences of individual differences in early reading acquisition. In P. Gough, L. Ehri, & R. Treiman (Eds.), *Reading acquisition* (pp. 307–342). Hillsdale, NJ: Lawrence Erlbaum.

Stanovich, K. (2000). *Progress in understanding reading: Scientific foundations and new frontiers.* New York, NY: Guilford Press.

Stanovich, K., Nathan, R., & Zolman, J. (1988). The developmental lag hypothesis in reading: Longitudinal and matched reading-level comparisons. *Child Development, 59*, 71–86.

Storch, S., & Whitehurst, G. (2002). Oral language and code-related precursors to reading: Evidence from a longitudinal structural model. *Developmental Psychology, 38*(6), 934–947.

Trezek, B., Wang, Y., & Paul, P. (2010). *Reading and deafness: Theory, research, and practice.* Clifton Park, NY: Cengage Learning.

Trezek, B., Wang, Y., & Paul, P. (2011). Processes and components of reading. In M. Marschark & P. Spencer (Eds.), *Handbook of deaf studies, language, and education* (2nd ed., Vol. 1, pp. 99–114). New York, NY: Oxford University Press.

Vellutino, F. (1979). *Dyslexia: Theory and research.* Cambridge, MA: MIT Press.

Vellutino, F. (2003). Individual differences as sources of variability in reading comprehension in elementary school children. In A. P. Sweet & C. E. Snow (Eds.), *Rethinking reading comprehension* (pp. 51–81). New York, NY: Guilford Press.

Wang, Y., Trezek, B., Luckner, J., & Paul, P. (2008). The role of phonology and phonological-related skills in reading instruction for students who are deaf or hard of hearing. *American Annals of the Deaf, 153*(4), 396–407.

Whitehurst, G., & Lonigan, C. (2002). Emergent literacy: Development from preschoolers to readers. In S. Neuman & D. Dickinson (Eds.), *Handbook of early literacy research* (pp. 11–29). New York, NY: Guilford Press.

Wilcox, J., & Tobin, H. (1974). Linguistic performance of hard-of-hearing and normal hearing children. *Journal of Speech and Hearing Research, 17*, 286–293.

Williams, C. (2004). Emergent literacy of deaf children. *Journal of Deaf Studies and Deaf Education, 9*(4), 352–365.

Williams, C. (2011). Adpated interactive writing instruction with kindergarten children who are deaf or hard of hearing. *American Annals of the Deaf, 156*(1), 23–34.

SUGGESTIONS FOR FURTHER READING

Bransford, J., Brown, A., & Cocking, R. (Eds.). (2000). *How people learn: Brain, mind, experience, and school.* Washington, DC: National Academy Press.

Huey, E. (1968). *The psychology and pedagogy of reading.* Cambridge, MA: MIT Press. (Original work published 1908)

Greene, R. (1992). *Human memory: Paradigms and paradoxes.* Mahwah, NJ: Lawrence Erlbaum.

Sternberg, R., & Ben-Zeev, T. (Eds.). (1996). *The nature of mathematical thinking.* Mahwah, NJ: Erlbaum.

Yuill, N., & Oakhill, J. (1991). *Children's problems in text comprehension: An experimental investigation.* Cambridge, UK: Cambridge University Press.

11

Educators Without Borders: A Metaparadigm for Literacy Instruction in Bilingual–Bicultural Education

Ye Wang

In 1981, Sweden became the first country in the world to officially recognize a sign language (i.e., Swedish Sign Language) as a bona fide language and proclaim the need for *bilingual–bicultural* (BiBi) education among d/Deaf individuals.[1] Two years later, special schools for students who are d/Deaf or hard of hearing implemented the first contemporary BiBi curriculum, which established languages of instruction as both Swedish Sign Language and Swedish, the latter of which was primarily intended to be acquired in its written form, and if possible, in its spoken modality for d/Deaf children (Svartholm, 2010). The underlying principles of the BiBi programs include "a heighted valuing of the language and culture of the Deaf community, a focus on equality of educational opportunity, the empowerment of Deaf people, and the recognition that d/Deaf children have the same potential for language and learning as their hearing peers" (Mayer & Leigh, 2010, p. 176). The Deaf community, meanwhile, gained increasing public visibility, and terms such as *Deaf culture, Deaf history, Deaf pride* (Lane, 1984), *Deafhood* (Ladd, 2003, 2008), *Deafnicity* (Eckert, 2005, 2010), and *deaf epistemologies* (see the review in Moores, 2010) have bloomed in the field of deaf studies and deaf education.

Forty-five years after the modern-day formal validation of sign languages as bona fide languages (Stokoe, Casterline, & Croneberg, 1965)[2] and 30 years after the contemporary implementation of BiBi education for children who are d/Deaf or hard of hearing, where are we today? In 2010, the *American Annals of the Deaf* devoted an issue (Vol. 154, No. 5) to deaf epistemologies, the *Journal of Deaf Studies and Deaf Education* dedicated its first issue of Vol. 15 to Deaf studies, and the *International Journal of Bilingual Education and Bilingualism* had a special issue (Vol. 13, No. 2) on sign bilingualism. This chapter continues the discussion on BiBi education for children who are d/Deaf or hard of hearing with the focus on the development of language and literacy.

MAPPING THE FIELD: EPISTEMOLOGY

Epistemology, also known as *theory of knowledge*, addresses the issues of not only the definition and nature of knowledge but also the way knowledge is acquired, that is, the relationship between the knower/inquirer and the known/knowledge (see also Paul & Moores, Chapter 1). Positivism and constructivism are two major umbrellas, each covering a range of epistemological beliefs.

Pure positivists believe in the existence of an external reality that consists of facts, which are obtainable with the appropriate methods, whereas *pure* constructivists consider reality as socially constructed through human interaction only. Furthermore, *pure* positivists believe in the separation of the knower/inquirer and the known/knowledge, that is, although knowledge, especially social knowledge, can be biased or subjective, regardless of the inquirer, the subjectivity can be and should be controlled or reduced through scientific methods such as hypothesis confirmation or Popperian falsification of theories (i.e., a hypothesis or theory is scientific only if it is, among other things, falsifiable—that is, there is the possibility of the theory being modified or even abandoned). Scientific inquiry is a never-ending refining process in which the scientific community is reaching closer and closer approximations of the external, knowable reality. In contrast, *pure* constructivists question the existence of "innocent" knowledge (Foucault, 1980) and assert that there is no separation between the knower/inquirer and the knowing because the knowing is socially and politically constructed by the knower. The term *knowing* is preferred over known or knowledge because of its fluidity (Denzin & Lincoln, 1994; Guba & Lincoln, 2005; Noddings, 1995, 2007; see also, the review in Wang, 2010).

Disciplinary matrices, or *paradigms* (Kuhn, 1962, 1996), which refer to "a fundamental image of the subject matter within a science" (Rizter, 2001, p. 60), are what differentiate positivism and constructivism. Why do we want to study paradigms in deaf education, or education in general? Because, similar to the patterns in general education, many of the so-called innovative "scientifically based approaches" for teaching children who are d/Deaf or hard of hearing are "re-creations of past innovations" (Rose, McAnally, & Quigley, 2004, p. 55). Chall (2000) famously claims:

> What is particularly striking about educational innovations is that most were considered successes long before they were actually sufficiently tried and tested. Seldom were they presented together with a rationale based on educational theory and research. Nor had they been tried first in small pilot studies before being offered as solutions to serious national educational problems.
>
> Why did so many intended reforms, undertaken with so much hope and enthusiasm, fail to fulfill their promise? And why did many result in even lower student achievement levels than those they replaced? Of even greater importance, why were the same reforms proposed again and again, under new labels, with little recognition that they were similar to practices or policies that had failed in the past? (Chall, 2000, p. 3)

Chall (2000) suggests that holding "a broad view of educational practices and preferences" (p. 5) is to be rational. That is, we need to explore the underlying philosophies (e.g., the related paradigms) within each educational practice and preference to look at the big picture. Education is a social and intellectual phenomenon that is, in turn, affected by a wide range of other social and cognitive phenomena. Therefore, like any other social and ideational entity, education can and should be studied theoretically and empirically.

BULL'S EYE: DEAF EPISTEMOLOGIES

Deaf epistemologies refer to a Deaf way or ways of thinking or viewing the world (Kelly, 2008; Ladd, 2003). The conceptualization of deaf epistemologies is comparable to the ones related with marginalized ethnic or cultural minority groups such as African American epistemologies, feminist epistemologies, or disability epistemologies. For example, Lane (1999) compares the colonization of the deaf body with the colonization of Africa. Deaf epistemologies are based on the belief that social conventions including research studies have traditionally favored the hearing perspective and have discriminated against d/Deaf individuals. It is one example of an antioppression or antidiscriminatory perspective. The binaries in the legitimate status of deaf epistemologies are largely related to the oppositions of two paradigms: positivism and constructivism, which represent a continuum of support for deaf epistemologies with the *pure* positivists as the strongest opponents of deaf epistemologies, who will not admit the existence of *deaf epistemologies* without empirical evidence, and *pure* constructivists as the strongest advocates of deaf epistemologies (Bauman, 2008; Kelly, 2008; Ladd, 2003; Wang, 2010).

The different perceptions of deaf epistemologies from positivists and constructivists are results of the fundamentally dissimilar philosophical approaches to viewing and interpreting reality. *Pure* constructivists believe that the way Deaf individuals construct reality is different from the way hearing individuals do because Deaf individuals have different values, traditions, cultures, rules of behavior, and language than hearing individuals (Bauman, 2008; Fernandes & Myers, 2010; Kelly, 2008; Ladd, 2003).

On the other side, although pure positivists deny the existence of what constitutes Deaf culture or even reject that a sign language is a bona fide language, many moderate positivists acknowledge the validity of Deaf culture and recognize sign languages as bona fide languages. Most positivists, however, disagree with the claim that the legality of Deaf culture consequentially leads to a Deaf way or ways of obtaining knowledge (see the discussion in Wang, 2010). *Pure* positivists recognize the standard epistemology as the single epistemology and the foundation for knowledge that transcends time, locations, and cultures (Lehrer, 2000; Noddings, 1995, 2007). Most positivists, including constructivists such as Piaget, believe that there is a parallel between the development of knowledge in the human race and the development exhibited in individuals (Noddings, 2007). That is, although every knower actively constructs his or her own knowledge, the process is not entirely idiosyncratic, and there are some qualitative similarities in the development of knowledge, regardless of race, gender, sexual orientation, or disabilities (Wang, 2010; see also, the discussion on the qualitative-similarity hypothesis in Paul & Lee, 2010, and Paul, Chapter 10). Otherwise, "since each human being is unique, reductio ad absurdum, there could be six billion categories" (Moores, 2010, p. 449).

The significance of this epistemological war becomes more outstanding when epistemological belief is connected with practice, particularly for pedagogical-uniformity-seeking educators who are searching for the "unitary, correct approach"

(Marschark, 2000, p. 275) to educate children who are d/Deaf or hard of hearing. For example, to keep the languages separate and distinct, the strongest supporters of Deaf epistemologies exclude the use of voice including sign and voice simultaneously, even if only for a certain group of people with a certain purpose (see the discussion in Fernandes & Myers, 2010). Similarly, they criticize the use of artificial Manually Coded English (MCE) systems with signs that are considered ungrammatical and phonologically impossible in any natural sign language (Chamberlain & Mayberry, 2008). Advocates of deaf epistemologies further maintain that d/Deaf students should be taught mostly by Deaf teachers and that Deaf history as well as Deaf culture should be important parts of the curricula for d/Deaf students (Gertz, 2008; Humphries, 2008).

In addition to the persistent argument that a sign language should be the natural language of a d/Deaf child from birth, advocates of deaf epistemologies also believe that d/Deaf individuals are visual learners, their brains are organized in ways different from those of the hearing individuals, and, most importantly, by virtue of their biology (e.g., different eye gaze behaviors from hearing individuals), d/Deaf individuals learn differently than hearing individuals (Hauser, O'Hearn, McKee, Steider, & Thew, 2010). Therefore, the general theories of instruction and research do not apply in deaf education. That is, institutional practices, such as schools, inherently reflect the values and norms of the dominant hearing culture, and d/Deaf students are marginalized by these institutional practices, although many teachers are not even aware of this marginalization. Consequently, Hauser and colleagues (2010) suggest that "deaf epistemology should be the lens through which auditory learners seek to expand their understanding of visual learners, in order, ultimately, to enhance learning and strive to create environments that value visual beings as much as auditory beings—environments that, in other words, embrace Deafhood and deafness as much as they embrace *hearinghood* and *hearingness*" (p. 490).

Alternatively, supporters of standard epistemology argue that although hearing and d/Deaf individuals, similar to male and female individuals, might have different brain structures to some degree, their brains function effectively in receiving and expressing information in a generally similar way; fundamentally different pedagogical approaches thus might not be required, although certain accommodations and adaptations in instructional strategies might be indispensable to meet the unique needs of d/Deaf learners (Moores, 2010; Paul & Lee, 2010; see also Paul, Chapter 10).

Language and literacy instruction in BiBi education for children who are d/Deaf or hard of hearing is one of the areas where the conflicts between deaf epistemologies and standard epistemology manifest.

LANGUAGE AND LITERACY INSTRUCTION IN BIBI EDUCATION AND DEAF EPISTEMOLOGIES

Although teachers might not necessarily share the epistemologists' concerns on the nature or scope of knowledge, they should be accustomed to epistemology because they must make decisions on the nature of material they teach as well as the strategies or communication modes for teaching these materials, evaluate the knowledge that comes to them from educational research, and decide whether certain knowledge should or can be made accessible to the students (Noddings, 1995, 2007). In the field of deaf education, different epistemological beliefs have led to radically dissimilar practices in the classrooms, although, often, the teachers or professionals themselves do not realize the epistemological underpinning of the disparity. This section discusses the theory, research, and practice of BiBi education, particularly in language and literacy instruction, and the relationship between BiBi education and deaf epistemologies.

Cummins's Linguistic Interdependence Theory and Literacy Instruction in BiBi Education

Cummins's linguistic interdependence theory (1978, 1979, 1980, 1981, 1984, 1989) is the most frequently cited theory in the field of sign bilingual education for both supporting and, interestingly, rejecting the assertion that literacy could be developed through reading and writing the print without exposure to, or proficiency in, the through-the-air (i.e., spoken or signed) form of the primary language. That is, meaning can be explained or negotiated via the use of American Sign Language (ASL) only in conjunction with English print, which is the predominant basis for using ASL to teach English as a second language or ASL/English bilingualism/biculturalism (see the review in Trezek, Wang, & Paul, 2010; Wang, Trezek, Luckner, & Paul, 2008).

Cummins's linguistic interdependence theory proposes a common proficiency underlying all languages allowing for transferring cognitive-academic skills or literacy-related skills from the first language (i.e., L1) to related skills in the second language (i.e., L2). One of the most cited quotations is as follows: "To the extent that instruction in Lx is effective in promoting proficiency in Lx, transfer of this proficiency to Ly will occur provided there is adequate exposure to Ly and adequate motivation to learn Ly" (Cummins, 1981, p. 29).

However, Cummins (2000) also acknowledge bilingual education for d/Deaf children as "high stakes, complex and controversial" (p. 29). Cummins considers it impossible for automatic linguistic transfer to happen in surface aspects of dissimilar languages, that is, lexical and grammatical knowledge in sign language cannot directly facilitate the acquisition of the lexical and grammatical knowledge in spoken/written language. He believes, however, the automatic transfer of conceptual knowledge as well as metalinguistic and metacognitive strategies between dissimilar languages such as a sign language and a spoken/written language might be possible.

Mayer and colleagues (Mayer, 2009; Mayer & Akamatsu 2003; Mayer & Leigh, 2010; Mayer & Wells, 1996) publish extensively on the implication of Cummins's linguistic interdependence theory in cross-modal bilingualism within the deaf community. She accentuates the importance of a threshold level L2 proficiency as a necessary condition for mediating L2 literacy development. Mayer asserts that the fundamental and crucial difference between hearing and d/Deaf L2 literacy learners is the various levels of L2 face-to-face or conversational (spoken or signed) proficiency that have been acquired before they have to use L2 in more cognitively and linguistically demanding situations. That is, without a basic conversational knowledge of the surface aspects of L2 (i.e., phonology, morphology, and syntax), it is difficult, if not impossible, for d/Deaf individuals, or any individuals, to make extensive use of L2 print in academic settings.

In addition to their limited proficiency in L2, Mayer believes that the second major obstacle to developing L2 literacy skills for many d/Deaf students is their inadequate proficiency in L1, partially because 95% of them were born to parent(s) who are hearing and utilize spoken communication (Mitchell & Karchmer, 2004). Most importantly, learning opportunities and quality of literacy instruction for children who are d/Deaf or hard of hearing are often restricted at academic settings, even in the BiBi programs. Next, the practice of language and literacy instruction in ASL/English BiBi programs is introduced.

The Practice of Language and Literacy Instruction in ASL/English BiBi Programs

Although research on BiBi is still in its infancy and there are few empirical data supporting or opposing its effectiveness (Moores, 2008; Spencer & Marschark, 2010; see the discussion on the correlation studies in the next section), some available survey studies and case studies offer pictures of how language and literacy is taught in ASL/English BiBi programs.

For example, LaSasso and Lollis (2003) conducted a survey study on BiBi programs at day and residential schools for d/Deaf students in the United States. Seventy-one out of 78 day and residential schools listed in the 1998 directory of the *American Annals of the Deaf* participated. Of the 19 schools self-identifying themselves as BiBi programs, 47% of them reported that no more than half of the instructional staff members were fluent in ASL, and 68% of them reported that no more than half of the support staff members were fluent. Furthermore, only 21% of the programs reported having an official BiBi curriculum with annual goals as well as recommended instructional materials and procedures for teachers. The difficulties of finding qualified personnel who were fluent in ASL and the absence of formulated BiBi curricula and teaching methods were almost identical to the research findings of Strong's (1995) pioneer study, in which seven BiBi residential programs in the United States were profiled.

Evans (2004) evaluated the instructional strategies used by BiBi programs for d/Deaf students in three elementary schools. The author identified three strategies that were inconsistent with a BiBi approach to educate d/Deaf student: (1) explicit teaching of grammatical structures and rules as well as word-based rather than discourse-based language structures; (2) small class size, which allowed more individualized teaching, but emphasized teacher-directed instruction that barely left any room for working group learning or other opportunities to learn from peers; and (3) inconsistent incorporation of Deaf culture in the classroom, that is, although a Deaf studies curriculum had been established at the school, the teachers did not implement it because academic subjects took precedence.

From the limited available data, we can conclude that BiBi curricula were implemented inconsistently in many programs and various instructional strategies were used in the classrooms to teach literacy. Such inconsistency in literacy instruction may be found in many oral-only and Total Communication programs for students who are d/Deaf or hard of hearing as well. However, one consistent theme at many BiBi programs in the United States is using ASL to teach written English directly without exposure to, or proficiency in, spoken or signed English.

Research on Literacy Instruction in BiBi Education

In 1817, Laurent Clerc, a deaf French teacher, initiated the first instructional use of sign language in the United States. However, the 1880 International Congress on Education of the Deaf held in Milan renounced the use of sign language in deaf education. Oralism, consequently, dominated the field of deaf education until the mid-1960s when the value of sign language started to be recognized (e.g., Stokoe, Casterline, & Croneberg, 1965) and oralism was under attack because of the chronically poor quality of deaf education. Meanwhile, various MCE systems appeared and mushroomed. They borrowed signs from ASL to represent the structure of English such as English words and word parts (see Paul, 2009, for a detailed description of various MCE systems).

Despite all these efforts, the third- or fourth-grade ceiling of reading achievement was consistently documented starting from the beginning of formal assessment (Pintner & Patterson, 1916) until today (Qi & Mitchell, 2007). Radical constructivists from Deaf culture disagree with this ceiling effect and claim that it is the product of positivist research on d/Deaf individuals. They assert that these research studies began with the premise that all d/Deaf individuals had problems with reading and writing and that the methodologies employed by the researchers might subconsciously challenge the abilities of the d/Deaf individuals (Ladd, 2003).

For example, Markowicz and Woodward (1982) claim that the literature on deafness was dominated by psychological studies explored the causal relationship between d/Deaf individuals' behavior and cognition without taking into account the potential influence of the Deaf cultural experience in the testing situation. Furthermore, the research results could be questionable, if the studies on deaf community membership are done by hearing researchers outside of the deaf community.

Eckert (2010) further claims:

> If teachers and parents prejudicially believe that Deaf adults read at a third-grade level, then they are less likely to assign challenging reading material for Deaf children. This results in lower reading scores, more prejudice, and further discrimination. Although applying Myrdal's vicious cycle to Deaf education oversimplifies complex pedagogical decisions made by teachers for individuals based on aggregate data, Myrdal's cycle of prejudice is important to Deaf studies because it informs us of the "cumulative causation" that reinforces and perpetuates individual, institutional, and metaphysical expressions of audism. (p. 312)

Deaf culture advocates turn to correlation studies on sign language proficiency and written language proficiency to support the use of ASL to teach English as a second language or ASL/English bilingualism/biculturalism.

Strong and Prinz (1997) conducted one of the pioneer studies on the correlations between linguistic proficiency in sign language and written language. Assessing the proficiency in ASL and written English of 160 d/Deaf children aged eight to 15 years, Strong and Prinz found that d/Deaf children with the higher two levels of

ASL significantly outperformed children in the lowest ASL ability level in written English after controlling for age and nonverbal intelligence. Additionally, although d/Deaf children with deaf mothers outperformed those of hearing mothers in both ASL and written English, when ASL level was held constant, no difference was identified between these two groups, except in the subgroup with the lowest level of ASL ability. Interestingly, the relationship between ASL level and English literacy was not significant for the subgroup of older children (aged 12–15) with deaf mothers; thus, the subgroup was excluded from subsequent analysis. They concluded that bilingual d/Deaf children could benefit from having even a moderate fluency in ASL. One of the limitations of this study was that it was unclear if the "higher" levels of literacy compared favorably with hearing age peers (Mayer & Akamatsu 2003; Mayer & Leigh, 2010). The second limitation of the study was that there was no analysis on the localization of the correlation, for example, whether the correlation between sign language and written language was at the grammatical or lexical level (Hermans, Ormel, & Knoors, 2010). Furthermore, additional research is needed to investigate the reason(s) for the insignificant correlation between ASL level and English literacy for older children with deaf mothers.

The first limitation of the study was repeated in many other similar studies as well. For example, with a small sample of students educated in MCE, Hoffmeister (2000) found that proficiency in ASL plural markers and knowledge of synonyms and antonyms correlated positively with reading achievement. Similarly, with a small sample of students educated in MCE or ASL, Padden and Ramsey (2000) found that recognition and memory of fingerspelled initialized signs within ASL sentences correlated positively with reading achievement. With a sample of 48 d/Deaf students aged six to 15 years, Chamberlain and Mayberry (2000) also found that both ASL and MCE narrative comprehension were best predictors of reading achievement. None of these studies reported the reading levels of the participants compared with their hearing peers.

In fact, comparing the written English vocabulary of 72 d/Deaf elementary school students of various proficiency levels in ASL with those of 60 hearing English-as-a-second-language (ESL) peers and 61 hearing monolingual peers of English, Singleton, Morgan, DiGello, Wiles, and Rivers (2004) found that although strong ASL signers outperformed the weaker signers in the quality of their written texts, neither of the deaf groups was commensurate with either the monolingual or ESL hearing peers.

Furthermore, Moores and Sweet (1990) found no correlation between reading or writing and ASL proficiency for two groups of congenitally deaf students 16 to 18 years of age, 65 of whom had hearing parents and 65 of whom had deaf parents. There were high correlations between reading and two measures of English grammar/structure (i.e., the Test of Syntactic Abilities and the Signed English Morphology Tests). The reading/ASL correlation, however, was .06 for deaf children of deaf parents and .04 for deaf children of hearing parents (see further discussions in Moores & Meadow-Orlans, 1990).

Most recently, Chamberlain and Mayberry (2008) assessed the linguistic comprehension skills of 31 d/Deaf adults in ASL, MCE, and written English and their syntactic skills in ASL, and they collected questionnaire data on their print exposure as well as speech use and comprehension. The participants were classified as skilled readers (SR) or less skilled readers (LSR) using an eighth-grade criterion. The assumption of the study was that

> if the grammatical structure of the reader's through the air language must match that of the written language for skilled reading to develop, then deaf signers who have high levels of ASL syntactic and narrative skills should more often be identified as LSR than those with low ASL syntactic and narrative skills. Alternatively, if the linguistic basis of reading is abstract and transcends language modality and grammatical form, as does the nature of language itself, then the reverse outcome should be observed. Skilled deaf readers should show high levels of ASL proficiency but less skilled deaf readers should not. (p. 370)

The study found that skilled d/Deaf readers demonstrated high levels of ASL syntactic ability and narrative comprehension, whereas less skilled d/Deaf readers did not. The authors concluded that ASL syntactic proficiency contributed significantly to the development of skilled reading of d/Deaf bilinguals. However, the assumption of the whole study was questionable. The study was based on the rationale that if the mismatch theory is correct, the mismatch between grammatical structure of ASL and that of written English means that d/Deaf signers who have high levels of ASL syntactic and narrative skills cannot be SRs. d/Deaf signers who had high levels of ASL syntactic and narrative skills turned out to be SRs; therefore, the mismatch theory is incorrect. Similarly, the authors considered a relationship between print exposure and sign language proficiency counterintuitive at first glance as well. However, as they explained in the discussion themselves, ASL signers are immersed in an English milieu and so their reading language is English—therefore how can the authors be so confident that ASL syntactic proficiency contributed to the development of written English, not the other way around or in both ways?

In sum, research studies supporting the use of ASL to directly teach written English without the spoken/signed form are primarily correlation studies on ASL proficiency and written English proficiency. To some degree, they validated Cummins's linguistic interdependence theory by providing evidence for correlations between ASL and written English on cognitive-academic and literacy-related skills. However, because of the nature of correlation studies, the direction of the relationship is indecisive; and most importantly, it is unknown if the "higher" literacy skills of more skilled ASL signer are sufficient.

What about BiBi sign education in other languages? The correlations between L1 sign language proficiency and L2 written language proficiency have been found with bilingual d/Deaf children aged six to 18 years on correlation of grammatical knowledge between German Sign Language and written German (Mann, 2007), bilingual d/Deaf children aged eight to 17 on correlation of grammatical knowledge between French Sign Language and spoken/written French (Niederberger, 2008), and bilingual d/Deaf children aged eight to 12 on correlation of lexical knowledge between Sign Language of the Netherlands (SLN) and written Dutch (Hermans, Knoors, Ormel, & Verhoeven, 2008).

Most recently, Hermans and colleagues (2010) assessed the expressive vocabulary and morphosyntactic skills in SLN and spoken Dutch (no assessments on written

Dutch) of 75 d/Deaf children, aged four to eight years, from bilingual education programs. The results showed significant overall correlations between SLN and spoken Dutch for the vocabulary tasks but not for the morphosyntactic tasks. Interestingly, scores on the expressive vocabulary test in SLN and spoken Dutch were correlated for the older children aged 5.7 to 8.10 years but not for the younger children aged 4.1 to 5.6. A similar pattern was found on the expressive morphosyntactic skill test as well. While confirming the Cummins's linguistic interdependence theory that automatic transfer between a sign language and a written language is limited to cognitive skills and conceptual knowledge, the authors proposed the concept of "cultivated transfer" to explain the apparent correlation of sign language linguistic skills and written language linguistic skills, particularly lexical and grammatical knowledge. The authors suggested that the signing skills of younger children might not have been developed to a level where cultivation actually could occur.

Menendez (2010) conducted a qualitative analysis on the written samples of 15 d/Deaf students, aged 13 to 17 years, in a bilingual school in Barcelona and found evidence of "language interaction" or "language contact phenomena" between written language and sign language at the lexical, morphological, and syntactic levels. The author concluded that "the pooling of resources that makes d/Deaf students use structures from Catalan Sign Language in written English is suggestive of linguistic transfer at a morphosyntactic level and that language contact is positive to students' bilingual development in this specific context" (p. 201).

Overall, the correlations between L1 sign language proficiency and L2 written language proficiency have been found with bilingual d/Deaf individuals using different languages; however, the direction and sufficiency of the linguistic transferring cannot be answered because of the limitation of the study design. Mere correlations between L1 sign language proficiency and L2 written language proficiency or evidence of L1 sign language influence in L2 written language do not necessarily mean that there is linguistic transfer from L1 sign language to L2 written language, let alone a positive transfer.

Conclusion

One of the very few things people in BiBi sign education agree upon (finally!) is that the reported low reading achievement of d/Deaf students is primarily a result of incomplete language acquisition, signed or spoken (e.g., Chamberlain & Mayberry, 2008; Mayer, 2009). However, one of the most controversial issues in BiBi sign education is whether complete sign language acquisition is enough for transferring from L1 sign language to L2 written language, without the exposure or proficiency in spoken or signed form of L2.

Supporters of the ASL / written English bilingual education often compare the literacy learning experiences of d/Deaf students with those of hearing English language learners (ELLs). What does the research on hearing ELLs say? The National Literacy Panel on Language-Minority Children and Youth (August & Shanahan, 2006), in the most recent and comprehensive synthesis of research on the literacy skills of ELLs, concludes that it is challenging for ELLs to achieve written language comprehension skills that are commensurable with those of English monolingual peers. Vocabulary knowledge, particularly school-based academic vocabulary, poses one of the biggest problems for ELLs. The best predictors of English written language comprehension skills of ELLs also include metalinguistic competence and other English oral proficiency variables such as listening comprehension, syntactic skills, and oral storytelling skills. Additional contributing factors include exposure to print, learning opportunities and quality of literacy instruction, first-language literacy development, the ability to navigate complex text and utilize prior knowledge to draw inferences, and use of cross-linguistic transfer strategies, particularly cognitive and metacognitive strategies (see the review in Paul & Wang, 2012).

In learning to read and write English, a language unfamiliar to many of them, children who are d/Deaf or hard of hearing will face similar challenges, if not more. For example, approximately 60% of the words considered important from a science curriculum review do not have sign representations (Lang, Hupper, Monte, Brown, Babb, & Scheifele, 2007), which makes acquiring school-based academic vocabulary knowledge even more challenging for children who are d/Deaf or hard of hearing. In contrast to hearing ELLs, children who are d/Deaf or hard of hearing generally have limited access to the phonology of English, although the role of which in literacy development is still controversial (see the discussion in Allen et al. 2009; Paul, Wang, Trezek, & Luckner, 2009; Wang et al., 2008).

It is naïve to believe that complete sign language acquisition is sufficient for automatic transferring from L1 sign language to L2 written language, never mind the fact that many d/Deaf children do not have a fully developed L1 sign language in the first place. Just as "there is much more to reading literacy than just phonological awareness" (Menendez, 2010, p. 204), there is much more to reading literacy than just sign language acquisition. There are many conflicting perspectives in the theory, research, and practice of literacy instruction in BiBi sign education, which require a metaparadigmatic view on understanding literacy and literacy education to unify the field.

METAPARADIGM AND LITERACY INSTRUCTION

Different paradigms lead to different definitions of literacy as well as to different practices in literacy education (Paul & Wang, 2012; Wang, 2005). Generally speaking, positivists espousing the standard epistemology view literacy as a traditional literacy, which is reading and writing. They commonly believe that everyone proceeds through similar developmental stages in learning to read and write, regardless of whether one is d/Deaf or hearing, man or woman, African American or Asian American (e.g., Chall, 1996). There are some fundamental components of effective reading instructions that should be applicable to everyone, including students who are d/Deaf. In contrast, most constructivists espousing deaf epistemologies advocate the use of ASL literacy and argue that d/Deaf individuals are visual learners; thus, mainstream literacy theories and research, particularly the ones based on a phonology of English, are inappropriate for d/Deaf individuals (Allen et al., 2009; Hauser et al., 2010; Kuntze, 2008).

How can we unify the field? Are different epistemological beliefs or paradigms commensurable? Do we have to select one from either/or dichotomies? The concept of a metaparadigm is introduced here as a mechanism to transform the destructive, competing forces into constructive, cooperative energy toward peace.

Metaparadigm

A *metaparadigm* is a hybrid paradigm that blurs the boundaries between different paradigms (Ritzer, 2001). Metaparadigms welcome multiple epistemological beliefs and include various methodologies. They are built upon the concept of *paradigmatic commensurability*, which claims that individuals from different paradigms can and should communicate with each other and make an effort to adjudicate and resolve the disagreement (Kuhn, 1996). Although pure paradigmatic harmony might be unrealistic, we need to move beyond either/or dichotomies that sparked the destructive interparadigmatic debates, and the point of departure is a core set of principles that we commonly value (Wang, 2010).

A distinction should be made between metaparadigm and *pragmatism*, which refers to the interpretation of material/knowledge based on its usefulness (Calderwood, 2002). Pragmatism is a paradigm that, in some cases, might disregard or relinquish the validity of other conflicting paradigms, whereas a metaparadigm considers paradigm borders as, in varying degrees, fluid, porous, and interactive, instead of stable and permeable. The shifting and contextual nature of a metaparadigm (Gieryn, 1995, 1999) allows its peace with multiple paradigms. Marschark (2000) warns about the danger of *pure* pragmatism:

> We often are channeled by how and where we were trained, by our pet theory, model or framework, or by our academic self-images. We may not be rigid, but we often do not appear to recognize the value of alternative possibilities. This is not to argue that holding a particular theoretical orientation with regard to deaf education is a bad thing. All too often, a focus only on the practicalities of "what works" results in the teaching of isolated facts or skills, leaving students without sufficient flexibility to adapt to novel concepts and tasks. An underlying understanding of the nature of learning and development is an important, if not essential, component to teaching children how to learn, and it does not matter if they are deaf or hearing. (p. 276)

Metaparadigm and Literacy Instruction in BiBi Education

Investigating the idiosyncratic formation of Deaf identity, Leigh (2009) claims that not all d/Deaf people's lives are alike. Most d/Deaf individuals were born into a non-Deaf world where the language of family and community is not fully accessible, which may preclude the complete resolution of their sense of who they are. The gray area between the Deaf world and the hearing world leads to their struggles in figuring out how they can fit in. Many people consider the Deaf community as "a community of 'converts' at least in large part" because of its "unorthodox pattern of socialization" (Bechter, 2008, p. 61). The heterogeneous nature of the Deaf community members requires us to explore issues through a metaparadigmatic lens to localize the problem. There should be multiple pathways in literacy education of children who are d/Deaf or hard of hearing.

When the goal of instruction is to discuss Deaf culture and/or Deaf history for students with strong Deaf background, the use of sign languages in the classroom might be appropriate. The benefits of using native sign language for the social-emotional well-being of these children are almost unquestionable. On the other hand, if the purpose of instruction is to teach English literacy skills, is it possible for d/Deaf students to use their knowledge of ASL to acquire adequate independent English literacy skills without any exposure to spoken or signed form of English? Such an assertion might be too naïve.

An emphasis on complete sign language acquisition in BiBi education for children who are d/Deaf or hard of hearing is unquestionably valuable for maintaining the language and culture of the Deaf community as well as for empowering its members; however, when the question at hand is to acquire written English skills, a fully developed sign language is necessary but not sufficient (see the discussion in Mayer, 2009). Similarly, phonemic awareness and phonics skills are necessary in learning to read English, a phonemic language that is more than 80% phonetic (Moats, 2001) but are not sufficient. Educators with different epistemological beliefs need to go across the borders and see what is on the other side of the fence. Standing alone, each paradigm is inadequate. To completely understand successful instructional practices, each paradigm needs insights from the others' "theoretical backyard" (Marschark, 2000). A metaparadigm makes it possible to walk in another's shoes.

In its comprehensive review of the literature on reading instruction, the National Reading Panel ([NRP], 2000; see also McGuinness, 2004, 2005; Snow, Burns, & Griffin, 1998) identified three broad reasons for reading difficulties: (1) problems in understanding and utilizing the alphabetic principle to acquire fluent and accurate word reading (i.e., decoding) skills, (2) failure to obtain the verbal knowledge and strategies that are exclusively required for comprehension of written materials, and (3) absence or loss of initial motivation to read or failure to develop a mature appreciation for the rewards of reading. Undoubtedly, a process as complex as reading can never be fully explained by such a simple decoding–language–motivation tripartite framework, which oversimplifies the range of difficulties children might encounter in learning to read. Categorizing reading difficulties into these three broad groups nevertheless avoids the pitfall of *one-size-fits-all* instructional practices (Paul & Wang, 2012).

A traditional BiBi sign program might be able to offer students who are d/Deaf or hard of hearing a sign language base and a rewarding motivation to read, but the negligence of the alphabetic principle might be one of the missing puzzles that prevent students from reading at a comparable level with their hearing peers. Within a metaparadigmatic model, educators in BiBi sign programs can teach phonemic awareness and phonics skills while celebrating Deaf culture and sign languages. Phonemic awareness and phonics skills are not necessarily speech skills that involve hearing or articulating each phoneme (Adams, 1990; Trezek et al., 2010; Trezek, Wang, & Paul, 2011; Wang, et al., 2008). As metalinguistic skills, phonemic awareness and phonics skills are mode independent; that is, the representation of phonemes can be in a speech or visual modality.

Two of the most promising techniques on developing phonology for children who are d/Deaf or hard of hearing are Cued Speech/Language and Visual Phonics (see the review in LaSasso, Crain, & Leybaert, 2010; Trezek et al., 2010; Trezek et al. 2011; Wang, et al., 2008). In contrast to MCE systems, which convey English inadequately at the morphological and syntactical levels, Cued Speech/Language, for instructional purposes, and Visual Phonics represent English at the phonemic level. Phonological processing does not necessarily have to be based on hearing (i.e., the use of audition), and children who are d/Deaf or hard of hearing can and should use alternative means such as Cued Speech/Language or Visual Phonics to acquire and develop their phonological knowledge, which might be one of the keys to ultimately improving their English reading skills (Paul & Wang, 2012).

In addition, many children who are d/Deaf or hard of hearing also have problems in two other critical forms of English, namely, morphology and syntax. Based on Cummins's linguistic interdependence theory, phonology, morphology, and syntax are language specific; that is, it is almost impossible to develop knowledge of these forms of English via the use of another language such as ASL. The content (i.e., semantics) and use (i.e., pragmatics) of English may be acquired via explanations in another language but not the forms. A rigid BiBi sign program without any exposure to the signed or spoken form of English might deprive the students of a required proficiency in the morphology and syntax of the language that they are trying to read. Through-the-air English-based systems, primarily MCE systems, have been proposed to bridge the gap between ASL and the written English (Stewart, 2006). Furthermore, spoken English, ASL, or any form of MCE can be a potential communication mode as long as good teaching practices are utilized in the classroom. The decision of a mode of communication should be based on the goal of the activity instead of the epistemological belief of the teacher or administrator. For example, spoken or signed English should be used in discussing English morphology and syntax, even in a BiBi sign program.

In sum, for a process as complex as reading, a successful literacy instruction program for children who are d/Deaf or hard of hearing should be based on a metaparadigmatical framework in which practices in all epistemological beliefs are valued and considered. Instead of embracing either an exclusive focus on promoting discourse-based sign language acquisition or an overwhelming emphasis on drilling English grammatical structures and rules at the word and/or syntactical levels, educators of the d/Deaf should be free from the constraints of epistemological beliefs and welcome effective instructional strategies across the borders. For example, explicit, direct instruction of syntactical skills should be conducted in meaningful contexts, maybe in discussion of a text on Deaf history. Additionally, instead of waiting for an equivalent level of L1 and L2 skills for children who are d/Deaf or hard of hearing, educators should teach higher levels of metalinguistic and metacognitive skills and more challenging content area knowledge through students' more skilled languages, most likely sign languages. Practices such as instructional strategies, materials, and modes of communication should not be limited to the philosophical beliefs that are adopted by the instructors or administrators.

CONCLUSION

Investigating deaf epistemologies through a metaparadigm enables us to employ multiple paradigms and/or approaches in the field of deaf education. Educators of the d/Deaf should be free from the boundaries of a certain paradigm commitment and welcome effective instructional strategies from the other side of the fence.

In closing, here are some recommendations for further theorizing, research, and practice:

- Theorizing in deaf education should not be limited to a particular epistemological commitment; rather, a metaparadigmatic approach should be applied to encourage paradigm integration. Advocates of standard epistemology should make special accommodations and/or adaptations in mainstreaming theories to reflect the unique needs of individuals who are d/Deaf or hard of hearing, whereas supporters of deaf epistemologies should often reference mainstreaming theories as a starting point before further investigation. Meanwhile, the heterogeneous nature of the Deaf community reminds us that there should be multiple pathways in literacy education of children who are d/Deaf or hard of hearing.
- In research, there are many conflicting perspectives in literacy instruction in BiBi sign education, which requires a metaparadigmatic framework in which research from all epistemological beliefs are valued and considered. Research should be evaluated by its relevance and quality, not the hearing status or the epistemological beliefs of the author(s). Educational or psychological research on individuals who are d/Deaf or hard of hearing should take into account the potential influence of Deaf cultural experience in the testing situation. More research on what works in BiBi sign education is needed.
- In practice, educators of the d/Deaf should embrace all effective instructional strategies across the borders. For example, although there may be certain fundamentals that apply to all children who are learning to read and write, how it is delivered via instruction should vary based on the individual differences in children. Depending on the instructional goal, the modes of communication in the classroom can be ASL, MCE, spoken English, Cued Speech/Language, or a combination of these. The efficiency of communication and teaching practices depends on the goal of the educational activity and the abilities of the students in the classroom, not the epistemological beliefs.

NOTES

1. The term *deaf* refers to the audiometric definition of deafness, whereas the term *Deaf* refers to identification with Deaf culture, which has its own set of values, social structure, forms of artistic expression, and language, such as American Sign Language (ASL).
2. In the first issue of the *American Annals of the Deaf* in 1847, T. H. Gallaudet wrote about the benefits of the natural sign language.

REFERENCES

Adams, M. (1990). *Beginning to read: Thinking and learning about print.* Cambridge, MA: MIT Press.

Allen, T., Clark, M. D., del Giudice, A., Koo, D., Lieberman, A., Mayberry, R., & Miller, P. (2009). Phonology and reading: A response to Wang, Trezek, Luckner, and Paul. *American Annals of the Deaf,* 154(4), 338–345.

August, D., & Shanahan, T. (Eds.). (2006). *Developing literacy in second-language learners: Report of the National Literacy Panel on Language-Minority Children and Youth.* Mahwah, NJ: Lawrence Erlbaum.

Bauman, H.-D. (2008). Introduction: Listening to Deaf studies. In H.-D. Bauman (Ed.), *Open your eyes: Deaf studies talking* (pp. 1–32). Minneapolis, MN: University of Minnesota Press.

Bechter, F. (2008). The deaf convert culture and its lessons for deaf theory. In H.-D. Bauman (Ed.), *Open your eyes: Deaf studies talking* (pp. 60–79). Minneapolis, MN: University of Minnesota Press.

Calderwood, K. (2002). Incorporating multiple epistemologies into teaching statistics to social work students. *Journal of Teaching in Social Work, 22*(1/2), 17–32.

Chall, J. S. (1996). *Stages of reading development* (2nd ed.). New York, NY: McGraw-Hill.

Chall, J. S. (2000). *The academic achievement challenge: What really works in the classroom?* New York, NY: Guilford Press.

Chamberlain, C., & Mayberry, R. I. (2000). Theorizing about the relationship between ASL and reading. In C. Chamberlain, J. Morford, & R. I. Mayberry (Eds.), *Language acquisition by eye* (pp. 221–260). Mahwah, NJ: Lawrence Erlbaum.

Chamberlain, C., & Mayberry, R. I. (2008). American Sign Language syntactic and narrative comprehension in skilled and less skilled readers: Bilingual and bimodal evidence for the linguistic basis of reading. *Applied Psycholinguistics, 29*, 367–388.

Cummins, J. (1978). Educational implications of mother tongue maintenance in minority language groups. *Canadian Modern Language Review, 35*, 395–416.

Cummins, J. (1979). Linguistic interdependence and the educational development of bilingual children. *Review of Educational Research, 49*(2), 222–251.

Cummins, J. (1980). The crosslingual dimensions of language proficiency: Implications for bilingual education and the optimal age issue. *TESOL Quarterly, 14*(2), 175–187.

Cummins, J. (1981). The role of primary language development in promoting educational success for language minority students. In *Schooling and language minority students: A theoretical framework* (pp. 3–49). Los Angeles, CA: Education, Dissemination, and Assessment Center, California State University.

Cummins, J. (1984). *Bilingual and special education: Issues in assessment and pedagogy.* San Diego, CA: College Hill Press.

Cummins, J. (1989). *Empowering minority students.* Sacramento, CA: California Association for Bilingual Education.

Cummins, J. (2000). *Language, power and pedagogy: Bilingual children in the crossfire.* Clevedon, UK: Multilingual Matters.

Denzin, N. K., & Lincoln, Y. S. (1994). Introduction: Entering the field of qualitative research. In N. K. Denzin and Y. S. Lincoln (Eds.), *Handbook of qualitative research* (pp. 1–17). Thousand Oaks, CA: Sage.

Eckert, R. C. (2005). *Deafnicity: A study of strategic and adaptive responses to audism by members of the Deaf American community of culture* (Unpublished doctoral dissertation). University of Michigan, Ann Arbor.

Eckert, R. C. (2010). Toward a theory of deaf ethnos: Deafnicity = D/deaf. *Journal of Deaf Studies and Deaf Education, 15*(4), 317–333.

Evans, C. J. (2004). Literacy development in deaf students: Case studies in bilingual teaching and learning. *American Annals of the Deaf, 149*(1), 17–27.

Fernandes, J. K., & Myers, S. S. (2010). Inclusive deaf studies: Barriers and pathways. *Journal of Deaf Studies and Deaf Education, 15*(1), 17–29.

Foucault, M. (1980). *Power/knowledge: Selected interviews and other writings, 1972–1977.* New York, NY: Pantheon Books.

Gertz, G. (2008). Dysconscious audism: A theoretical proposition. In H.-D. Bauman (Ed.), *Open your eyes: Deaf studies talking* (pp. 219–234). Minneapolis, MN: University of Minnesota Press.

Gieryn, T. (1995). Boundaries of science. In S. Jansanoff, G. Markle, J. Petersen, & T. Pinch (Eds.), *Handbook of science and technology studies* (pp. 393–443). Thousand Oaks, CA: Sage.

Gieryn, T. (1999). *Cultural boundaries of science*. Chicago, IL: University of Chicago Press.

Guba, E. G., & Lincoln, Y. S. (2005). Paradigmatic controversies, contradictions, and emerging confluences. In N. K. Denzin & Y. S. Lincoln (Eds.), *The Sage handbook of qualitative research* (3rd ed., pp. 191–215). Thousand Oaks, CA: Sage Publications.

Hauser, P. C., O'Hearn, A., McKee, M., Steider, A., & Thew, D. (2010). Deaf epistemology: Deafhood and deafness. *American Annals of the Deaf, 154*(5), 486–492.

Hermans, D., Knoors, H., Ormel, E., & Verhoeven, L. (2008). The relationship between the reading and signing skills of deaf children in bilingual education programs. *Journal of Deaf Studies and Deaf Education, 13*(4), 518–530.

Hermans, D., Ormel, E., & Knoors, H. (2010). On the relation between the signing and reading skills of deaf bilinguals. *International Journal of Bilingual Education and Bilingualism, 13*(2), 187–199.

Hoffmeister, R. (2000). A piece of the puzzle: ASL and reading comprehension in deaf children. In C. Chamberlain, J. Monford, & R. Mayberry (Eds.), *Language acquisition by eye* (pp. 143–164). Mahwah, NJ: Lawrence Erlbaum.

Humphries, T. (2008). Talking culture and culture talking. In H.-D. Bauman (Ed.), *Open your eyes: Deaf studies talking* (pp. 35–41). Minneapolis, MN: University of Minnesota Press.

Kelly, A. B. (2008). Where is Deaf herstory? In H.-D. Bauman (Ed.), *Open your eyes: Deaf studies talking* (pp. 251–263). Minneapolis, MN: University of Minnesota Press.

Kuhn, T. S. (1962). *The structure of scientific revolutions*. Chicago, IL: University of Chicago Press.

Kuhn, T. S. (1996). *The structure of scientific revolutions* (3rd ed.). Chicago, IL: University of Chicago Press.

Kuntze, M. (2008). Turning literacy inside out. In H.-D. Bauman (Ed.), *Open your eyes: Deaf studies talking* (pp. 146–157). Minneapolis, MN: University of Minnesota Press.

Ladd, P. (2003). *Understanding Deaf culture: In search of deafhood*. Tonawanda, NY: Multilingual Matters.

Ladd, P. (2008). Colonialism and resistance: A brief history of deafhood. In H.-D. Bauman (Ed.), *Open your eyes: Deaf studies talking* (pp. 42–59). Minneapolis, MN: University of Minnesota Press.

Lane, H. (1984). *When the mind hears*. New York, NY: Random House.

Lane, H. (1999). *The mask of benevolence: Disabling the Deaf community*. San Diego, CA: DawnSignPress.

Lang, H., Hupper, M., Monte, D., Brown, S., Babb, I., & Scheifele, P. (2007). A study of technical signs in science: Implications for lexical database development. *Journal of Deaf Studies and Deaf Education, 12*(1), 65–79.

LaSasso, C., Crain, K. L., & Leybaert, J. (2010). (Eds.). *Cued speech and cued language for deaf and hard of hearing children*. San Diego, CA: Plural Publishing.

LaSasso, C., & Lollis, J. (2003). Survey of residential and day schools for deaf students in the United States that identify themselves as bilingual–bicultural programs. *Journal of Deaf Studies and Deaf Education, 8*(1), 79–91.

Lehrer, K. (2000). *Theory of knowledge* (2nd ed.). Boulder, CO: Westview Press.

Leigh, I. W. (2009). *A lens on deaf identities*. New York, NY: Oxford University Press.

Mann, W. (2007). German deaf children's understanding of referential distinction in written German and German Sign Language. *Educational and Child Psychology, 24*(4), 59–76.

Markowicz, H., & Woodward, J. (1982). Language and the maintenance of ethnic boundaries in the Deaf community. In J. Woodward (Ed.), *How you gonna get to heaven if you can't talk with Jesus: On depathologizing deafness* (pp. 3–10). Silver Spring, MD: T. J. Publishers.

Marschark, M. (2000). Education and development of deaf children—Or is it development and education? In P. E. Spencer, K. P. Meadow-Orlans, & C. Erting (Eds.), *The deaf child in the family and at school* (pp. 275–291). Mahwah, NJ: Lawrence Erlbaum.

Mayer, C. (2009). Issues in second language literacy education with learners who are deaf. *International Journal of Bilingualism and Bilingual Education, 12*(3), 325–334.

Mayer, C., & Akamatsu, C. T. (2003). Bilingualism and literacy. In M. Marschark & P. Spencer (Eds.), *Oxford handbook of deaf studies, language, and education* (Vol. 1, pp. 136–147). New York, NY: Oxford University Press.

Mayer, C., & Leigh, G. (2010). The changing context for sign bilingual education programs: Issues in language and the development of literacy. *International Journal of Bilingual Education and Bilingualism, 13*(2), 175–186.

Mayer, C., & Wells, G. (1996). Can the linguistic interdependence theory support a bilingual–bicultural model of literacy education for deaf students? *Journal of Deaf Studies and Deaf Education, 1*(2), 93–107.

McGuinness, D. (2004). *Early reading instruction: What science really tells us about how to teach reading.* Cambridge, MA: MIT Press.

McGuinness, D. (2005). *Language development and learning to read: The scientific study of how language development affects reading skill.* Cambridge, MA: MIT Press.

Menendez, B. (2010). Cross-modal bilingualism: Language contact as evidence of linguistic transfer in sign bilingual education. *International Journal of Bilingual Education and Bilingualism, 13*(2), 201–223.

Mitchell, R. E., & Karchmer, M. A. (2004). Chasing the mythical 10%: Parental hearing status of deaf and hard of hearing students in the United States. *Sign Language Studies, 4*, 138–163.

Moats, L. M. (2001). *Speech to print: Language essentials for teachers.* Baltimore, MD: Paul H. Brookes.

Moores, D. (2008). Research on bi–bi instruction. *American Annals of the Deaf, 153*(1), 3–4.

Moores, D. (2010). Epistemologies, deafness, learning, and teaching. *American Annals of the Deaf, 154*(5), 447–455.

Moores, D., & Meadow-Orlans, K. (Eds.). (1990). *Educational and developmental aspects of deafness.* Washington, DC: Gallaudet University Press.

Moores, D., & Sweet, C. (1990). Relationships of English grammar and communicative fluency in reading in deaf adolescents. *Exceptionality, 1*, 97–106.

National Reading Panel (NRP). (2000). *Report of the National Reading Panel: Teaching children to read—An evidence-based assessment of the scientific research literature on reading and its implications for reading instruction.* Jessup, MD: National Institute for Literacy.

Niederberger, N. (2008). Does the knowledge of a natural sign language facilitate Deaf children's learning to read and write? Insights from French Sign Language and written French data. In C. Plaza-Pust & E. Morales-Lopez (Eds.), *Sign bilingualism: Language development, interaction, and maintenance in sign language contact situations* (pp. 29–50). Amsterdam, the Netherlands: John Benjamins.

Noddings, N. (1995). *Philosophy of education.* Boulder, CO: Westview Press.

Noddings, N. (2007). *Philosophy of education* (2nd ed.). Boulder, CO: Westview Press.

Padden, C., & Ramsey, C. (2000). American sign language and reading ability in deaf children. In C. Chamberlain, J. Morford, & R. Mayberry (Eds.), *Language acquisition by eye* (pp. 165–189). Mahwah, NJ: Lawrence Erlbaum.

Paul, P. (2009). *Language and deafness* (4th ed.). Sudbury, MA: Jones & Bartlett.

Paul, P., & Lee, C. (2010). The qualitative similarity hypothesis. *American Annals of the Deaf, 154*(5), 456–462.

Paul, P., & Wang, Y. (2012). *Literate thought—Understanding comprehension and literacy.* Sudbury, MA: Jones & Bartlett.

Paul, P., Wang, Y., Trezek, B., & Luckner, J. (2009). Phonology is necessary, but not sufficient: A rejoinder. *American Annals of the Deaf, 154*(4), 346–356.

Pintner, R., & Patterson, D. (1916). A measure of the language ability of deaf children. *Psychological Review, 23*, 413–436.

Qi, S., & Mitchell, R. E. (2007, April). *Large-scaled academic achievement testing of deaf and hard-of-hearing students: Past, present, and future.* Paper presented at the Annual Meeting of the American Educational Research Association, Chicago, IL.

Ritzer, G. (2001). *Explorations in social theory: From metatheorizing to rationalization.* London, UK: Sage.

Rose, S., McAnally, P. L., & Quigley, S. P. (2004). *Language learning practices with deaf children* (3rd ed.). Austin, TX: PRO-ED.

Singleton, J. L., Morgan, D., DiGello, E., Wiles, J., & Rivers, R. (2004). Vocabulary use by low, moderate, and high ASL-proficient writers compared to hearing ESL and monolingual speakers. *Journal of Deaf Studies and Deaf Education, 9*(1), 86–103.

Snow, C., Burns, S., & Griffin, P. (Eds.). (1998). *Preventing reading difficulties in young children.* Washington, DC: National Academy Press.

Spencer, P. E., & Marschark, M. (2010). *Evidence-based practice in educating deaf and hard-of-hearing students.* New York, NY: Oxford University Press.

Stewart, D. (2006). Instructional and practical communication: ASL and English-based signing in the classroom. In D. Moores & D. Martin (Eds.), *Deaf learners: Developments in curriculum and instruction* (pp. 207–220). Washington, DC: Gallaudet University Press.

Stokoe, W., Casterline, D., & Croneberg, C. (1965). *A dictionary of American Sign Language on linguistic principles.* Washington, DC: Gallaudet College Press.

Strong, M. (1995). A review of bilingual–bicultural programs for deaf children in North America. *American Annals of the Deaf, 140*(2), 84–94.

Strong, M., & Prinz, P. M. (1997). A study of the relationship between ASL and English literacy. *Journal of Deaf Studies and Deaf Education, 2*(1), 37–46.

Svartholm, K. (2010). Bilingual education for deaf children in Sweden. *International Journal of Bilingual Education and Bilingualism, 13*(2), 159–174.

Trezek, B., Wang, Y., & Paul, P. (2010). *Reading and deafness: Theory, research, and practice.* Clifton Park, NY: Cengage Learning.

Trezek, B., Wang, Y., & Paul, P. (2011). Processes and components of reading. In M. Marschark & P. Spencer (Eds.), *Handbook of deaf studies, language, and education* (Vol. 1, part 2, pp. 99–114). New York, NY: Oxford University Press.

Wang, Y. (2005). *Literate thought: Metatheorizing in literacy and deafness* (Unpublished doctoral dissertation). Ohio State University, Columbus, OH.

Wang, Y. (2010). Without boundaries: An inquiry of Deaf epistemologies through a metaparadigm. *American Annals of the Deaf, 154*(5), 428–434.

Wang, Y., Trezek, B., Luckner, J., & Paul, P. (2008). The role of phonology and phonological-related skills in reading instruction for students who are deaf or hard of hearing. *American Annals of the Deaf, 153*(4), 396–407.

SUGGESTIONS FOR FURTHER READING

Bornstein, H. (Ed.). (1990). *Manual communication: Implications for education.* Washington, DC: Gallaudet University Press.

Bragg, L. (Ed.). (1999). *Deaf world: A historical reader and primary sourcebook.* New York, NY: New York University Press.

Brueggemann, B. (Ed.) (2004). *Literacy and deaf people: Cultural and contextual perspectives.* Washington, DC: Gallaudet University Press.

Heiling, K. (1995). *The development of deaf children: Academic achievement levels and social processes.* Hamburg, Germany: Signum.

Parasnis, I. (Ed.). (1998). *Cultural and language diversity and the Deaf experience.* Cambridge, UK: Cambridge University Press.

12

Collaborative Knowledge Building for Accessibility in Academia

Antti Raike

Learning opportunities for students with hearing impairments[1] in higher education have increased in recent decades. For an individual Deaf student, the challenge of entering academia is the equivalent of Bruce Lee's challenges in the film *Enter the Dragon*. Indeed, scientific thinking, multiple viewpoints, and diversity of the student body in higher education are arduous tasks to every student's epistemological assumptions. Consequently, university faculties need more evidence-based information about how Deaf students as a cultural and linguistic subgroup of students with hearing impairment make sense of the curricula and cultural diversity of academia.

This chapter discusses the development of a personal epistemology by Deaf students and the issue of valid and legitimate knowledge production in higher education. In philosophy, the term *epistemology* means a theory of knowledge. In sociology (and other fields), the term refers to the use of scientific methods, which lead to the acquisition of sociological knowledge. Here *epistemology* refers to the nature and justification of socially shared knowledge (i.e., social constructivism) and is associated with the structure of meaning. The term *ontology* is interpreted as the expression of ideas in artifacts; nevertheless, the distinction between ontology and epistemology is blurred.

I investigate connections between Deaf students' evolving epistemological beliefs, terming them *personal epistemology* (PE) and *collaborative knowledge building* (KB). PE is difficult to evaluate, whereas the KB can be evaluated to some extent by the artifacts produced by students during knowledge-building activities. The knowledge artifacts that students learn to use, modify, or create are laden with social and cultural values; once established, these artifacts (technical tools, signs, language, machines, websites, and script activities) persist as the structures of mediation.

The metaphor of a cable illustrates the connection or integration between PE and KB (Lewis-Williams, 2002), where each strand of the cable represents one research-supported explanation to connect the two facets of human knowledge as seen in the form of artifacts. To support this description, I integrate the latest "foundations and outcomes of Deaf cognition" (Marschark & Hauser, 2008) and recent theories of cognitive psychology and development with design research methodologies (Krippendorff, 2006). This integration is grounded in the major concepts of theorists such as Popper, Polanyi, and Vygotsky, as well as in modern activity theory.

Furthermore, recent social constructivist theories of knowledge emphasize situational dependence and continuous evolution along active interference with the world and its subjects and objects (Heylighen, 2000). An actor constructs reality socially with peers, and this process is value laden; the objective and value-free actor does not exist. The processes of perception and thinking are individually oriented, but the construction process involves cultural artifacts and therefore becomes social. The social constructions of reality are neither personal nor technical. The patterns of externalization and internalization constitute the social construction of reality as the shared epistemology (Boyer, 1997; Crossman & Devisch, 2002).

The view of knowledge as abstract conceptual artifacts created by humans to specify the relationships of other objects, in the form of explanations or theories, originates from Popper (1972, 1973; in Bereiter, 2002, and Champion, 2010, respectively). Our main focus is on world 3 artifacts, the products of the human mind; however, to provide a context, it is important to introduce Popper's idea of three ontological worlds or domains:

- World 1 (W1): the world of physical objects and events, including biological entities
- World 2 (W2): the world of mental objects and events
- World 3 (W3): the world of the products of the human mind

A physical object, such as a published academic paper, belongs to W1 and contains information that belongs to W3. Two documents with identical contents are two separate W1 objects containing identical W3 contents. When read by two people, they give rise to two distinct and private sets of W2 events, based on W1 brain processes. If two people attempt to communicate their understanding of the document (in spoken, signed, or written form), the contents of their speech, signing, or text/print belong to W3. However, the communication involves W2 in the form of thoughts and intentions and W1 in the form of brain processes and the sound waves, visual gestures, or the marks on paper. The contents of the communication may differ from the original contents of the document (e.g., because of imperfect understanding); nevertheless, there will be objective relationships between the original contents and the modified contents (Popper 1972, 1973; in Bereiter, 2002, and Champion, 2010, respectively). In sum, approaches to knowledge start with knowledge seen as mental states and gradually develop to view knowledge as W3 objects that students can evaluate and improve.

Hence, the development of knowledge involves epistemological changes where the PE of a novice student matures to higher stages of reflective judgment. The path of epistemological development may begin with an objectivist and a dualistic view of knowledge (Hogan, 2000), followed by multiplicity as the student begins to accept the uncertainty of knowledge (Hogan, 2000; Ryan, 1984; Zadeh, 2005), which is the cornerstone and starting point for scientific thinking (Hawkins & Pea, 1987).

The process is enacted by the challenges of diverse academic tasks that promote the evolving understanding of students, who should be the experts of their own motivation, whereas the faculty's role is to turn the motivation into agency. This complex process can be supported by collaborative KB activities and formative interventions with students. Hofer (2002) concludes that we need to know more about the type of academic tasks that might be the most conducive to fostering intellectual development, how they might best be sequenced, and when they can most effectively be offered to students. This is challenging because of the internal characteristics of the mostly unobservable process of learning, which is expected to result in changes in beliefs, attitudes, or skills while a student grows from a novice to an expert (Dreyfus & Dreyfus, 1980).

THE EPISTEMIC CHALLENGE: ENTER THE ZONE OF ACADEMIA

Inquiry into the individual development of conceptions of knowledge and knowing was central to the work of Vygotsky (1978) and Piaget (1954, 1963) and has grown in recent decades. An extensive body of research demonstrates that epistemological beliefs about learning and knowing influence student approaches to learning and KB (Marschark & Hauser, 2008; Martin, 1991; Moores, 2001, Moores & Martin, 2006; Paul, 2010). In addition, high-level language skills are necessary in collaboration, typically carried out in the form of dialogue to guide the learning process of students by using knowledge objects such as problems, hypotheses, theories, explanations, or interpretations (Muukkonen, Hakkarainen, & Lakkala, 1999; Scardamalia & Bereiter, 1996). Walker et al. (2009) show how first-year students' epistemological beliefs are related to their course of study, previous education experiences, family experiences, gender, and age.

However, there is a lack of research on the development of Deaf university students as actors and knowledge creators in an academic community (Raike, 2005; Raike & Hakkarainen, 2009). The challenge is to consider how university educators can maintain a previously launched *developmental trajectory* leading from the natural curiosity of a child to the disciplined creativity of the Deaf expert and knowledge producer. This leads us to ask what kinds of learning experiences foster epistemological understanding. Should we also consider whether the experiences that enhance epistemological thinking could be provided at earlier points (i.e., age), and if so, how early? Thus, individuals invested in the higher education of Deaf students can benefit from reflection on how general and discipline-specific beliefs of hearing impairment and Deaf studies operate together to produce more meaningful knowledge artifacts.

Fortunately, a large body of research evidence on early childhood and language acquisition is available for researchers and educators. Results suggest that by three months of age, infants are sensitive to a number of cues from social partners that are required for the later engagement in joint attention (Cleveland & Striano, 2007). According to Tomasello (1999), the more *joint attentional engagement* children receive after about nine months of age, the faster their comprehension and production of language becomes. In general, the major infrastructure of language is completed by age six to eight. Most important, the acquisition of a language as early as possible cannot be overemphasized.

Further, within the framework of Vygotsky (and other socioculturalists), we note that children will invent a language on their own in a community with other children in a single generation, if they have some source for individual words (Pinker, 1995). This phenomenon has been observed among children in past slave colonies, who were often exposed to a crude pidgin that served as the lingua franca and grew up to speak expressive "creoles" with their own complex grammars (Bickerton, 1984), as well as with the sign languages that arise in similar ways spontaneously in a community of deaf children (Senghas, 1994; Kegl, 1994).

Vygotsky applied cultural–historical theory to disabilities such as deafness, emphasizing that the child's social deprivation is liable for defective development in knowledge and understanding (Gredler & Shields, 2008). There is much anecdotal and commonsense evidence for this; for example, a Deaf orphan in a refugee camp and one that is a member of an academic family in Western Europe are in different psychological situations because their social situations differ. Hence, to address the difficulties faced by disabled learners, Vygotsky suggested that societies continue developing psychological tools that provide opportunities for social and cultural interactions, which are essential for cognitive development (Gredler & Shields, 2008).

In contrast to Piaget, Vygotsky maintained that, through a dialectical transformation, external self-focused speech during activities becomes inner speech that in turn guides planning and other emerging thought processes. The *zone of proximal development* (ZPD) is determined by the cognitive tasks the learner can first complete in collaboration with an adult or an advanced peer but later is able to accomplish alone; ZPD is the move from the present level of development to the new potential level of development.

Clearly, Vygotsky discussed the teacher–student collaboration in the classroom when higher cognitive functions develop and students learn to control their attention, to think conceptually, and to develop logical networks of advanced concepts in long-term memory. However, in the university setting, context intelligence can be seen as an index of what a novice can do and is capable of doing while interacting with experts either in a classroom or using the tools of social media providing flexible opportunities for advanced collaboration.

To contextualize this development or the developmental trajectory, one can use *activity theory* (AT) to explain the cable-metaphor continuum from PE to collaborative KB. AT is a set of basic principles that constitute a general conceptual system rather than a highly predictive theory. The challenge is to connect human knowledge, actions, and W3 artifacts with *activity* in knowledge production and learning.

Briefly, the basic principles of AT include the hierarchical structure of activity, object orientation, internalization/externalization, tool mediation, and development (Engeström, 2009). The beginner's tentative conceptions and first learning experiences influence later navigations through inclusive studies. Academic activity intensifies at the beginning of university studies when students start to develop existing PE into academic PE to meet the needs of collaborative KB with the assistance of faculty. Translating AT into the language and practice of academia involves exposing the PE of the novice for peer review in discussions, joining the academic discourse by learning the necessary argumentation skills, conceptualizing the discipline in question, and gradually improving knowledge production and academic writing skills.

AT (Leontiev, 1978; Vygotsky, 1978) addresses the problem of connecting epistemological meanings with ontological forms. The dynamic relationship between "knowledge realms" is an iterative loop where personal (i.e., tacit) and social thoughts constitute the realm of practical consciousness (epistemology), while objectification belongs to the realm of practical knowledge (ontology). The main argument of AT is that socially embedded activity precedes the development of individual consciousness, and learning by doing must be considered.

In a university setting, some Deaf students experience difficulty in advancing their knowledge and understanding. A Deaf student may be unable to articulate PE or personal tacit knowledge explicitly through language and conceptual artifacts, but this does not necessarily mean that it cannot be communicated in other ways, such as action. According to Polanyi (1966), tacit knowledge is knowledge of which the actor is not explicitly conscious, and it is based within the W2 domain of Popper (1972). The term *tacit* is an appeal to a form of knowledge with which we are all intimately familiar, the kind of knowledge that is reliable when we join a new community or activity.

EXPANDING PERSONAL EPISTEMOLOGY INTO KNOWLEDGE BUILDING

Schön (1983) maintains that knowledgeable professionals know more than they can put into words. Humans have the capacity to learn from instruction with tools, and the teacher plays a central role. Apprentices are often taught for a profession without formal instruction. The traditional process of apprenticeship in education is called *scaffolding*, in which a teacher helps a student proceed beyond his or her current level of competence via dialogue and demonstrations.

In this context, the distinction between objective (W3) and tacit knowledge (W2) should be noted, especially when addressing issues of expanding the PE of Deaf students into KB. Faculty in higher education tend to favor the use of rhetoric; nonverbal behavior and learning by doing have not been in focus until recently. Thus, the implications of the *reflective practitioner* for educators seem obvious: The effectiveness of tuition depends less on degrees or years of experience and more on how effectively an expert can help novices to learn (Schön, 1987). Experts rely less on formulas learned in graduate school than on the kind of improvisation learned in practice.

Dreyfus and Dreyfus (1980) remarked that students normally pass through five developmental stages: novice, advanced beginner, competent, proficient, and expert. They concluded that any skill-training procedure must be based on some model of skill acquisition so that it can address, at each stage of training, the appropriate issues involved in facilitating advancement.

To become experts, it is necessary for Deaf students to construct qualitative models, which are essential for a deep understanding about their own field of study. This deep understanding, that is, domain-specific knowledge, consists of facts, concepts, propositions, and theories (W3). The structural organization of the domain-specific knowledge base essentially differentiates novices from experts; and advanced cognitive development requires the constant reorganization of domain-specific knowledge structures (Honkela, Leinonen, Lonka, & Raike, 2000). A novice may treat knowledge as individuated mental states that reflect reality as facts. Later knowledge is not considered as facts in the head, but as mental representations that are shared and interpreted from different perspectives by community members.

According to Bereiter (2002), knowledge objectification is a process where knowledge is treated as improvable personal artifacts and even semiautonomous artifacts that can take on a life of their own. Individuals see themselves as constructors of provisional solutions to theoretical problems instead of as constructors of knowledge representations such as opinions or interpretations as in earlier levels. At higher levels, students consider whether their knowledge artifacts are up to the standards commonly accepted in the specific knowledge domain (e.g., scientific requirements) in order for the artifact to be recognized as significant to the community.

KB addresses the need to educate Deaf students for a world in which knowledge creation and innovation are incessant. KB may be defined as the production and continual improvement of ideas of value to a community, through means that increase the likelihood that what the community accomplishes will be greater than the sum of individual contributions and part of broader cultural efforts. Hence, KB is not limited to educational settings.

As applied to higher education, the KB approach means engaging novice learners in the full process of knowledge creation from an early stage. The basic premise of this approach is that although achievements may differ, the *process* of building knowledge is essentially the same from early childhood to the most advanced levels of theorizing, invention, and design and across the spectrum of knowledge-creating organizations, within and beyond academia. Hence, students are not engaged in KB in a broad sense if they are engaged in processes suitable only for university activities.

As mentioned previously, understanding PE involves the study of people's beliefs about the nature of knowledge and the knowing process and how these beliefs affect engagements in different learning situations. PE manifests itself in the external actions of a student and can be verified and corrected in KB communities. Research on PE addresses students' thinking and beliefs about knowledge and knowing and typically includes beliefs about some or all of the following: the definition of knowledge, how knowledge is constructed, how knowledge is evaluated, where knowledge resides, and how knowing occurs. According to Hofer (2002), several research programs with disparate names have targeted the ideas that individuals hold about knowledge and knowing; epistemological beliefs, reflective judgment, epistemological reflection, epistemological theories, epistemic beliefs, and epistemological resources. Thus, Hofer (2002) suggests that the term *personal epistemology* is a possible umbrella term for those research programs that address individual conceptions of knowledge and knowing.

Perry (1970, 1981) focused on the development of individuals during their college years and constructed PE as a student's views on diversity and uncertainty with respect to new learning. Perry showed that "a revolution in the very definition of knowledge confronted by freshmen in a college of liberal arts" by graphing the increase in examination topics that required two or more frames of reference. He also noted that college students were confronted with a pluralism of values, not only in courses but also in their interaction with a diverse student body. Perry's model of PE describes the critical intertwining of cognitive and affective perspectives as a student develops more complex forms of thought about the world, discipline, and self during college years.

According to Yuen (2009), Perry's model of PE does not take learning into account. Excluding learning as one of the theoretical constructs in models of PE accords with KB's claim that learning is only a side product of KB processes. Hofer (2002) has argued that we need a better understanding about these processes and how they are related to the educational process because of a growing body of evidence that the concept of PE is a significant component of understanding student learning. My educated guess is that Deaf students' PE is highly challenged in academia by the academic environment itself and by models of knowledge production.

Vygotsky (1978) claims that the new mental tools are developed through a teaching–learning process that involves social exchange where shared meanings are developed through joint activity. Learning at the collective level is the outcome of the interplay between the individual and collective types of knowledge as they interact through the social processes of the community such as teamwork and other collaborative activities. This is related to the model of the social construction of reality developed by Berger and Luckmann (1966).

The shift from a novice relying entirely on PE to an expert capable of KB with peers involves psychological resistance and a gradual restructuring of the novice's belief system (Niiniluoto, 1991). According to Hofer (2002), a period of extreme subjectivity is followed by the ability to acknowledge the relative merits of different points of view and to begin to distinguish the role that evidence plays in supporting one's position. In the final stage, knowledge is actively constructed by the knower, knowledge and truth are evolving, and knowing is coordinated with justification.

The results of a study by Walker et al. (2009) provide support for courses that explicitly focus on the nature of learning and knowledge to help students reflect on and possibly reconstruct their beliefs. These scholars are not advocating for the movement of students along a developmental trajectory. Rather, they suggest that we need to promote a view that, in order to function in increasingly complex learning environments, both professional and personal, students need to understand that sometimes it is necessary to see knowledge as complex, evolving, effortful, tentative, and evidence based. These epistemological beliefs are at the core of deep approaches to learning (Walker et al., 2009).

Thus, it is essential to clarify the relationship between the PE of novice Deaf students in higher education and advanced students participation in collaborative KB activities as follows:

- PE refers to the study of how the individual develops a conception of knowledge and how the same individual uses that to understand the world, and
- KB is a creation or modification of available public or academic knowledge and refers to the process of creating new cognitive and cultural artifacts as a result of common goals, group discussions, and synthesis of ideas.

In the next section, I discuss the developmental trajectory of Deaf students as novice learners to that as experts in KB, especially with the assistance of information and communication technology (ICT).

LEARNING PRACTICES TO CREATE KNOWLEDGE

To promote sophisticated epistemological beliefs, educators need to encourage Deaf students to actively reflect upon their beliefs and to see knowledge as a problematic epistemic discourse. In universities, KB takes place typically in student groups, academic teams, and faculty communities of practice, using physical and virtual learning environments. Both *networked learning* (NL) and *computer-supported collaborative learning* (CSCL) include the wide range of mobile and social media tools with university services.

Engeström (2009) argues that the notion of *learning environment* is not a theoretical concept that can serve as the centrepiece and unit of analysis in CSCL (NL) research. In addition, he argues that the preoccupation with the implementation of digital learning environment is a largely misguided consequence of the unquestioned expectation that technology will radically change learning. Thus, I suggest activity systems as an alternative unit of analysis and a focus on expansive learning instead of implementation.

Engeström (2008) asserts that Vygotsky's methodological principle of double stimulation implies that the subjects gain agency and take charge of the process. In general, students construct certain entrenched beliefs that are based on their everyday experience. Depending on the domain, the knowledge acquisition and construction processes require a revision of some of those beliefs and replacement with a new explanatory structure. This challenging process is called *conceptual change* (Vosniadou, 1994).

With respect to conducting research in this area, there are challenges with the collection of data. Artifacts such as concept maps and self-organizing maps with other electronic objects serve as items for data collection in a complex design research project. The concept maps are explicit descriptions of the concepts the student has acquired (Novak & Gowin, 1984). Besides being learning tools, concept maps can also be produced to visualize interactions. Thus, knowledge artifacts such as concept maps, questionnaires, e-mail messages, and diaries can be collected to track conceptual change.

Furthermore, concept maps illustrate complex structures and processes and function as flexible instruments when designing interactive user interfaces for NL (Raike & Hakkarainen, 2009). With concept maps, it is possible to discuss whether a certain statement is valid or to identify the missing connections between the concepts, which in turn demonstrates a need for further study. The resulting data corpus can be further encoded and visualized using, for example, *self-organizing maps* (SOMs, Kohonen, 2001). SOMs provide statistical visualizations of how students' conceptualizations evolve during the investigations.

However, students are not able to demonstrate their tacit knowledge in the concept maps (Choo, Detlor, & Turnbull, 2000; Polanyi, 1966). In addition, Raike and Hakkarainen (2009) observed that Deaf students need tutoring and on-location teaching to collaborate effectively on a complicated project. Students should be almost continuously assisted and tutored especially at the novice phase to keep them on the developmental trajectory. The meetings with tutors and peer groups provide an opportunity for students to reflect on their own learning skills and methods. Implications for creating more accessible learning environments are discussed in detail elsewhere (Honkela, Leinonen, Lonka, & Raike, 2000; Raike, 2000, 2005, 2006; Raike & Hakkarainen, 2009).

Raike and Hakkarainen (2009) conclude that design research increases our understanding of proper use of CSCL and NL. They propose that similar methods can be applied in the production of multimodal web courses, interfaces, and services that promote inclusive higher education. In addition, design methodologies and theories assist learning by doing in higher education and can be used in formative interventions.

Some scholars have argued that to be legitimate, design research should imitate traditional scientific inquiry. Recently, others have disputed this on the basis of the unique nature of design knowledge (Bratteteig & Stolterman, 1997; Lawson, 2005; Nelson & Stolterman, 2003). For example, Bereiter and Scardamalia (2003) assert that the essence of the design mode is idea improvement. From another perspective, Gibbons et al. (1994) map changes in the modes of knowledge production. Mode 1 is identified as "traditional knowledge" generated within a specific disciplinary (i.e., Deaf education), cognitive, and primarily academic context. Mode 2 is knowledge generated outside academic institutions in broader, transdisciplinary social and economic contexts. The process of transition from mode 1 to mode 2 has been precipitated mainly by a dramatic expansion of possibilities in higher education in the past few decades that created a surplus of highly skilled Deaf graduates who could not be absorbed into traditional academic settings.

COLLABORATION AS A SOCIAL TOOL TO PRODUCE KNOWLEDGE ARTIFACTS

The collaborative KB (Bereiter, 2002; Bereiter & Scardamalia, 1993; Scardamalia & Bereiter, 2003) refers to an epistemic discourse where concerted communal efforts at continual improvement of understanding lead to the creation and refinement of new knowledge valuable to a community. At the same time, participants "learn" (analogous with scientific discovery and theory formation; Hakkarainen, Lipponen, & Järvelä, 2002) as a result of their efforts to obtain a more comprehensive understanding (Bereiter, 2002). Hence, a KB discourse is the formulation of ideas (PE, W2) used to refine knowledge artifacts (W3) and address the authentic and complex problems of the world (W1). By simulating the culture and practices of expert communities, such as a scientific research community or a film production team, novice students may engage in problem- and explanation-driven inquiry (Bratteteig & Stolterman, 1997; Cagan & Vogel, 2002; Engeström, 2008; Kuutti, 2007; Raike, 2005, 2009).

Maturana and Varela (1987) see knowledge as a necessary component of the processes of autopoiesis ("self-production") characterizing living organisms. They argue that the nervous system of an organism cannot in any absolute way distinguish between a perception (caused by an external phenomenon) and a hallucination (a purely internal event). The only basic criterion is that different mental entities or processes within or between individuals should reach some kind of equilibrium. Lewis-Williams (2002) accepts the notion of primary and higher order consciousness and explains how higher-order consciousness permits a socially constructed self, complex language, the recognition of one's own acts and emotions, and long-term storage of symbolic relations. In addition, higher order consciousness enables individuals to remember and to socialize their dreams and visions.

According to memetics (Blackmore, 1999; Dawkins, 1976; Hofstadter, 1985; see Miller, Chapter 8), knowledge can even be transmitted from one subject to another and thereby loses its dependence on any single individual. Similar to social constructivism, memetics is the study of communication and social processes in the development of knowledge, but instead of seeing knowledge as constructed by the social system, memetics scholars see social systems as constructed by knowledge processes. Thus, the concept of *self*, which distinguishes a person as an individual, can be considered as a piece of knowledge constructed through social processes and hence a result of memetics or memetic evolution (Heylighen, 2000).

The *adequacy* of knowledge depends on many different criteria, none of which has an absolute priority over the others. Popper (1972) breaks with a traditional commonsense theory of knowledge that can be traced back to Aristotle and argues that scientific knowledge, once stated in human language, is no longer part of us but a separate entity that grows through critical selection. Recent theories and research have provided more detailed insights into how students represent knowledge and develop competence in specific domains (Lonka, Joram, & Bryson, 1996). In the constructivist approach, learning is viewed as an active, constructive process rather than a passive, reproductive process (Glaser & Bassok, 1989). Students are portrayed as intentional individuals primarily responsible for their own learning and knowledge construction; knowledge is not passively received either through the senses or by way of communication but is actively built up by the cognizing subject.

Moreover, representations are highly situational (Brown, Collins, & Duguid, 1989), and knowledge is socially shared and constructed (Salomon, 1993). In problem-based learning processes, information is treated as something that needs to be explained. Instead of the direct assimilation of the information, students construct knowledge through solving problems in the communities of practice (Wenger, 1998). Performance on problem-solving tasks and explanations of such tasks are often accounted for by the nature of students' mental representations and prior knowledge.

Pure constructivism may lead to relativism, the idea that all models constructed by students are equal and that there are no ways to decide between adequate and inadequate knowledge (Heylighen, 2000). Furthermore, constructivism can lapse into absolute relativism if any model is as adequate as any other. Thus, individual constructivism assumes that a student seeks coherence among pieces of knowledge; inconsistent constructions with the body of other personal knowledge will be rejected, and constructions used to successfully integrate earlier incoherent knowledge parts will be maintained. Further, Berger and Luckmann (1966) claim that a culture is socially constructed; any given culture does not reside solely in forms of knowledge but also in social practices and objectifications. Hence, social constructivism sees consensus between different subjects as the vital criterion to judge knowledge; truth will be accorded to only those constructions on which most students of a community agree and knowledge is seen as the product of the social processes of communication and negotiation.

To summarize, I agree with Bereiter and Scardamalia (1993) that collaborative KB is a continuous creation and refinement of knowledge artifacts through collaborative intentional efforts. Apart from addressing discourse characteristics, one distinctive feature of the KB is that it sees knowledge not as something to be stored in one's mind but as knowledge artifacts "existing out there," which have a certain value or function (Bereiter, 2002). So far there is lack of effective methods to help Deaf novices develop into the experts and active producers of knowledge artifacts. This presents a challenge for educators: How to help Deaf students who are able and willing to participate in the creation of new knowledge develop into active members of academia?

DISCUSSION: LEARNING TO COLLABORATE AND REFLECT IN ACADEMIA

Universities use more NL (CSCL), which in turn increases the possibilities of using double-stimulation methods in education (Vygotsky, 1978). Research on the pedagogical implementation of KB has been conducted at various educational levels over the past two decades. However, utilizing CSCL should not become a lecturer's personal device for structuring learning activities and obtaining information about learners, for example, in a situation where a more verbal teacher simply does not know how to teach less verbal students or those who rely more on a visual sense and learning by doing. This could lead to categorical divisions of students as "with special talents (or needs)" or just "different" and thus subtly separate groups of students from collaboration with a larger student community.

According to Lund and Rasmussen (2008), the center of attention has shifted from approaching a task as a controlled variable in an individual's learning experience toward an understanding about the task as an object that needs to be interpreted and negotiated by learners. Thus, what individual students can do alone is losing importance; what matters more is what students can do with others (i.e., collaboration), especially with the use of technology.

One of the most persistent issues has been knowledge (Cagan & Vogel, 2002; Pullin, 2009; Schön, 1983, 1987): What is the nature of the knowledge needed? The traditional epistemological theories of knowledge have been based to some extent on predicate logic and related methodologies and frameworks. Quite often, the basic assumption is that the world consists merely of objects, events, and relationships. Moreover, some researchers presume that language and conceptual structures reflect rather straightforwardly the perceived ontological structures of the world. In this view, learning is a means to memorize the connections of the aspects of the epistemological domain (i.e., concepts, terms, words, or signs) with those of the ontological domain (objects, events, and relationships).

The question of knowledge has further generated the question of the nature of design research. Researchers such as Collins, Joseph, and Bielaczyc (2004) and Collins (1992) argue for the need to investigate how different designs of ICT affect variables in teaching and learning. According to Kuutti (2007), an interesting development has occurred within academia itself; that is, existing disciplines seem to reflect the activity of a design approach for producing knowledge. Hence, researchers and practitioners need to consider models that advocate for a more contextual, situated, and nuanced understanding of personal Deaf epistemology. This in turn would help educators and developers improve tools for collaborative KB in communities of academia involving Deaf students.

To foster KB among students, both the PE and an approach to knowledge should be promoted concurrently (Bereiter & Scardamalia, 1993). In practice, a collaborative KB or formative intervention will happen in a community as a participatory codesigned project for a novel artifact. Contemporary designers, working in information-technology areas, participate in hybrid networks of mind and matter rather than just creating products (Ehn & Badham, 2002). Within such networks, the activity of design involves the *orienteering* of situated practices within the already existing academic communities of practice (CoP) such as Deaf students and (mainly) hearing faculty. Nelson and Stolterman (2003) describe design activity as being "of service" to others. Krippendorff (2006) argues the need for a semantic turn in design, and he proposes that design involves an "understanding of the understanding of others." Understanding others remains a challenging cognitive task for researchers, students, and faculty, especially when new communities of Deaf experts arise inside academia.

Williams Woolley, Chabris, Pentland, Hashmi, and Malone (2010) believe that *collective intelligence* stems from how well the group works together. They conducted studies at MIT's Center for Collective Intelligence and at Carnegie Mellon of 699 participants, who were placed in groups of two to five. The findings revealed that groups whose members had greater levels of "social sensitivity" were more collectively intelligent. Moreover, the researchers found that the performance of groups was not primarily due to the individual abilities of the group's members. Williams Woolley et al. (2010) hypothesize that it is possible to improve the intelligence of a group by changing the members of a group, teaching members better ways of interacting, and giving the members better electronic collaboration tools.

Engeström (2008) argues that students are the best judges (i.e., experts) of their own motivations, including critical awareness of factors that prevent or distort their motivation to learn. Thus, formative interventions reveal the social, cultural, and political character of the design process, can give voice to this expertise, and open up new ways to build motivation, or more appropriately, to turn motivation into agency. The aim of any codesigned project, discussed previously, is to refocus the diverse objects of activity within collaborative KB practices toward shared outcomes and communal artifacts, such as a website for basic film studies (Raike, 2005; Raike & Hakkarainen, 2009).

There are only a few Deaf individuals entering academia; thus, they must learn to collaborate with other student groups. In addition, within a university setting, it is essential to understand what is considered valid knowledge and how learners and teachers can be made accountable for this knowledge (Ludvigsen, 2008). One of the pillars of deaf epistemologies could be formed by the new sciences of cognition influenced by the information-processing approach to psychology, artificial intelligence, and design research as an attempt to develop computer programs and computer-supported services that mimic the humans' capacity to use knowledge in an intelligent way. Whatever the truth, possibly a model of culture at least needs to take into consideration both mental models (epistemology) and the cultural products (ontology).

CONCLUSION

In this chapter, I emphasized that a learning environment is not a simple entity that exists independently of its users or stakeholders. Within the learning environment, individuals construct new knowledge, especially in their role as a necessary contributing partner in collaborative design processes. A Deaf student does not simply exist in a university; every student is a unique individual, a learning novice growing to become a master with peers (Sen, 2006).

Effective collaborative KB needs a high level of motivation from the student as well as diverse levels of tutoring from the university. Well-designed intensive networked learning is promising for Deaf students. However, evidence indicates that higher education for Deaf students might not be successful with a virtual education model alone. Instead, the on-location instruction must also be taken into account as well as interactions and collaborations among the teachers, tutors, interpreters, and students. In essence, on-location instruction seems to be critical in light of utilizing Vygotsky's (1978) construct of a zone of proximal development—nothing is more important than a true facilitative interaction between the novice and the expert. Finally, the joint activity of KB in codesigned projects and the use of traditional research might be effective for producing sustainable learning artifacts.

It is essential to understand how Deaf students conceive of learning, knowing, and collaborating to promote efficient approaches in universities. Data-based research would enhance our evidence-based understanding of the epistemological beliefs of Deaf students in diverse educational, social, and linguistic contexts. The construct of Deaf epistemologies is not simple, and individuals in higher education should consider the role of learners' *activity* in the KB process as an essential part of developing a PE of Deaf students. Hence, educators and scholars need to be concerned about the possible insufficiency of epistemological understanding, given the difference such understanding makes in Deaf students' abilities to interpret and evaluate information and to make decisions vis-à-vis the multifaceted problems of the world.

Obviously two constructs, KB and PE, capture the complementary aspects of a student's beliefs in the nature of knowledge, including knowledge objectification, the likelihood of modification of understanding, and the structure of justification. With respect to recommendations for further theorizing and research, I present the following ideas:

- We need to know more about the types of academic tasks that might be most conducive to fostering intellectual development, how they might best be sequenced, and when they can most effectively be offered to Deaf students.
- There is a need to understand events in the earlier years of life in a Deaf individual and how these experiences affect later learning within a university.
- We need more field-based research, especially to obtain data on Deaf students within technologically enhanced learning environments prior to university experiences.

NOTE

1. The term *hearing impairment* here covers *deaf, Deaf,* and *hard of hearing. Deaf* with a capital D refers to a member of a sociological group or culture.

REFERENCES

Bereiter, C. (2002). *Education and mind in the knowledge age.* Mahwah, NJ: Lawrence Erlbaum.

Bereiter, C., & Scardamalia, M. (1993). *Surpassing ourselves: An inquiry into the nature and implications of expertise.* Chicago, IL: Open Court.

Bereiter, C., & Scardamalia, M. (2003). Learning to work creatively with knowledge. In E. De Corte, L. Verschaffel, N. Entwistle, & J. Merriënboer (Eds.), *Powerful learning environments: Unraveling basic components and dimensions* (pp. 55–68). Oxford, UK: Elsevier Science.

Berger, P. L., & Luckmann, T. (1966). *The social construction of reality: A treatise in the sociology of knowledge.* Garden City, NY: Anchor Books.

Bickerton, D. (1984). The language bioprogram hypothesis. *Behavioral and Brain Sciences, 7*(2), 173–188. doi:10.1017/S0140525X00044149

Blackmore, S. (1999). *The meme machine.* New York, NY: Oxford University Press.

Boyer, D. R. (1997). *Narratives of teenage addiction: A thematic unfolding of shared epistemology through multiple levels of cognitive development* (Doctoral dissertation). Retrieved from http://scholarworks.umass.edu/dissertations/AAI9721434

Bratteteig, T., & Stolterman, E. (1997). Design in groups—and all that jazz. In M. Kyng & L. Mathiassen (Eds.), *Computers and design in context* (pp. 289–315). Cambridge, MA: MIT Press.

Brown, J. S., Collins, A., & Duguid, P. (1989). Situated cognition and the culture of learning. *Educational Researcher, 18,* 32–42. doi:10.3102/0013189X018001032

Cagan, J., & Vogel, C. M. (2002). *Creating breakthrough products: Innovation from product planning to program approval.* Upper Saddle River, NJ: Prentice Hall.

Champion, R. (2010). *Popper's theory of objective knowledge* Retrieved from http://www.the-rathouse.com/popobjectknow.html

Choo, C. W., Detlor, B., & Turnbull, D. (2000). *Web work—Information seeking and knowledge work on the World Wide Web.* Dordrecht, the Netherlands: Kluwer Academic.

Cleveland, A., & Striano, T. (2007). The effects of joint attention on object processing in 4- and 9-month-old infants. *Infant Behavior and Development, 30*(3), 499–504.

Collins, A. (1992). Toward a design science of education. In T. O'Shea & E. Scanlon (Eds.), *New directions in educational technology.* Berlin, Germany: Springer-Verlag.

Collins, A., Joseph, D., & Bielaczyc, K. (2004). Design research: Theoretical and methodological issues. *Journal of the Learning Sciences, 13*(1), 15–42.

Crossman, P., & Devisch, R. (2002). Endogenous knowledge in anthropological perspective. In C. A. Odora Hoppers (Ed.), *Indigenous knowledge and the integration of knowledge systems* (pp. 96–128). Cape Town, South Africa: New Africa Books.

Dawkins, R. (1976). *The selfish gene*. Oxford, UK: Oxford University Press.

Dreyfus, S. E., & Dreyfus, H. L. (1980). *A five-stage model of the mental activities involved in directed skill acquisition*. University of California, Berkeley. Unpublished report supported by the Air Force Office of Scientific Research, USAF (contract F49620-79-C0063). Retrieved from http://www.dtic.mil/cgi-bin/GetTRDoc?Location=U2&doc=GetTRDoc.pdf&AD=ADA084551

Ehn, P., & Badham, R. (2002). Participatory design and the collective designer. In T. Binder, J. Gregory, & I. Wagner (Eds.) *PDC 2002. Proceedings of the Participatory Design Conference* (pp. 1–10). Palo Alto, CA: CPSR. Retrieved from http://cpsr.org/issues/pd/pdc2002/index_html/

Engeström, Y. (2008). From design experiments to formative interventions. In *ICLS '08: Proceedings of the Eighth International Conference on the Learning Sciences* (pp. 3–24). Utrecht, the Netherlands: International Society of the Learning Sciences. Retrieved from http://portal.acm.org/citation.cfm?id=1599814&CFID=27802588&CFTOKEN=20459821

Engeström, Y. (2009). From learning environments and implementation to activity systems and expansive learning. *Actio: An International Journal of Human Activity Theory, 2*, pp. 17–33. Retrieved from http://www.chat.kansai-u.ac.jp/english/publications/actio/pdf/no2-2.pdf

Gibbons, M., Limoges, C., Nowotny, H., Scott, P., Schwartzman, S., & Trow, M. (1994). *The new production of knowledge: The dynamics of science and research in contemporary societies*. London, UK: Sage.

Glaser, R., & Bassok, M. (1989). Learning theory and the study of instruction. *Annual Review of Psychology, 40*, 631–666.

Gredler, M. E., & Shields, C. (2008). *Vygotsky's legacy: A foundation for research and practice*. New York, NY: Guilford.

Hakkarainen, K., Lipponen, L., & Järvelä, S. (2002). Epistemology of inquiry and computer-supported collaborative learning. In *CSCL 2: Carrying forward the conversation* (pp. 129–156). Mahwah, NJ: Lawrence Erlbaum.

Hawkins, J., & Pea, R. D. (1987). Tools for bridging the cultures of everyday and scientific thinking. *Journal of Research in Science Teaching, 24*(4), 291–307. Retrieved from http://halshs.archives-ouvertes.fr/docs/00/19/05/49/PDF/A45_Hawkins_Pea_87.pdf

Heylighen, F. (2000). Referencing pages in Principia Cybernetica Web. In F. Heylighen, C. Joslyn, & V. Turchin (Eds.), *Principia Cybernetica Web*. Brussels, Belgium: Principia Cybernetica. Retrieved from http://cleamc11.vub.ac.be/epistemi.html

Hofer, B. (2002). Personal epistemology as a psychological and educational construct: An introduction. In B. Hofer & P. Pintrich (Eds.), *Personal epistemology: The psychology of beliefs about knowledge and knowing* (pp. 3–15). Mahwah, NJ: Lawrence Erlbaum.

Hofstadter, D. R. (1985). *Metamagical themas*. New York, NY: Basic Books.

Hogan, K. (2000). Exploring a process view of students' knowledge about the nature of science. *Science Education, 84*, 51–70. doi:10.1002/(SICI)1098-237X(200001)84:1<51::AID-SCE5>3.0.CO;2-H

Honkela, T., Leinonen, T., Lonka, K., & Raike, A. (2000). Self-organizing maps and constructive learning. In D.H. Benzie & D. Passey (Eds.), *Proceedings of Conference on Educational Uses of Information and Communications Technologies: 16th IFIP World Computer Congress* (pp. 339–343). Beijing: Publishing House of Electronics Industry (PHEI). Retrieved from http://citeseerx.ist.psu.edu/viewdoc/download?doi=10.1.1.117.2706&rep=rep1&type=pdf

Kegl, J. (1994). The Nicaraguan Sign Language project: An overview. *Signpost, 7*(1), 24–31.

Kohonen, T. (2001). *Self-organizing maps*. Berlin, Germany: Springer.

Krippendorff, K. (2006). *The semantic turn: A new foundation for design*. Boca Raton, FL: Taylor and Francis.

Kuutti, K. (2007). Design research, disciplines, and the new production of knowledge. In S. Poggenpohl (Ed.), *Proceedings of the International Association of Societies for Design Research (IASDR) Conference: Emerging trends in design research* (paper 39). Retrieved from http://www.sd.polyu.edu.hk/iasdr/proceeding/papers/Design%20Research%20Disciplines%20and%20New%20Production%20of%20Knowledge.pdf

Lawson, B. (2005). *How designers think: The design process demystified* (4th ed.). Oxford, UK: Architectural Press.

Leontiev, A. N. (1978). *Activity, consciousness, and personality*. Hillsdale, NJ: Prentice-Hall.

Lewis-Williams, D. (2002). *The mind in the cave: Consciousness and the origins of art*. London, UK: Thames & Hudson.

Lonka, K., Joram, E., & Bryson, M. (1996). Conceptions of learning and knowledge—Does training make a difference? *Contemporary Educational Psychology, 21*, 240–260.

Ludvigsen, S. (2008). What counts as knowledge: Learning to use categories in computer environments. In R. Säljö (Ed.), *ICT and transformation of learning practices*. Oxford, UK: Pergamon. Retrieved from http://www.intermedia.uio.no/kal/readings/supplementary-reading/stenversjonfinal.pdf

Lund, A., & Rasmussen, I. (2008). The right tool for the wrong task? Match and mismatch between first and second stimulus in double stimulation. *International Journal of Computer-Supported Collaborative Learning, 3*(4), 387–412. doi: 10.1007/s11412-008-9050-8

Marschark, M., & Hauser, P. C. (Eds.). (2008). *Deaf cognition: Foundations and outcomes*. New York, NY: Oxford University Press.

Martin, D. S. (Ed.). (1991). *Advances in cognition, education, and deafness*. Washington, DC: Gallaudet University Press.

Maturana, H. R., & Varela, F. J. (1987). *The tree of knowledge: The biological roots of human understanding*. Boston, MA: Shambhala.

Moores, D. F. (Ed.). (2001). *Educating the deaf: Psychology, principles, and practices* (5th ed.). Boston, MA: Houghton Mifflin.

Moores, D. F., & Martin, D. S. (Eds.). (2006). *Deaf learners: Developments in curriculum and instruction*. Washington, DC: Gallaudet University Press.

Muukkonen, H., Hakkarainen, K., & Lakkala M. (1999). Collaborative technology for facilitating progressive inquiry: Future learning environment tools. In C. Hoadley & J. Roschelle (Eds.), *The Proceedings of the CSCL '99 Conference*, pp. 406–415. Mahwah, NJ: Lawrence Erlbaum. Retrieved from http://www.gerrystahl.net/proceedings/cscl1999/A51/A51.HTM

Nelson, H. G., & Stolterman, E. (2003). *The design way: Intentional change in an unpredictable world*. Englewood Cliffs, NJ: Educational Technology.

Niiniluoto, I. (1991). Realism, relativism, and constructivism. *Synthese, 89*(1), 135–162. doi: 10.1007/BF00413803

Novak, J., & Gowin, B. (1984). *Learning how to learn*. Cambridge, UK: Cambridge University Press.

Paul, P. V. (Ed.). (2010). Deaf epistemologies [Special issue]. *American Annals of the Deaf, 154*(5).

Perry, W. G. (1970). *Forms of intellectual and ethical development in the college years: A scheme*. New York, NY: Holt, Rinehart, and Winston.

Perry, W. G. (1981). Cognitive and ethical growth: The making of meaning. In A. Chickering (Ed.), *The modern American college* (pp. 76–116). San Francisco, CA: Jossey-Bass.

Piaget, J. (1954). *The construction of reality in the child* (M. Cook, Trans.). New York, NY: Basic Books.

Piaget, J. (1963). *Origins of intelligence in children*. New York, NY: Norton.

Pinker, S. (1995). Language acquisition. In L. R. Gleitman, M. Liberman, & D. N. Osherson (Eds.). *An invitation to cognitive science: Vol. 1. Language*. Cambridge, MA: MIT Press.

Polanyi, M. (1966). *The tacit dimension*. New York, NY: Doubleday & Company.

Popper, K. (1972). *Objective knowledge: An evolutionary approach*. Oxford, UK: Oxford University Press.

Popper, K. (1973). Indeterminism is not enough. *Encounter, 50*(4), 20–26.

Pullin, G. (2009). *Design meets disability*. Cambridge, MA: MIT Press.

Raike, A. (2000). Hypermedia and the sense of cinematic expression: Deaf students and distance learning of fine arts in higher education. In *Proceedings of the XIII World Congress of the World Federation of the Deaf* (Vol. 2, pp. 660–675). Sydney, Australia: Australian Association of the Deaf.

Raike, A. (2005). *Löytäjät Elokuvantajua rakentamassa—yhteisöllinen WWW-palvelun tuotanto* (Doctoral dissertation). Helsinki: University of Art and Design. Retrieved from http://www.uiah.fi/ISBN/951-558-172-9/

Raike, A. (2006). Searching knowledge: CinemaSense as a case study in collaborative production of a WWW service in two universities. In A. Miesenberger et al. (Eds.), *Computers Helping People With Special Needs: 10th International Conference, ICCHP 2006, Linz, Austria, July 2006 Proceedings* (pp. 568–574). doi:10.1007/11788713_84

Raike, A., & Hakkarainen, K. (2009). Concept maps in the design of an accessible CinemaSense service. *Art, Design, and Communication in Higher Education, 8*(1), 27–55. doi:10.1386/adch.8.1.27_1

Ryan, M. P. (1984). Monitoring text comprehension: Individual differences in epistemological standards. *Journal of Educational Psychology, 76*, 248–258. Retrieved from http://www.eric.ed.gov:80/PDFS/ED233300.pdf

Salomon, G. (Ed.). (1993). *Distributed cognitions: Psychological and educational considerations.* New York, NY: Cambridge University Press.

Scardamalia, M., & Bereiter, C. (1996). Adaptation and understanding: A case for new cultures of schooling. In S. Vosniadou, E. De Corte, R. Glaser, & H. Mandl (Eds.), *International perspectives on the psychological foundations of technology-based learning environments.* Mahwah, NJ: Lawrence Erlbaum.

Scardamalia, M., & Bereiter, C. (2003). Knowledge building. In *Encyclopedia of education* (2nd ed., pp. 1370–1373). New York, NY: Macmillan.

Schön, D. (1983). *The reflective practitioner: How professionals think in action.* New York, NY: Basic Books.

Schön, D. (1987). *Educating the reflective practitioner.* San Francisco, CA: Jossey-Bass.

Sen, A. (2006). *Identity and violence: The illusion of destiny.* London, UK: Allen Lane.

Senghas, A. (1994). Nicaragua's lessons for language acquisition. *Signpost, 7*(1).

Tomasello, M. (1999). *The cultural origins of human cognition.* Cambridge, MA: Harvard University Press.

Vosniadou, S. (1994). Capturing and modeling the process of conceptual change. *Learning and Instruction, 4*, 45–69. Retrieved from http://www.cs.phs.uoa.gr/en/staff/32.%20vosniadou%201994.pdf

Vygotsky, L. (1978). Interaction between learning and development. In M. Cole (Trans.), *Mind in society* (pp. 79–91). Cambridge, MA: Harvard University Press.

Walker, S., Brownlee, J., Lennox, S., Exley, B., Howell, K., & Cocker, F. (2009). Understanding first year university students: Personal epistemology and learning. *Teaching Education, 20*(3), 243–256.

Wenger, E. (1998). *Communities of practice: Learning, meaning, and identity.* Cambridge, UK: Cambridge University Press.

Williams Woolley, A., Chabris, C. F., Pentland, A., Hashmi, N., & Malone, T. W. (2010, September 30). Evidence for a collective intelligence factor in the performance of human groups. *Science.* doi:10.1126/science.1193147

Yuen, J. (2009). Fostering collaborative knowledge building through advancing students' personal epistemology. In *CSCL'09: Proceedings of the Ninth International Conference on Computer Supported Collaborative Learning* (pp. 273–275). Rhodes, Greece: International Society of the Learning Sciences.

Zadeh, L. (2005). Toward a generalized theory of uncertainty (GTU): An outline. *Information Sciences, 172*(1–2), 1–40. doi: 10.1016/j.ins.2005.01.017

SUGGESTIONS FOR FURTHER READING

Krippendorff, K. (2006). *The semantic turn: A new foundation for design*. Boca Raton, FL: Taylor and Francis.
Marschark, M., & Hauser, P. C. (Eds.). (2008). *Deaf cognition: Foundations and outcomes*. New York, NY: Oxford University Press.
Pullin, G. (2009). *Design meets disability*. Cambridge, MA: MIT Press.
Raike, A., & Hakkarainen, K. (2009). Concept maps in the design of an accessible CinemaSense service. *Art, Design, and Communication in Higher Education, 8*(1). doi:10.1386/adch.8.1.27_1
Tomasello, M. (1999). *The cultural origins of human cognition*. Cambridge, MA: Harvard University Press.

13

Can It Be a Good Thing to Be Deaf?

Rachel Cooper

In this chapter, I ask whether it can be a good thing to be deaf. Before the philosophical work begins, a note regarding terminology is necessary. It has become commonplace for writers to distinguish between *Deaf* people, with a capital *D*, and *deaf* people, with a lowercase *d*. Capital-D Deaf people self-ascribe to Deaf culture, think of themselves as part of the Deaf community, and typically communicate using a sign language. Lowercase-d deaf is less standardized, but I use it to describe people who are physically deaf but who may or may not consider themselves to be part of the Deaf community. Some writers have used the term only for people who do not identify with the Deaf community (Ladd, 2003). I reject this usage because it leaves no term to refer to people who are physically deaf but whose cultural affiliation is unclear. The hearing status and communication modalities employed by people who are "physically deaf" are heterogeneous. People may have different degrees of hearing loss, they may have been deaf from birth or become deaf later, and they may use speech, a sign language, or a mixture. In this chapter, I focus on people who have been physically deaf from birth, use a sign language, and are fully involved in the Deaf community.

It is increasingly common for activists associated with the Deaf community to claim that it can be a good thing to be Deaf. They mean not only that deafness might be a blessing in some cases (as, for example, in the case of a draftee whose deafness excuses him from service) and that one might have a good life despite being deaf, but also that deafness in and of itself can be a good thing. Deafness is not pathological but merely another way of being normal, or possibly even a way of being better than normal, they claim. Despite such assertions, however, much of the hearing world remains unconvinced and continues to think of deafness in negative terms.

This chapter is based on my 2007 article "Can it be a good thing to be deaf? in the *Journal of Medicine and Philosophy, 32,* 563–583. This paper also has been presented at seminars at Bristol University and Lancaster University, and I am grateful for the comments of those present. Mike Gulliver and Kearsy Cormier, in particular, have been generous with advice. I expect that both will continue to think much of the final version of this paper wrong-headed, but while we disagree on much, I am very grateful for their help.

Whether it can be good to be deaf is an important question, as it has practical consequences. Many philosophers of medicine hold that a condition should be considered pathological only if it is a bad thing (Cooper, 2002; Englehardt, 1974; King, 1954; Reznek, 1987), although what they qualify as "bad" may differ. Assuming they are right, if and when deafness is a good thing, it is not pathological. This implies that it does not need "fixing" by medical experts. Following this line of thought, some Deaf parents have refused cochlear implants for their children, and others have refused genetic testing designed to enable the detection and abortion of deaf fetuses.[1] There have also been cases where Deaf couples have purposefully conceived deaf babies, in the belief that it is good to be deaf.[2] Whether such actions should be encouraged or permitted depends at least in part on whether it can be good to be deaf.

IS IT ACCEPTABLE FOR HEARING PEOPLE TO ASK WHETHER IT CAN BE A GOOD THING TO BE DEAF?

Judging the quality of others' lives is often considered ethically dubious. However, there are multiple areas in which such questions cannot be avoided. To list just a few examples, when considering whether to have children ourselves or to help others to have children, we are frequently forced to question what kinds of people should be brought into existence. When deciding whether to undergo medical treatments or other alterations we have to consider what kinds of people we wish to become. At a societal level, we have to make decisions as to which people deserve compensation or help because through no fault of their own their lives are not as good as others' lives.

Even if it is necessary to determine whether it can be good to be deaf, some activists associated with the Deaf community have claimed that such questions can only be appropriately considered by Deaf people. For example, Paddy Ladd, Mike Gulliver, and Sarah Batterbury have claimed that

> Research affecting Deaf people and their lives must be Deaf-led; originating with Deaf people, coordinated by Deaf people and disseminated by Deaf people for the empowerment of the Deaf community. Any other level of involvement, especially within an academy whose stated aim is the attainment of "full knowledge" simply renders the research invalid. (2003, pp. 27)

The idea that minority groups should only be studied by members of those groups is also commonplace in other areas. For example, in women's studies some literature considers the "men problem"—the problem that some men wish to do research in women's studies (Klein, 1983; Philips & Westland, 1992). Similarly, in disability studies (which has developed separately from Deaf studies because many Deaf people do not consider themselves to be disabled), the "emancipatory" research paradigm proposed by Mike Oliver and others suggests that all research on disabilities should be controlled by people with disabilities and that disability research should be "part of the struggle by disabled people to challenge the oppression they currently experience in their daily lives" (Oliver, 1992, p. 102). The idea that minority groups should be studied only by members of those groups potentially can be supported in two ways. First, there is the thought that members of the minority group are in an epistemically privileged position: They have first-hand knowledge of what it is like to be a member of the group. Second, some theorists are inspired by the idea that knowledge is power and claim the right for minorities to study themselves as a political statement.

Whatever the motivation, the claim that only the members of a minority group should study that group becomes problematic. Such a stance rules out the possibility of making many comparative judgments, and often when we evaluate a way of being, what we are really after is a comparative judgment. Suppose, for example, we are trying to decide whether fetuses with Down syndrome should be aborted. When we ask whether people with Down syndrome have a poor life, what we really need to know is whether they have a poor life compared to those without Down syndrome. We want to know whether one way of being is better or worse than another. However, if only those who are a certain way can judge it, then many comparative judgments are ruled out.

The belief that for political reasons only the members of minority groups should study such groups leads to an endless fragmentation of areas of study. Neither women nor disabled people nor Deaf people form homogeneous classes. Thus, if one thinks that it is unjustifiable for men to write about women, one should also think it unjustifiable for white women to write about black women, and so on. However, claiming that only black bisexual women should study black bisexual women, and only prelingually Deaf people should study prelingually Deaf people, is problematic, as in many cases one will be left with very few people who are "qualified" to study a way of being. When few people work on a problem, the chances of any of them being able to solve it are reduced.

For these reasons, I reject the suggestion that only the members of minority groups should study such groups. In saying this, however, I do not mean to imply that the viewpoints of deaf people can be ignored when asking whether it can be good to be deaf. Of course, what deaf people have to say about the advantages or disadvantages of being deaf is important. Through being deaf, deaf people are likely to notice consequences of deafness that others would not. Still, once deaf people have said why they like or dislike being deaf, much work to be done in evaluating their claims can be done by hearing researchers as easily as it can be done by deaf researchers. As an example, a deaf person may suspect that deaf people have enhanced visual awareness, but it still takes a psychologist to find out whether deaf people really do see things differently and a philosopher to work out whether any such enhanced vision is necessarily a good thing. While the psychologist and philosopher may be deaf, I see no reason why they need to be.

CAN IT BE A GOOD THING TO BE DEAF? ATTEMPTED EASY ANSWERS THAT WILL NOT WORK

Ask Deaf People

When hearing people become deaf, they typically experience this as a loss. A deafened person becomes unable to participate in activities that he or she used to take for granted. That person can no longer chat with friends on the phone or listen to music.

The ways in which the person has learned to deal with the world no longer work. All things being equal, it is a bad thing to become deaf.

It is tempting to think that because it is a bad thing to become deaf it must also be a bad thing to be deaf from birth. This, however, does not necessarily follow. The temptation comes from thinking of congenitally deaf people merely in terms of deficiency, as people who cannot do various things, while forgetting that deaf people develop skills and abilities that other people do not have. Those who claim that it can be a good thing to be deaf normally have congenitally deaf people in mind. In asking whether deafness can be a good thing, I too mainly am concerned with congenitally deaf people. From now on, when talking about Deaf or deaf people, I am referring to people who have been deaf from birth.

One might think that one can determine whether it is a good thing to be born deaf by asking someone who has been deaf all their life. Indeed, based on their experience of what it is like to be deaf, some deaf people will claim that being deaf is a good thing.[3] Unfortunately, the matter is not so simple. When we ask whether being deaf from birth is a good thing, we really want to know whether it is better, or at least as good, as being hearing from birth, but no one can possibly be in a position to answer this question. No one can be born both hearing and deaf.

Admittedly, some deaf people try using cochlear implants and then choose to abandon them because they like being deaf better. However, such individuals have tried hearing with a brain that has become adapted to deafness. As a consequence, the experience of being deaf and using a cochlear implant may be unlike the experience of having been hearing from birth.

Other deaf people find cochlear implants useful and report that being able to hear is better than being deaf. However, plausibly, those deaf people who seek implants are disproportionately likely to be unhappy about being deaf (as it is more rational to accept the risks and costs of operation if one is unhappy with one's present state). As the sample of such individuals is likely to be biased, we cannot conclude that it is generally better to be hearing based on their reports.

The Appeal to the Natural

Often people assume that it must be a bad thing to be deaf because they consider being deaf to be a biological dysfunction and therefore "unnatural." However, even if being deaf is a biological dysfunction, to think that this implies that it is a bad thing is simply to make a mistake. The natural is good only in children's hymns. In actuality. "Mother Nature" does not care about her offspring, and some conditions that are bad for the individual organism are selected because they increase an organism's inclusive fitness. To take some concrete examples, evolutionary psychologists have been struck by the fact that some mental disorders, including bipolar disorder, obsessive–compulsive disorder, and sociopathy, seem to have a genetic cause but occur at rates too high to be the result of random mutations (Wilson, 1997). Such disorders can only occur at the rates that they do because they are evolutionarily advantageous in some way. Maybe sufferers take better care of their children or their disorder benefits other close kin. Whatever the exact mechanism, in evolutionary terms these conditions are not dysfunctions, but still they are bad conditions to suffer from. There may also be states that are biological dysfunctions but not harmful. Homosexuality is a possible example (Ruse, 1981). There is no necessary link between an organism functioning properly in a biological sense and being in a good state. As such, asking whether deafness is a biological dysfunction will not help determine whether it is a bad thing to be deaf.

WHAT DOES IT MEAN TO SAY THAT A CONDITION IS A GOOD THING FOR AN INDIVIDUAL?

What does it mean to say that a condition is a good thing for an individual? This is a very difficult question, and I cannot answer it fully here. Various accounts of the good for an individual have been proposed, but all are problematic (for an overview, see Griffin, 1986). The problems can best be understood by thinking of the possible ways of determining what is good for an individual as varying along a scale. At one end of the scale, one might rely on asking actual people what they want (the "subjective" or "desire satisfaction" approach). At the other end of the scale, one might claim that something is good for an individual if it helps that individual meet some ideal standard of human flourishing (the "objective" or "Aristotelian" approach). Between these extremes are methods that claim that something is good for an individual if that individual would judge it to be good in ideal circumstances, for example, if he or she were calmer, wiser, and better informed than in reality.

Relying on asking actual people runs into problems: People often do not know what is in their own best interest. They may make mistakes because they lack essential information. Thus, I may take great delight in my win of a free holiday to some exotic-sounding city but only because I have failed to realize that it is in the middle of a war zone. Actual people are also notoriously prone to self-deception. Surveys repeatedly find that the vast majority of people believe they are brighter and more attractive than average (for a review, see Alicke, Vredenburg, Hiatt, & Govorun, 2001). Self-deception is particularly likely to arise when people are faced with making judgments regarding their bodily states, as within our culture how we evaluate our bodies is closely linked to how we evaluate ourselves.

Given such difficulties, it is tempting to move to the opposite end of the scale and claim that something is good for someone if it helps that person to meet some ideal standard of human flourishing. Here, too, there are problems. Relying on the judgements of actual people to determine what is good is satisfyingly down to earth: We only have to ask actual people to find out whether a condition is good. In contrast, appeals to "ideal standards of human flourishing" seem disturbingly abstract. It is not clear how the ideal standards are fixed, nor is it clear how we can find out about them.

To a greater or lesser extent, all other methods on the scale are beset by the problems of the extreme methods. Methods that require idealization run into epistemic problems. As I am not ideal, it is hard for me to find out what an idealized version of myself would value. Methods that make use of the judgments of actual people risk giving the wrong answers; after all, actual people make mistakes.

Here, in seeking to determine what is good for an individual, I adopt the following strategy: I go through potential alleged benefits and disadvantages of being deaf one by one, and see if they survive scrutiny.[4] I make use of our commonplace intuitions as to what kinds of thing are good or bad. Thus, I take it that advantages include having a language, having friends, and experiencing pleasant sensations and that drawbacks are things like being in pain and being lonely. While such a method may seem crude, I take it that no one seriously doubts such commonplace intuitions, and so it is worth seeing how far we can get in assessing whether it can be good to be deaf by using them alone.

WEIGHING THE COSTS AND BENEFITS

The most striking differences between those who have been deaf from birth and sign and people who hear are that they experience different sensations and make use of different language modalities.

Differences in Sensations

Deaf people necessarily miss out on certain sensations that others find intensely pleasurable. A deaf person will never get to hear symphonies or birdsong. Surely, this is at least one aspect of being deaf that must be admitted to be a bad thing? Unfortunately, things are not so simple. Of course, to have no sensations in any sensory modalities at all would be awful; such a person would be entirely cut off from the world. However, plausibly, there is a limit to the volume of sensations that our brains can process. As such, we will be able to appreciate only so much, and there must be a point where having an additional sense would not be a blessing but merely produce confusion.

Some might suggest that this cannot be the case with being able to hear—natural selection has fitted us with five senses, and so our brain must be able to make use of that amount of data. Remember, however, we now live in environments unlike those in which humans evolved. Maybe present environments contain more stimuli, and as a consequence most of us now live in states of sensory overload.

I suggest that there are no senses that are necessarily a blessing. With luck, we will live in an environment where many of our sensations are pleasant, but this need not be so. Take smells. If pollution increases, then people who lack a sense of smell may come to be considered unusually fortunate. Similarly, there are environments in which deaf people miss out on few pleasant sensations. If one lives under a railway, with neighbors who play novelty pop records at full volume, then not hearing noises is a benefit.

Not only is it possible that sounds might on balance be unpleasant, but people who are deaf from birth experience sensations that hearing people do not. Deaf people may become more sensitive to vibrations and to visual stimuli than hearing people are (Bahan 2008; Bavelier et al., 2000). Such sensations bring their own pleasures, which might make up for those lost. (This possibility is nicely explored in Michael Dowse's 2004 film *It's All Gone, Pete Tong,* which is about a DJ who becomes deaf and gradually comes to a greater appreciation of visual sensations and vibrations.) I conclude that the fact that deaf people miss out on auditory sensations that many enjoy does not show that deafness is a bad thing.

Auditory sensations may have other benefits than producing pleasure: They give us information about our environment. Thus, a fire alarm may warn hearing people of danger, for example. However, as deaf people may become more sensitive in other sense modalities, it is not clear that hearing people will always have the edge when it comes to finding out about the environment.

Differences in Language

It is extremely difficult for congenitally deaf people to learn to speak. Even after years of voice tuition, many never manage to speak intelligibly (Lane, Hoffmeister, & Bahan, 1996, p. 361). As a consequence, deaf people are often cut off from the hearing population. In addition, many deaf people fail to learn to read and write well.[5] Theorists are divided as to whether this is because the amount of time some deaf children spend trying to learn to speak leaves little time for other activities, whether this is because the structure of sign language is so different from that of English that learning to read is difficult, or whether there is some other explanation.

Some activists associated with the Deaf community claim that this does not matter.[6] Deaf people have their own languages in which they can become fluent. Sign languages enable Deaf people to communicate with other Deaf people and form the basis for vibrant Deaf cultures. There are signed poems, jokes, and plays. According to many scholars, the problems experienced by those who use sign languages when seeking to communicate with the hearing population are no different in kind from those experienced by members of other linguistic minorities (Ladd, 2003; Lane, 1992; Lane, Hoffmeister, & Bahan, 1996).

In assessing such claims, we must ask two questions. First, is the situation of a Deaf person analogous to that of the members of other linguistic minorities? Second, is it true that sign languages are as good as any other language and that Deaf culture is as good as any other culture?

Is the situation of a Deaf person analogous to that of a member of another linguistic minority? There are some similarities. Many members of other linguistic minorities are unable to speak the majority language and experience difficulties communicating with the rest of the population. However, there are also important differences. Members of other linguistic communities can learn to speak the majority language. In contrast, for congenitally deaf people, it may not be a viable possibility. This difference is important and means that deaf people are disadvantaged relative to the members of other linguistic communities in this respect.

Are sign languages as good as other languages? Often scholars claim that all languages and all cultures are equally good. To take a typical example, in his book *Seeing Voices*, Oliver Sacks claims that

> all languages, whether signed or spoken, no matter how new, or how limited their geographical distribution, have the same potential, the same range of possibility—none can be dismissed as "primitive" or "defective". Thus British Sign Language (BSL) is fully the equal of ASL; Irish Sign Language is fully the equal of both; and so too is Icelandic Sign Language (even though there are only seventy deaf people in Iceland). (Sacks, 1991, p. 165)

Sacks makes these claims without supporting them. In some cases, such claims seem to be motivated by a beneficent liberalism. The thought seems to be that one must claim that all languages are equal, or else one will soon be led to claim that some peoples are better than others, and that from that point fascism is but a small step away. In other cases, the claim that all languages are equal is made by linguists who mean to assert that all languages are equally languages and as such are equally worthy of linguistic study (see, for example, Burns, Matthews, & Nolan-Conroy 2001; Evans, 1998). This may be true, but we should remember that here "equal" is being used in a technical sense. When linguists say that all languages are equal in the sense of all being equally languages, they are moving away from the question of whether all languages are equal as a layperson might pose it. All languages might be equally languages, but the question of whether they are equally good for expressing ideas remains. When one asks whether sign languages are as good as other languages, one wants to know whether one can communicate as many ideas as easily, as precisely, as elegantly, and so on as one can in a spoken language. I argue that, at least in this vernacular sense, plausibly some languages are better than others. There is thus no a priori reason for thinking that sign languages and spoken languages will be equal.

My starting point is that some languages have resources that others do not. Some languages have a written form; others do not. Some have tenses that others lack. In some one can build up complex words easily; in others one cannot. One might hope that benefits will balance out, but a moment's reflection suggests that there is no reason to expect things to even out. Plausibly one might expect those languages that have been used for the longest time, or by the most people, or in the greatest variety of settings, to end up being better all round at enabling humans to formulate and communicate ideas.

On occasion, linguists say that all languages are equal because they all have the same potential (see, for example, Harlow, 1998). Here the idea seems to be that a group of language users who find themselves with a need that their language cannot currently fulfill will simply add new resources to their language so that it becomes adequate to the task. To take a simple case, suppose a group of language users only have words for the numbers up to 10 but are faced with the necessity of counting 15 cows. Here, the language users may simply invent new words and so expand their language so that it meets their needs. However, although languages clearly can sometimes be expanded, to think that this implies that they are all potentially equal betrays a rather odd view of language use. It suggests that all people are capable of having the same ideas irrespective of their language. The picture is one of people having ideas in some nonlinguistic medium and then searching about for a way to convey these ideas in words. It is more likely that our thoughts are at least shaped, if not determined, by our language. (For a useful introduction on the ways in which language shapes thought, see Devitt and Sterelny, 1999, chap. 10.) Thus, once one learns to make use of the jargon of music theory, for example, one is able to have different thoughts about music, not just able to express more clearly the very same thoughts that one always had. As our language plausibly shapes our thoughts, I suggest that it is not true that all languages are even potentially equal. Language users whose language lacks the resources needed to express a particular range of thoughts are less likely to have those thoughts. Thus, they cannot be relied on to simply expand their language once the thoughts occur to them.

If it is accepted that one language may be better than another in a certain respect, and it is accepted that there is no reason to expect things to even out so that all languages are equally good, then there is no a priori reason to claim that sign languages will be as good as other languages. Rather, working out how the resources of a sign language compare to those of a spoken language will be a matter for empirical research.

There is some research that suggests that sign languages are superior to spoken languages in a variety of ways. Less muscle control is required to make signs than to form the right mouth movements to make phonemes. As a consequence, deaf infants who have been exposed to a sign language from birth can often form the sign for "milk" at four months (Lane et al., 1996, p. 46; Sacks, 1991, p. 30), while their hearing contemporaries can only cry. Harlan Lane claims that sign languages are intrinsically better than oral languages for providing information regarding spatial relations: In a sign language, one can sign so as to show where objects are placed relative to each other (Lane, 1992, pp. 124–125; Lane et al., 1996, pp. 104–111). Some have claimed that the four-dimensional nature of sign languages makes them more expressive than oral languages (Sacks, 1991, pp. 89–90). Others suggest that the iconographic nature of sign languages enables users to think more concretely and thus in many cases more clearly (although there is also resistance to this idea, as some see it as stemming from the notion that sign languages are systems of mime rather than proper languages) (Sacks, 1991, pp. 122–124).

Investigating the net importance of these various factors would take empirical research. I do not know whether sign languages can be expected to be poorer, richer, or the equal to oral languages. The key point is there is no a priori justification for the claim that sign languages are equal to other languages. Sign languages may be relatively impoverished, in which case signers will be restricted in their ability to communicate. On the other hand, sign languages may be richer than oral languages, in which case signers will be at an advantage in these respects.

It is worth emphasizing that having a rich or poor language plausibly affects more than one's ability to communicate. Having a rich language can enhance one's ability to think. This means that whether sign languages are rich or poor compared to oral languages will play a huge role in determining whether it can be a good thing to be deaf.

If sign languages turn out to be poorer than oral languages, this will be a disadvantage to being deaf. However, the converse does not follow. If sign languages are richer than oral languages, this is not an advantage to being deaf. Sign language use is not restricted to deaf people, and so if sign languages are rich compared to oral languages this would be a reason for all infants to be taught sign, not a reason for people to remain or become deaf.

Problems Regarding Communication

Even if sign languages are as good as other languages, deaf people may face other problems. Humans need others in order to communicate. If only a small number of people use a language, then the chances of finding other language users interested in discussing the subjects one is interested in are reduced.

Some may claim that the small size of the Deaf community results in other benefits that outweigh this difficulty. The Deaf community, they may say, is unusually close knit, warm, and supportive (see, for example, Ladd, 2003, pp.360–361). As opposed to the hearing community, it offers the benefits of the village over the city. Of course, some people like living in villages. However, a deaf person, who cannot communicate with hearing people, has no choice. (See Nyman, 1991, for a discussion of the problems faced by gay members of the Deaf community, for example.)

For those deaf people who would rather belong to a large community, being limited in their ability to communicate with the hearing population is a major disadvantage But is it a disadvantage for those who are quite happy communicating with mainly other deaf people? I suggest that it is a disadvantage to *have* to belong to a small community even if one likes small communities, although the disadvantage is only slight. This is because in general it is a good thing to have worthwhile opportunities, even if one does not presently want to take advantage of them. Thus, I benefit, slightly, from there being a sports center at my university even if I do not presently foresee ever wishing to go there. People generally value "leaving their options open," mainly because they might want to make use of an opportunity in the future. In addition, even if someone never actually makes use of an opportunity, they may dream of making use of it in the future, an activity that in itself is often of value. Thus, I can enjoy talking and thinking about vacations that I may one day take, even if I never actually take a vacation. It is a slight disadvantage for a deaf person to be limited to the Deaf community, even if that person would choose to belong that community.

At this point it might be suggested that deaf people often have problems communicating with hearing people because there is a lack of interpreters or because hearing people cannot sign, rather than because they are deaf per se. If there were the facilities, deaf people could communicate with hearing people if they wanted and avoid the problems associated with belonging to a small community.

It is certainly true that the extent to which deafness restricts someone's ability to function socially depends on the kind of environment within which a deaf person lives. There have been communities in which everyone, hearing and deaf, could use sign language, and in such societies deaf people experience no problems with communication (see, for example, Groce's description of Martha's Vineyard [1985]). Changes in the material and social environments can make a difference. In the late 18th century, it was claimed that one of the major disadvantages of sign language compared to oral language is that sign language cannot be used to communicate in the dark.[6] Today, widespread lighting means that there is almost always enough light to see signs. As such, a disadvantage that may have existed in the past no longer exists.

Biological conditions can be a bad thing in some environments but not in others. For example, dyslexia may have some kind of biological root, and there may well have been people with dyslexic brains throughout history. Still, it is only a bad thing to be dyslexic in societies that use writing. As a consequence, stone-age dyslexics did not suffer from a bad condition whereas present-day dyslexics do. Similarly, deafness limits a deaf person's ability to function socially only in certain societies. If communication difficulties were the only negative consequences of being deaf, then being deaf would be a bad thing only in certain societies.

On occasion, this point has been taken to show that deaf people have problems with communication only from a certain "point of view" and that from another point of view the problem lies with the hearing population. Thus, Wendell (1996) writes,

> From a medical and rehabilitative point of view (which is also the point of view of most hearing people), a deaf child is disabled by her inability to hear, and so the child becomes the focus of efforts to "normalize" her as far as possible within the hearing community. But from another, equally valid point of view, the same child is handicapped by hearing people's (often including her parents') ignorance of Sign. (Wendell, 1996, p. 29)

This way of describing things is unhelpful. Rather than the communication problems stemming from the child's inability to hear, or from her parents' inability to sign, the communication problems suffered by deaf people are relational problems—the problem stems from the fact that the child cannot hear coupled with the fact that her parents cannot sign. As such, the communication difficulties of deaf people can be solved either by hearing people learning sign language, or, potentially, through altering the deaf person (e.g., through cochlear implantation).

Relational problems faced by people who are physically or mentally different are not uncommon. Consider the following cases:

1. Black people suffer discrimination.
2. A gay man regrets having no children.
3. An ugly person cannot find a partner.

All these problems are relational in that they can potentially be solved either by changing the individual or by changing society. Black people could have their skin bleached, or society could stop being racist. The gay man could have sex with a woman, children could be obtained via artificial insemination, or changes in adoption law could permit him to adopt a child. The ugly person can have plastic surgery, or social notions of the beautiful or of qualities requisite in a partner could shift.

Despite all these problems being relational, in the sense that they can be solved either by altering the individual or by making social changes, we tend to think about them very differently. Least controversially, the problems faced by black people, we say, should be solved via changing society, not through altering black people's skin color. In contrast, many people think that the problems faced by the ugly person can best be alleviated by making the ugly person more attractive. In the case of the gay man, many people will split when locating the source of the problem. Some will say that childlessness is a natural consequence of being gay; others believe that people who are childless for whatever reason should be helped to have children.

These examples illustrate that whether a problem is thought of as being caused by the individual's condition or by society depends on the politics of the situation. All the difficulties are relational in the sense that they could be solved either by changing society or by changing the individual. However, when we think that the individual *should* change, if possible, we tend to locate the problem as being "in" the individual. Thus, we see ugliness as being an intrinsic problem, and say that it is bad to be ugly. In contrast, when we think that society should change, we locate the problem elsewhere. Thus, we see the problems faced by black people as stemming from racist prejudice. We say that it is bad that society is racist, not that it is bad to be black.

Homosexuality is an especially interesting case in this respect. In the 1970s, it was usual to consider homosexuals who were unhappy about being gay to suffer from a disease, ego-dystonic homosexuality, and this disease could be treated by psychiatrists either through counselling to help the patient accept his sexual orientation or through therapy aimed at changing it. More recently, it has become socially unacceptable for therapists to aim to change their clients' sexual orientation, even at their clients' request.[7] At the same time, homosexuality is increasingly seen as a condition that is not in itself a bad thing. The problems faced by gay people are instead considered to be caused by a homophobic society. Here we have an example of a condition that ceased to be considered a bad thing as people came to think that the problems faced by homosexuals should be solved by changing society rather than by changing the homosexuals.[8]

Providing a descriptive account of how, in general, we decide whether problems faced by an individual should be changed by altering the individual or by altering society is too large a task for this essay. Providing a normative account of how such decisions should be made is even more problematic. Very briefly, whether society or the individual should change will depend on the following kinds of factors, among others: (a) what changes are practically possible, (b) whether it is easier for society or the individual to change, and (c) the history that resulted in the problem in the first place. (If, for example, I have intentionally messed up your life, it only seems fair that I should bear the burden of fixing the problem. If self-destructive behavior on your part has produced your difficulties, it seems right that you should bear more responsibility for resolving them.)

Those who adopt social models of disability claim that the source of disabilities lies in society rather than in the individual, and that society should change to fix the resulting problems. (Classic formulations of the social model are given by Oliver, 1990, and Finkelstein, 1980.) For example, those who adopt a social model of disability commonly claim that people in wheelchairs are disabled not by their inability to walk but by a society that builds stairs. This claim should not be understood as a purported description of fact but as a political claim. In themselves, the problems faced by wheelchair users are relational. They can be fixed either by enabling the wheelchair user to walk or by changing the material environment. When the social model of disability claims that society causes disabilities, this should be understood as a political claim, asserting that society and not disabled individuals should change to solve the problems faced by disabled people.

While these political claims are frequently plausible, this will not always be the case. Whether society or the different individuals should change depends on highly contingent factors. In a population with a large percentage of deaf people, it may be reasonable for hearing people to learn to sign. However, it is not the case that the problems faced by atypical people should always and necessarily be solved by changing society.

This can be seen by considering an extreme and hypothetical example. Suppose in the future cochlear implant technology improves greatly. It comes to be the case that deafness can be cured completely, and the operation itself advances to the stage where it is almost completely safe and painless. Suppose furthermore that most deaf people have been implanted. Sign languages cease to be living languages, as no one learns them and those who can sign die. Eventually, only one non-oral, signing deaf person remains in the world. I suggest that it is not at all clear that the hearing community would have a duty to learn to sign in order to communicate with this person.

CONCLUSION

Finally, we are in a position to conclude the discussion of whether it can be a good thing to be deaf. We have gone through the potential costs and benefits associated with being deaf and are now in a position to try to sum these together. First, certainly deaf people miss out on sound sensations. However, this is not necessarily a bad thing, as deaf people may have more sensations in other sensory modalities, and in any case having more sensations is not necessarily better. Second, deaf people may well be unable to speak and so be limited to sign language. Whether sign languages are as rich as other languages cannot be established a priori but instead depends on empirical facts. However, even if sign languages are richer than other languages this would not be something good about being deaf per se. Rather it would be an advantage to be a signer, and hearing people can also learn sign language. Third, depending on the society within which they live, deaf people may be limited to a fairly small Deaf community. Some will claim that this limitation should be thought of as being caused by a society that will not sign, rather than by being caused by deafness itself. I claim that in themselves communication problems are relational. Whether they are said to be located in society or the individual depends on whether we think society or the individual should change. The solution to this normative question is not straightforward and depends on numerous contingent factors.

I conclude that whether it is a good or bad thing to be deaf is hard to determine. Plausibly, being deaf may be a bad thing for some deaf people but not for others. Deaf people who would like to communicate with hearing people but cannot are more greatly disadvantaged than those who are happy sticking to the Deaf community. In addition, deaf people have different sensations than hearing people. Whether deaf sensations are better than hearing sensations will likely be largely a matter of taste.

If being deaf is good for some people but not for others, this would not be a surprising conclusion. Commonly, the same biological condition can affect people differently because different people have different aims, different abilities, and different preferences. The case is no different for deafness.

Further research might consider a number of questions:

- How exactly does the lived experience of deaf people differ from that of hearing people? How do the sensory abilities of deaf and hearing people differ? How do sign languages differ from oral languages in their capacity to serve various types of human need?

- It is becoming increasingly common for a wide variety of differently abled persons to claim that it is good to be like them. To give just some examples, such claims have been made by some of those with Asperger's syndrome, anorexia, dwarfism, intersex conditions, and schizophrenia. Further research of a historical and sociological nature might consider the conditions under which such claims are made, and further philosophical research might usefully consider the normative question of when such claims are justified.
- What, in general, are the components of a good life? Can an adequate philosophical account of the good life be developed? How important is it to have friends, meaningful work, or linguistic capabilities?

NOTES

1. Tucker (1998) reports that many of the Deaf families seen by the genetic counselling service offered at Gallaudet University (an American university for the Deaf) want deaf rather than hearing babies. However, in a study of the preferences of 100 Deaf students at Gallaudet, Moores, Miller, and Sicoli (2001) found that 97% reported that the hearing status of a child would make no difference to them. For a study of attitudes in the United Kingdom, see Middleton, Hewison, and Mueller (2001).
2. See Mundy, 2002. Discussing this case, Sparrow (2002) argues that it might be justifiable for Deaf parents to choose to have deaf babies even if deafness is not generally a good because a Deaf parent may be able to be a better parent to a deaf child.
3. Lane, Hoffmeister, and Bahan (1996, p. 405) claim that Deaf people are not impaired because "Deaf people themselves, who surely must know whether they have a grave impairment, say they do not."
4. My list of potential advantages to being deaf is taken from a survey of the literature. Almost certainly it is not an exhaustive list. A potential worry is that my list of goods in itself builds in "hearing" biases. Deaf people might value different goods, and if so judging deafness against a list of goods complied from commonplace hearing intuitions would be unfair. I accept that it is possible that deaf people value goods that hearing people overlook. However, in the absence of a competing list of "deaf goods," these hypothetical goods cannot be factored into the discussion here. If in the future someone proposes such a list, I would be happy to add them to my list of potential goods.
5. In 1996, U.S. 17- and 18-year-old deaf and hard of hearing students could on average only read as well as an average fourth-grade student (Gallaudet Research Institute, 1999).
6. Crouch (1997) claims that "considered in the proper light, the decision to forgo cochlear implantation for one's child, far from condemning a child to a world of meaningless silence, opens the child up to membership in the Deaf community, a unique community with a rich history, a rich language, and a value system of its own." The richness of Deaf culture is discussed in Lane et al. (1996), especially chap. 5.
7. Desloges (1984) discusses objections to sign language made by Deschamps. As Desloges explains, sign languages can in fact be used in the dark, although the method of using them is cumbersome. To use sign language in the dark, the "speaker" takes the hands of the "listener" and places the listener's fingers in the position for the signs that the speaker wishes to communicate.
8. For discussion of the changing conceptions of homosexuality, see Bayer (1981). For statements by professional organizations condemning "reparative therapy" (therapy that attempts to change the sexual orientation of homosexuals), see Robinson (2000).

REFERENCES

Alicke, M., Vredenburg, D., Hiatt, M., & Govorun, O. (2001). The "better than myself" effect. *Motivation and Emotion, 25,* 7–22.

ASL-Info. (2003). Untitled. Retrieved from http://www.ASL-info.com

Bahan, B. (2008). Upon the formation of a visual variety of the human race. In H.-D. Bauman (Ed.), *Open your eyes: Deaf studies talking* (pp. 83–99). Minneapolis, MN: University of Minnesota Press.

Bavelier, D., Tomann, A., Hutton, C., Mitchell, T., Corina, D., Liu, G., and Neville, H. (2000). Visual attention to the periphery is enhanced in congenitally Deaf individuals. *Journal of Neuroscience,* 20 (17), RC93. Retrieved from http://www.jneurosci.org/cgi/content/full/20/17/RC93

Bayer, R. (1981). *Homosexuality and American psychiatry.* New York: Basic Books.

Burns, S., Matthews, P., and Nolan-Conroy, E. (2001). Language attitudes. In C. Lucas (Ed.), *The sociolinguistics of sign language* (pp. 181–216). Cambridge, UK: Cambridge University Press.

Cooper, R. (2002). Disease. *Studies in History and Philosophy of Biological and Biomedical Sciences, 33,* 263–282.

Crouch, R. (1997). Letting the deaf be Deaf: Reconsidering the use of cochlear implants in prelingually deaf children. *Hastings Center Report, 27,* 14–21.

Desloges, P. (1984). A deaf person's observations about "An elementary course of education for the Deaf." In H. Lane (Ed.), *The Deaf experience,* 28–48. Cambridge, MA: Harvard University Press.

Devitt, M., & Sterelny, K. (1999). *Language and reality* (2nd ed.). Cambridge, MA: MIT Press.

Engelhardt, H. (1974). The disease of masturbation: Values and the concept of disease. *Bulletin of the History of Medicine, 48,* 234–248.

Evans, N. (1998). Aborigines speak a primitive language. In. L. Bauer & P. Trudgill (Eds.), *Language myths.* London, UK: Penguin.

Finkelstein, V. (1980). *Attitudes and disabled people.* New York, NY: World Rehabilitation Fund.

Gallaudet Research Institute. (1999). *What is the reading level for deaf and hard of hearing people?* Retrieved from http://gri.gallaudet.edu/Literacy/

Griffin, J. (1986). *Well-being.* Oxford, UK: Clarendon Press.

Groce, N. (1985). *Everyone here spoke sign language.* Cambridge, MA: Harvard University Press.

Harlow, R. (1998). Some languages are just not good enough. In L. Bauer & P. Trudgill (Eds.), *Language myths.* London, UK: Penguin.

King, L. (1954). What is disease? *Philosophy of Science, 21,* 193–203.

Klein, R. (1983). The "men-problem" in women's studies: The expert, the ignoramus, and the poor dear. *Women's Studies International Forum, 6,* 413–421.

Ladd, P. (2003). *Understanding Deaf culture.* Clevedon, UK: Multilingual Matters.

Ladd, P., Gulliver, M., & Batterbury, S. (2003). Reassessing minority language empowerment from a Deaf perspective: The other 32 languages. *Deaf Worlds, 19,* 6–32.

Lane, H. (1992). *The mask of benevolence: Disabling the Deaf community.* New York, NY: Alfred A. Knopf.

Lane, H., Hoffmeister, R., & Bahan, B. (1996). *A journey into the Deaf-World.* San Diego, CA: DawnSignPress.

Middleton, A., Hewison, J., & Mueller, R. (2001). Prenatal diagnosis for inherited deafness—What is the potential demand? *Journal of Genetic Counselling, 10,* 121–131.

Moores, D., Miller, M., & Sicoli, D. (2001). Preferences of deaf college students for the hearing status of their children. *Journal of the American Deafness and Rehabilitation Association, 32,* 1–8.

Mundy, L. (2002, March 31). A world of their own. *Washington Post,* p. W22.

Nyman, D. (1991). A deaf-gay man. In G. Taylor & J. Bishop (Eds.), *Being deaf: The experience of deafness.* London, UK: Pinter.

Oliver, M. (1990). *The politics of disablement.* Houndmills, Basingstoke, UK: Macmillan.
Oliver, M. (1992). Changing the social relations of research production? *Disability and Society, 7,* 101–114.
Philips, D., & Westland, E. (1992). Men in women's studies classrooms. In H. Hinds, A. Phoenix, & J. Stacey (Eds.), *Working out: New directions for women's studies.* London, UK: Falmer Press.
Reznek, L. (1987). *The nature of disease.* London, UK: Routledge.
Robinson, B. (2000). *Statements by professional associations about reparative therapy.* Retrieved from http://www.religioustolerance.org/hom_expr.html
Ruse, M. (1981). Are homosexuals sick? In A. Caplan, H. Engelhardt, & J. McCartney (Eds.), *Concepts of health and disease: Interdisciplinary perspectives.* Reading, MA: Addison-Wesley.
Sacks, O. (1991). *Seeing voices.* London, UK: Macmillan.
Sparrow, R. (2002). *Better off deaf?* [CAPPE Working Paper]. Retrieved from http://www.csu.edu.au/faculty/arts/cappe/wps.htm
Steinbock, B. (2000). Disability, prenatal testing, and selective abortion. In E. Parens & A. Asch (Eds.), *Prenatal testing and disability rights.* Washington, DC: Georgetown University Press.
Tucker, B. (1998). Deaf culture, cochlear implants, and elective disability. *Hasting's Center Report, 28,* 6–14.
Wendell, S. (1996). *The rejected body: Feminist philosophical reflections on disability.* New York, NY: Routledge.
Wilson, D. (1997). Evolutionary epidemiology: Darwinian theory in the service of medicine and psychiatry. In S. Baron-Cohen (Ed.), *The maladapted mind.* Hove, UK: Psychology Press.

SUGGESTIONS FOR FURTHER READING

Amundson, R. (2000). Against normal function. *Studies in History and Philosophy of Biological and Biomedical Sciences, 31,* 33–53.
Griffin, J. (1986). *Well-being.* Oxford, UK: Clarendon Press.
Lane, H., Hoffmeister, R., & Bahan, B. (1996). *A journey into the Deaf-World.* San Diego, CA: DawnSignPress.
Sacks, O. (1991). *Seeing voices.* London, UK: Macmillan.
Sacks, O. (1995). *An anthropologist on Mars.* New York, NY: Alfred A. Knopf.

PART V

CONCLUSION

14

Retrospectus and Prospectus

Donald F. Moores and Peter V. Paul

This book is the third step of a journey with no discernable final destination. The journey began over dinner at a national convention in 2008 in which we discussed various worldviews, or epistemologies, related to deafness and the diverse perspectives of professionals in our field. Because we had received our doctoral training at the same institution, the University of Illinois, to a large extent we shared an orientation to the scientific method and some variation of the standard epistemology. At the same time, as pragmatic educators, we were well aware and accepting of the diversity within the d/Deaf or hard of hearing (d/Dhh) population and the existence of one or more deaf epistemologies.

As we discussed different perspectives, it became clear to us that there were a few treatments of deaf epistemologies, mostly in book form, but that each one presented only a single position on the subject. We agreed that it would be exciting, challenging, and informative—in that order—to put together a publication in which d/Dhh and hearing professionals from different disciplines could present their worldviews on deafness, Deafhood, and related topics within the framework of the standard epistemology and/or deaf epistemologies.

The second step was the publication of a special issue on deaf epistemologies in the *American Annals of the Deaf* (see Paul & Moores, 2010). Although quite diverse, the contributors were professionals sharing an interest in the reality, nature, and epistemology of deafness/Deafhood either through direct experience or through professional and social interactions. In the final remarks of that special issue, we stated that our intention was not to provide a summary or conclusion but rather a few remarks on the end of the beginning of a long journey in which we might provide some clarification of the constructs of *deafness*, *epistemology*, and particularly *deaf epistemologies*, leading to a deeper understanding of the complexities and challenges with respect to the teaching/learning situations of individuals who are d/Dhh.

Reactions to the special issue were quite positive, and we were encouraged to continue our efforts. Fortunately, contributors to each of the original *Annals* articles agreed to update, expand, and treat their original work in more detail. In one case, an article was expanded to include two chapters. We were also fortunate to include additional authors, thus expanding the diversity of our contributors. In this publication, we have representatives from education, medicine, psychology, anthropology, literature, the arts, and philosophy. They provide a plethora of knowledge, expertise, and insight, and we are grateful to each and every one of them. We encourage the reader to avail him- or herself of all of the information available. This is especially germane in that we do not see consensus as the goal of this publication. As stated in our introductory chapter, several theorists and philosophers contend that the goal is understanding, not consensus. What happens *after understanding* is another matter.

It is not the purpose of this concluding chapter to address in detail all of the issues raised in the individual chapters, especially given the range of epistemologies and the nuances of the discussions. However, a few general comments are called for from our perspective. Several authors have endeavored to describe or define terms such as *epistemology, Deaf World, Deafhood, deafness, audism, objectivism,* and *relativism.* In some cases, the terms mean different things to different people. For example, we may state that epistemology is the philosophical study of a construct labeled knowledge (e.g., Chapter 1); however, in reality, *epistemology* is also a construct, as are *philosophy, deafness, Deafhood, audism,* and so on. The meanings and implications of constructs are open to debate (e.g., Pring, 2004; Ritzer, 2001).

In essence, *reality* itself is a construct. There are numerous philosophical—actually metaphysical—discussions on the construct of reality (e.g., Blackburn, 1999, 2005; Noddings, 2007; Pring, 2004). For example, nominalism is the metaphysical view that general or abstract terms may exist but that abstract objects do not; that is, abstract labels cannot stand for objectively existing entities. The basic argument is that we may acquire or develop abstract constructs cognitively, which may be individually or socially shared, but these ideas may or may not correspond to an objective reality. Thus, with nominalism, we might reject the notion of universals (or even fundamentals) or reject the notion of abstract objects. In short, nominalism is a position on the problem of universals, which dates as far back as Plato and perhaps even longer (Copleston, 1985).

Reification, which refers to the fallacy of treating a theoretical abstraction as something concrete, is a related concept. An example is the construct *intelligence,* which many theorists, researchers, and others treat as a real entity. Of course, this leads to the question of what intelligence tests really measure, how intelligence might be related to cognition, and the intertwinement, if any, of intelligence, cognition, and rationality (Stanovich, 2009).

We come down to one existential question: Is there an external, knowable, objective reality that can be apprehended only or predominantly through the scientific method? Of course, this represents a version of the standard epistemology that has existed in one form or another for centuries (Blackburn, 1999, 2005; Noddings, 2007; Ritzer, 2001; see also Chapter 1). If the answer is *yes,* then we concentrate our efforts in our perpetual, unending search for truth (i.e., a form of objective reality). If the answer is *no,* then we encounter other questions, which engender a range of different knowledge-seeking approaches. Of the multitude of potential nonstandard epistemologies, how do we decide which ones are most salient for our particular purposes? Do we still use the scientific method? If knowledge is local, how is it situated?

The law of parsimony states that when there are alternate explanations of events, the simplest (and most elegant) one is superior and should be preferred (e.g., see Copleston, 1985). In this case, a version of the standard epistemology would seem to be preferred—or perhaps the use of the scientific method is the real issue. However, this would be true only if it was as effective as the alternative explanations, assuming that we can agree on the nature of the ends or the outcomes (e.g., Pring, 2004; see Chapter 1). Despite the risk of oversimplification, we assert that the majority of contributors to this text prefer alternative, relativistic, or multiple epistemologies, and their arguments are similar to those offered by professionals in feminist studies, African American studies, and gay/lesbian/bisexual/transgender studies.

We have only begun the journey into understanding—having not reached a consensus—on the constructs of epistemology and deafness/Deafhood. We are faced with the challenge of proceeding beyond understanding and proffering recommendations for professionals. Nevertheless, several of us argue that an adequate understanding might be elusive at best and incomplete at least. At the least, a number of issues need to be explored.

- What is the role of a standard epistemology in the lives of d/Dhh individuals? Ideally, versions of the standard epistemology represent a search for objective, verifiable universal truths. In this case, the findings should apply to deaf, Deaf, hard of hearing, and hearing individuals regardless of age, gender, race, ethnicity, education, nationality, and so on. There are arguments that the standard epistemology represents an oppressive white, male, Western worldview that ignores the reality of gender, race, ethnicity, sexual orientation, and deafness/disability, among others. Of course, there are counterarguments that this is not the case or, rather, this is a mischaracterization of the standard epistemology.
- Are there or should there be separate deaf epistemologies? Put another way, are d/Deaf and hearing people more different than they are alike? We have read that d/Deaf people are visual learners and that their life experiences are different, often because of the negative effects of audism and negative stereotypes. Terms such as *deaf culture, Deafhood,* and *Deaf-World* have been coined to express the uniqueness of deafness or, rather, the uniqueness of d/Dhh individuals. Are these terms developed by an elite group or do they reflect the day-to-day lives of a majority of d/Dhh individuals?
- Can and should a comprehensive and inclusive epistemology be developed and agreed on that accounts for the tremendous diversity of the human race? There are more than seven billion human individuals on the planet. As human beings, we all share certain characteristics. A single epistemology is, by definition, weak and superficial in its explanatory power. Seven billion epistemologies are unmanageable. We need to identify universal and unique characteristics.
- What are the relative contributions of adult Deaf children of deaf parents (DCDP) and of adult Deaf children of hearing parents (DCHP) to d/Deaf epistemologies? Although they comprise less than 5% of the d/Dhh population, it has been assumed that DCDPs are the major contributors to Deaf culture or the Deaf World. This may be true, but the far more numerous DCHP population has shared experiences that may be of at least equal importance.

- As with a standard epistemology, can and should a comprehensive and inclusive deaf epistemology be developed that accounts for the tremendous diversity of the d/Dhh population? On first examination, a standard deaf epistemology has primarily been developed by highly educated, white, male Americans and Europeans. As such, it is open to the same criticism as the standard epistemology. Does the present deaf epistemology have the flexibility to accommodate diversity? Can or should non-d/Dhh individuals contribute to the development of deaf epistemologies?
- Given the global push for inclusion of d/Dhh children in general education classrooms with hearing children and standardized instruction and testing, what are the implications for deaf epistemologies in the future? Until the recent past, residential schools for d/Dhh children were the major sources of enculturation into a Deaf community. In a majority of countries now, most d/Dhh children are educated contiguous to hearing peers and may have little or no contact with other d/Dhh children or adults. What will be the impact?

Given the continuing development of assistive devices such as digital hearing aids and cochlear implants (and more to come), perhaps we might have new perspectives on the question (Cooper, Chapter 13): Can it be a good thing to be deaf? In fact, we contend that the construct of deaf epistemologies will also evolve as a result of the changing demographics of d/Dhh individuals. We end this journey, for now, with a passage from Blackburn (1999):

> I believe the process of understanding the problems is itself a good. If the upshot of what Hume called a "mitigated scepticism" or sense of how much a decent modesty becomes us in our intellectual speculations, that is surely no bad thing. The world is full of ideas, and a becoming sense of their power, their difficulty, their frailties, and their fallibility cannot be the least of the things it needs. (p. 298)

REFERENCES

Blackburn, S. (1999). *Think: A compelling introduction to philosophy*. New York, NY: Oxford University Press.

Blackburn, S. (2005). *Truth: A guide*. New York, NY: Oxford University Press.

Copleston, F. (1985). *A history of philosophy*, Vol. 1 New York, NY: Image.

Moores, D., & Paul, P. (2010). Summary and prologue. *American Annals of the Deaf, 154*(5), 493–496.

Noddings, N. (2007). *Philosophy of education* (2nd ed.). Boulder, CO: Westview.

Paul, P., & Moores, D. (2010). Toward an understanding of epistemology and deafness. *American Annals of the Deaf, 154*(5), 417–420.

Pring, R. (2004). *Philosophy of educational research* (2nd ed.). New York, NY: Continuum.

Ritzer, G. (2001). *Explorations in social theory: From metatheorizing to rationalization*. Thousand Oaks, CA: Sage.

Stanovich, K. (2009). *What intelligence tests miss: The psychology of rational thought*. New Haven, CT: Yale University Press.

Index

Figures, notes, and tables are indicated by f, n, and t following page numbers.